This book provides an up-to-date look at the complex interplay between women's psychological and physical health. Central to the discussion is evidence that – in addition to genetic endowment – hormonal balance and environmental influences contribute significantly to how disorders are expressed in women. The book takes note of the growing literature on sexually dimorphic brain structures and how these might mediate cognition, behavior, and emotions. It contains information on the safety and use of psychotropic drugs for women, including alcohol and nicotine during pregnancy and nursing, and about ongoing trials in which drugs or hormones are used to improve functioning or delay aging.

This monograph reviews data on the interaction between hormonal activation and individual and environmental influences in health and disease in women. The book provides useful information and background material important for treating problems related to the reproductive cycle, depression and anxiety disorders, eating disorders, and drug treatment of women and discusses clinical issues in coronary artery disease and breast cancer.

This is a medically oriented book written mainly for practicing physicians in primary care, psychiatry, internal medicine, and gynecology and obstetrics. It takes a broad view, considering a range of psychological and physical disorders affecting women, and discussing treatment issues.

WOMEN'S HEALTH: HORMONES, EMOTIONS, AND BEHAVIOR

PSYCHIATRY

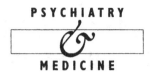

MEDICINE

Over recent years, the extent of psychiatric morbidity among patients seen in general hospital practice and primary care has been well established. Physicians and surgeons are becoming increasingly aware of the importance of recognizing and treating the psychiatric problems that their patients experience, and consultation–liaison psychiatry has become a distinct field for research and clinical practice. In the context of general medicine and its specialties, psychiatric morbidity may coexist with definite organic pathology or present largely with somatic symptoms in the absence of organic disease. This area is receiving more attention in postgraduate and undergraduate teaching, but there are few specialist textbooks that cover the topic.

This series is introduced to review particular areas of medicine in which psychological factors and psychiatric morbidity are especially significant. Each volume is written or edited by a clinician with extensive experience in the area and combines clinical insight with a discussion of relevant research. The series is aimed at senior clinicians and trainees, particularly in psychiatry, internal medicine, and primary care, and individual volumes will interest a wider audience in the health professions.

WOMEN'S HEALTH: HORMONES, EMOTIONS, AND BEHAVIOR

REGINA C. CASPER

Department of Psychiatry and Behavioral Sciences
Stanford University School of Medicine

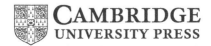

CAMBRIDGE UNIVERSITY PRESS
Cambridge, New York, Melbourne, Madrid, Cape Town, Singapore, São Paulo

Cambridge University Press
The Edinburgh Building, Cambridge CB2 8RU, UK

Published in the United States of America by Cambridge University Press, New York

www.cambridge.org
Information on this title: www.cambridge.org/9780521563413

First published 1998
This digitally printed version 2008

A catalogue record for this publication is available from the British Library

Library of Congress Cataloguing in Publication data

Women's health : hormones, emotions, and behavior / edited by
Regina C. Casper.
p. cm. – (Cambridge studies in medicine)
Includes bibliographical references.
ISBN 0-521-56341-0 (hardcover)
1. Women – Mental health. 2. Women – Health and hygiene.
3. Psychoneuroendocrinology. I. Casper, Regina C. II. Series.
RC451.4.W6W659 1997
616.89'0082 – DC21   97-3022
                                                      CIP

ISBN 978-0-521-56341-3 hardback
ISBN 978-0-521-06020-2 paperback

To our families

CONTRIBUTORS

Gail Anderson, M.D.
Clinical Assistant Professor
Department of Psychiatry and Behavioral Sciences
Emory University School of Medicine
Woodruff Memorial Research Building
1639 Pierce Drive, Suite 4000
Atlanta, GA 30322

Kathleen A. Berra, R.N., N.P., M.S.N.
Nurse Educator Medicine and Cardiovascular Medicine
Stanford Center for Research in Disease Prevention
Stanford University School of Medicine
730 Welch Road
Stanford, CA 94305-0113

Regina C. Casper, M.D.
Professor of Psychiatry, Director, Women's Wellness Clinic
Department of Psychiatry and Behavioral Sciences
Stanford University School of Medicine
401 Quarry Road
Stanford, CA 94305-5546

Joan M. Fair, R.N., Ph.D.
Clinical Trials Director
Center for Research and Development
730 Welch Road, Suite B
Stanford, CA 94304

Kaye Hermanson, Ph.D.
Professor of Psychiatry
Department of Psychiatry and Behavioral Sciences
Stanford University School of Medicine
401 Quarry Road
Stanford, CA 94305-5544

Jennifer L. Kelsey, Ph.D.
Professor of Health Research and Policy
Professor of Medicine, Immunology and Rheumatology
Departments of Health Research and Policy Medicine
Stanford University School of Medicine
Redwood Building, T223
Stanford, CA 94305-5092

Peter T. Loosen, M.D.
Professor of Psychiatry and Medicine
Chief, Division of Psychoneuroendocrinology
Vanderbilt University
Nashville, TN 37212
and
Chief of Psychiatry
VA Medical Center (116A)
1310 24th Avenue South
Nashville, TN 37212-2637

Robert Marcus, M.D.
Professor of Medicine, Endocrinology, Gerontology, and Metabolism
Department of Medicine
300 Pasteur Drive
Stanford University Medical Center
Stanford, CA 94305-5109
and
Geriatrics Research, Education, and Clinical Center
Palo Alto VA Hospital
Palo Alto, CA 94304

Laura Marsh, M.D.
Assistant Professor of Psychiatry
Department of Psychiatry and Behavioral Sciences
Stanford University School of Medicine
401 Quarry Road
Stanford, CA 94305-5546

Dominique L. Musselman, M.D.
Assistant Professor
Department of Psychiatry and Behavioral Sciences
Emory University School of Medicine
1639 Pierce Drive, Suite 4400
Atlanta, GA 30322

Charles B. Nemeroff, M.D., Ph.D.
Chairman, Department of Psychiatry and Behavioral Sciences
Reunette W. Harris Professor of Psychiatry
Emory University School of Medicine
Woodruff Memorial Research Building
1639 Pierce Drive, Suite 4000
Atlanta, GA 30322

Maryfrances R. Porter, B.A.
Lab Manager, Relationship Center
Department of Psychology
University of Denver
2155 South Race Street
Denver, CO 80208

Domeena C. Renshaw, M.D.
Professor of Psychiatry, Director, Sexual Dysfunction Clinic
Department of Psychiatry
Loyola University Chicago
2160 South First Avenue
Maywood, IL 60153

Naseem Ahmed Smith, M.D.
Child Psychiatry Fellow
Department of Child Psychiatry
University of Colorado Health Science Center
4200 East 9th Avenue
Denver, CO 80262

David Spiegel, M.D.
Professor of Psychiatry
Department of Psychiatry and Behavioral Sciences
Stanford University School of Medicine
401 Quarry Road
Stanford, CA 94305-5544

Sara L. Stein, M.D.
Research Fellow
Department of Psychiatry and Behavioral Sciences
Stanford University School of Medicine
401 Quarry Road
Stanford, CA 94305-5544

Katherine E. Williams, M.D.
NIH Research Fellow
Department of Psychiatry and Behavioral Sciences
Stanford University School of Medicine
401 Quarry Road
Stanford, CA 94305-5544

CONTENTS

PREFACE

The term "women's health" is now commonly used to describe all the efforts under way to improve women's soundness of mind and body. Self-evidently, women experience health problems that differ from those of men – an old idea alive in classical times when Hygeia, the daughter of Asklepios, the god of medicine and healing, was venerated as the goddess of health. To return to the present, the workplace is increasingly the defining element in the lives of women, as it has always been for men, yet the care of the family and the task of raising children – often as a single parent – remain the woman's domain, a dual role that may have unknown long-term health consequences.

Fortunately, and this allows us to take a fresh look at women's health, or rather at those conditions that interfere with it, women's health has become a scientific discipline. The research literature, and in particular studies on hormones, reveal ever more complex findings which show that biologic factors are interwoven with and altered by human behavior, environmental influences, and social forces. There is, we think, an urgent need to draw on the results of new research to protect the health of women. This book is a first step, and it is designed to make visible the conditions and changes – some long familiar, others newly recognized – that affect women's health in various ways.

The chapters in the first part of the book describe psychopathology unique to women or more commonly observed in women than in men. Early chapters first discuss research findings, then the clinical phenomenology, and briefly the treatment of sexual dysfunction, disorders related to the reproductive cycle, and depressive, anxiety, and eating disorders. Sex differences in disease incidence and symptomatology are reviewed. Chapters on cardiovascular disease and breast cancer illustrate the complex interaction of physiological, emotional, and behavioral elements in the disposition to disease and disease progression. The last part of the book considers psychopharmacological issues relative to women and reviews ongoing intervention trials concerned with disease prevention in women.

Regina C. Casper

CHAPTER ONE

GROWING UP FEMALE

REGINA C. CASPER

Population statistics consistently record more male than female human births (Babb, 1995), the outcome of a significantly higher conception rate for males (McMillen, 1979). Such sex ratio bias occurs in several species, where research is now examining environmental and physiologic conditions as well as maternal effects that influence the sex ratio at conception and at birth (Bacon and McClintock, 1994). This higher birth rate notwithstanding, beginning at birth and throughout life, male mortality tends to be significantly higher. In the first year of life, 25 percent more male than female infants die, and in adult life the male:female mortality ratio exceeds 2:1 (U.S. Bureau of the Census, 1990).

This phenomenon of women outranking men in survival is relatively new. Until the last century, before the discovery of antisepsis and antibiotics, many young women died in their child beds as a result of birth complications, hemorrhages, and postpartum infections. In 1868, maternal mortality rates were 84.4:1,000 births as opposed to 5:1,000 births in 1986 (O'Dowd and Philipp, 1994). Furthermore, some illnesses are unique to women. Medical complications and pathology associated with the female reproductive system, with pregnancy, and with child rearing confer increased risks of physical and psychological morbidity.

This first chapter presents a necessarily abbreviated account of normal female somatic and psychological development as an introduction to the material in the following chapters, which cover disorders that are known to affect women uniquely or disproportionately.

Postnatal growth

Sexual differentiation and hormonal regulation of behavior

Sex determination for some time has been known to be under the control of an X-specific gene (German et al., 1978). It appears now that a region of chromosome Xp21 affects sexual differentiation (Bardoni et al., 1994). The mechanisms through which these genes operate are not fully understood, yet work in developmental neurobiology and neuroendocrinology is providing new information about the processes through which gonadal hormones pattern sexual differentiation. Early hypotheses about the action of gonadal hormones on the development of reproductive physiology and behavior, which proposed that hormones in early fetal life produce "organizational," that is, permanent, changes and in postnatal life "activate" sex-specific behaviors have been amended. Current theories hold that steroid hormones effect sexual differentiation by gaining control over certain key maturational processes in the brain by influencing cell proliferation, cell migration, ontogenetic cell death, and synaptogenesis at critical prenatal periods and in postnatal life (MacLusky and Naftolin, 1981; Kelley, 1986).

McEwen's studies (McEwen, 1981) in rats have mapped and identified estrogen-sensitive cells in many brain areas, one example being neurons in ventromedial hypothalamic regions critical for the female rat's sexual receptivity. Based on research in the female spotted hyena, which exhibits malelike genitalia and dominance over males, yet gives birth, Glickman et al. (1992) have proposed that female sexual differentiation may also be influenced by naturally circulating androgens. Many examples of sexual dimorphic neurons or cell groups in different species now exist; most were identified because they regulate conspicuous male evolutionary characteristics, such as bright plumage, frog croaking, and bird song. In some birds, estradiol may establish the capacity for growth in song-control nuclei, whereas dihydrotestosterone may control the number of neurons that innervate syringeal muscle groups for male song. A particularly telling example is the remarkable and seasonally varying differences in the volume of cell groups that innervate muscles controlling song in male canaries and finches (Nottebohm and Arnold, 1976). Structural differences in female and male brains are reviewed in Chapter Four.

Maternal and attachment behavior

Behavioral endocrinology – how hormones affect behavior and are affected by behavior – was an emerging field 20 years ago (Beach, 1975) and is still in its infancy. Nearly all research has been conducted in nonhuman species. The neurochemical determinants that facilitate recognition and bonding in the infant to the mother have not been clarified, although it is known that physical contact and other cues, for example, visual, auditory, and sensory ones, are necessary conduits (Bowlby, 1982). Conversely, the agents and neuronal pathways that promote affiliative and maternal behavior from the parents to the infant are incompletely understood. Early investigations established the permissive and necessary role of the gonadal hormones, estradiol and progesterone, for maternal behavior (Bridges, 1984). It appears now that central neuropeptide pathways are indispensable for some social behaviors and that oxytocin, a cyclic octapeptide secreted by the paraventricular and supraoptic nuclei and stored in the neurohypophysis, is involved in activating maternal behavior in rodents and many other species (Pedersen and Prange Jr., 1987; Insel, 1990).

Based on studies into the neural correlates of pair bond formation in prairie voles, a mammalian species exhibiting monogamy – unlike rats and mice, which do not pair bond – Insel and co-workers (Carter et al., 1992) have reported that oxytocin release follows sexual behavior and leads to strong selective heterosexual social preferences. Because in the prairie vole physical contact, for instance, sharing a nest, outside of sexual activity is a major component of monogamous behavior, it can be used to characterize social preferences. It appears that oxytocin may be critical for social and sexual bond formation in the female prairie vole; by contrast, vasopressin seems to be more important for pair bonding in the male prairie vole and for inducing paternal behavior in the presence of testosterone (Wang and de Vries, 1993). Vasopressin has also been reported to facilitate social recognition and memory in the male rat by Dantzer and co-workers (Dantzer et al., 1988). Social recognition in rats is based on chemosensory cues and is dependent on circulating androgen levels. By using vasopressin antagonists, Bluthé and Dantzer (1990) demonstrated that vasopressin did not mediate social recognition in female rats, which suggests sexually dimorphic processing of social olfactory stimuli and bond formation in these rodents. On a molecular genetic level, Insel and co-workers (Kirkpatrick, Kim, and Insel, 1994) reported by measuring increased *fos* expression that the medial nucleus of the amygdala of the prairie vole was involved in paternal and maternal behavior. Greenberg's group (Brown et al., 1996) has shown in mice that the capacity to react with an immediate postpartum nurturing response to the young is genetically controlled by *fosB*. *FosB* is one of the early immediate genes uniquely activated by environmental stimuli, and its cellular and behavioral effects would complement the hormonal regulation of nurturing behavior.

In humans, oxytocin has long been known to be released during parturition and during suckling to facilitate milk ejection, whereas vasopressin has been reported to promote learning and memory (Kovacs and Telegdy, 1985). During the long period of human gestation, estrogen and progesterone act as priming agents. It is likely, although it has not been established, that oxytocin and vasopressin not only play a role in rodents but also mediate human parental and social behavior (Rosenblatt, 1994).

Somatic growth

Speed of growth is fastest from the beginning of conception to birth and thereafter declines gradually, except during the adolescent growth spurt. Whereas growth in height is fairly steady until adolescence, 80 percent of the postnatal growth of the skull, the brain, the eyes, and the ears is completed by the end of the second or third year of life (Marshall and Tanner, 1969). The size of the head approaches adult size by age 10, but changes in the jaw and other parts of the face and overlying soft tissues are apparent during and after puberty.

The trunk develops earlier than the legs, and the feet are more developed than the calf or thigh. Interestingly, at birth the male forearm is already longer than that of the female, whereas in females, as opposed to males, the second finger is more often longer than the fourth finger. Growth velocity is quite different in lymphoid tissues, which reach "adult" size by age 6, double in size by puberty, and under the influence of sexual hormones shrink back to half this size. Subcutaneous fat thickness increases rapidly in the first through the second year and gradually declines until the age of 6 or 7, when children tend to look thin. From age 8 or 9 onward, fat thickness on the trunk and arms increases until the time of puberty. Prepubertal children of both sexes have the same range of heights and equal body and skeletal mass and body fat; therefore, in childhood girls and boys actually have similar body dimensions.

Constitutional factors: temperament and personality

Chess and Thomas (1968) were the first among developmental psychiatrists to record systematically individual styles in infants and children. These individual behaviors came to be known as temperaments. Behavioral observations in a sample of children who were part of the New York Longitudinal Study, begun in 1956, showed that two fifths of the children displayed an easy temperament, about 10 percent were difficult, and about 15 percent were slow to warm up, with the remainder not clearly belonging to either group. The child's sleep and feeding patterns and the reaction to the environment provided further behavioral constructs – the biologically regular or irregular infant, high or low activity levels, high or low sensory thresholds, high persistence–low distractability, and varying combinations of each. Besides identifying temperamental characteristics, the investigators were interested in helping parents understand their children's individual differences and using this knowledge to respond to and guide their children. Kagan and his group (Kagan, Reznick, and Snidman, 1987) have continued this work on inherited profiles and have focused on a temperamental category called inhibited or uninhibited to the unfamiliar, for example, children who are timid, shy, and inhibited in response to novel stimuli as opposed to children who are affectively spontaneous, sociable, and fearless in new situations. They have shown that in a certain proportion of children these behavioral tendencies are stable and that a relationship exists between behavioral inhibition and biologic indexes such as plasma cortisol levels and heart rate responses, suggesting inherent differences in arousal and reactivity, perhaps influenced by hypothalamic activity. So far, most studies on temperament have not analyzed sex differences.

Environmental factors: sexual and female identity

In any society, a child lives with individuals of all types and ages, classified into female and male, who are conspicuous by their primary sex characteristics. For children, the clearest distinctions are of the two sexes and the role of each sex within the family; hence, femaleness or maleness is a child's first identification (Mead, 1949). Once this identification is made, the child begins to compare and define herself with respect to other characteristics and abilities and to learn how others view and relate to her. If children understand first in the family and in their culture that their sensations, feelings, reactions, and actions are meaningful and effective, they memorize these experiences and integrate them into Children and adults continuously reinterpret their experiences as their minds and bodies mature. In every society girls learn early not only about their bodily differences but how such differences fit into the social organization. If prestige is accorded to women, girls will be more likely to value feminity.

Each female child grows up in her own cultural tradition. Despite marked differences in appearance and temperament, no universal characteristics or behaviors are exclusively associated with either sex across cultures. Divisions of labor are present in any society, not only between the sexes. What counts is whether bearing children is considered not only an activity unique to women but also enough for women, and whether talented and gifted women have access to activities in science or the arts and to public life. As long as women cannot own property or cannot vote – for instance, Swiss women gained suffrage only in 1971 – or are denied the opportunity to train and use their minds, they are likely to suffer a loss in their sense of self.

Puberty and adolescence

Puberty in females

Puberty reflects maturation of the hypothalamic-pituitary-gonadal axis, a process that begins early in fetal life. Hypothalamic luteinizing hormone-releasing hormone (LHRH) neurons originate in the olfactory epithelial placode and from there migrate via the forebrain to the hypothalamus. Primordial follicles appear during the fourth and fifth months of fetal life. Follicular growth occurs during fetal life, and in childhood, yet before puberty, all developed follicles undergo atresia (Grumbach and Kaplan, 1990). In the fetus and at birth estrogen levels are high because of the conversion of fetal and maternal steroids by the placenta. In the newborn, plasma estradiol levels drop precipitously in the first days of life and remain low until puberty. By contrast, plasma levels of luteinizing hormone (LH) and follicle-stimulating hormone (FSH) rise intermittently to adult values during the first 2 years after birth. Subsequently, LH and FSH levels decline and remain low until puberty (Jakacki et al., 1982). FSH levels rise during the early stages of puberty, and in late prepuberty augmented release of LH during sleep is observed. During puberty, the amplitude and frequency of gonadotropin pulses increase, leading to episodic LH secretion during the day, rising in total over a hundred-fold. These events lead eventually to the appearance of secondary sexual characteristics, the adolescent growth spurt, and fertility.

Adolescent growth spurt

On average, girls begin the adolescent growth spurt 1–2 years earlier than boys, and therefore girls are typically taller than boys around age 12. Because girls reach peak height velocity about 1.3 years before menarche, most girls grow no more than 1–7 cm after menarche. Menarche usually occurs as growth in height is slowing down. The hormonal mechanisms involved in growth at puberty are not well understood. Estrogens may stimulate growth by increasing production of insulin-like growth factor-1 (IGF-1). Prolonged delay of puberty can prolong growth in stature, but only under conditions of good nutrition and normal activity levels. If delayed puberty is due to low body fat and excessive exercise, prepubertal growth is not assured, but catch-up growth has been reported with weight recovery (Prader, Tanner, and von Harnack, 1963). During puberty, boys in contrast to girls lose fat on limbs and on the trunk, and they usually become leaner, whereas girls on average accumulate nearly twice as much body fat as boys. Shape differences are produced by the widening of boys' shoulders and the enlargement of girls' hips. Ultimately, boys have more muscle mass, larger bones, and therefore higher bone-density measurements than girls. Skeletal maturation can be assessed by comparing radiographs of the hand, the knee, or the elbow with standards of maturation in a reference normal population. Bone age, an index of ossification and epiphyseal fusion, is useful for predicting the age of menarche. In delayed puberty, bone age correlates better with the appearance of secondary sexual characteristics than with chronologic age.

Skeletal growth is not complete by the end of adolescence because the vertebral column can continue to grow until about age 30. Tanner's growth charts (Tanner, Whitehouse, and Marshall, 1975) from longitudinal and cross-sectional data of British children have been updated and estimated for populations in other countries – in the United States by the National Center for Health Statistics (Hamill et al., 1979). Surveys of workers and military recruits indicate that the average age for attaining adult height was much later in past centuries (Tanner, 1981). Better nutrition and improved health in childhood and adolescence largely explain the earlier growth and the growth acceleration in U.S. and West European young adults. Fogel (1993) has calculated that around 1855 about two thirds of young adult males in Holland, a country with a fairly genetically homogeneous population, were below 5 feet 4 inches (168 cm), whereas in 1980 a mere 2 percent of males remained below this height. There is clear evidence that emotional factors affect growth; for instance, emotional dwarfism is a well-described phenomenon in childhood (Powell, Brasel, and Blizzard, 1967), and Pine, Cohen, and Brook (1996) have reported from a prospective epidemiologic study that anxiety disorders in childhood appear to predict relatively short stature in young adulthood in females, but not in males.

Endocrinology of puberty

The episodic FSH and LH secretion that occurs during early puberty, mainly at night, gradually increases in amplitude and frequency, and by late puberty daytime secretory peaks reach a plateau (Reiter et al., 1987). Amplified FSH pulses lead to secretion of estradiol from the ovary. About 10 percent of circulating estradiol arises from extraglandular conversion of testosterone and androstendione (Grumbach and Kaplan, 1990). Plasma estradiol concentrations rise steadily through the stages of puberty until they reach mean levels of 50 pg/ml in the follicular phase, 220 pg/ml at midcycle, and 150 pg/ml in the luteal phase at maturity. Anovulatory cycles are common in the first year after menarche (Apper and Vikho, 1977). Estradiol and testosterone are highly (95–97 percent), yet reversibly, bound to sex steroid–binding globulin (SBG) present in equal levels in boys and girls during prepuberty. SBG decreases with puberty in girls less than in boys (Lindstedt et al., 1985). Beginning at age 8, there is an increase in adrenal steroids, dehydroepiandrosterone (DHEA) and its sulfate (DHEAS) – a phenomenon called adrenarche – which continues through ages 13 to 15 years. The circadian rhythm of DHEA release parallels the diurnal rhythm of cortisol secretion.

Secondary sex characteristics

Puberty for girls is unmistakable and dramatic, whereas for boys the events unfold slowly. In the majority of U.S. girls (95 percent) the first signs of puberty, either breast or pubic hair growth, appear between the ages of 8 and 13 years (mean 10.5 years) (Fig. 1.1) (Marshall and Tanner, 1969). Actually, increase in

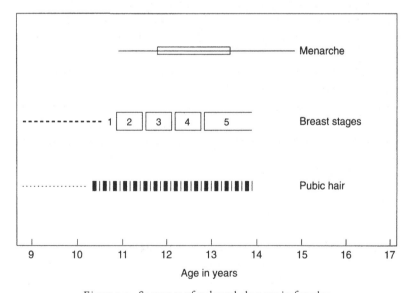

Figure 1.1. Sequence of pubertal changes in females.

height velocity rather than breast development may be the first sign of puberty in girls. The development of the breast is primarily under the control of estrogens secreted by the ovaries, whereas growth of pubic and axillary hair is mainly under the influence of androgens secreted by the adrenal gland and the ovary (Drife, 1986). Axillary hair appears at approximately age 13 in U.S. girls. Breast development may be asymmetrical for several months and may cause unfounded concerns for the girl and the parents. Marshall and Tanner (1969) have provided the most widely used classification of the stages of breast development, based on specific characteristics common to the female breast:

Stage 1: elevation of papilla only.
Stage 2: breast bud stage.
Stage 3: elevation of breast and papilla as a small mound, enlargement of the areola.
Stage 4: projection of areola and papilla from a secondary mound above the level of the breast.
Stage 5: mature stage, recession of areola to the general contour of the breast.

The stage of breast development usually corresponds to the stage of pubic hair development.

Menarche

Historical documents provide evidence that in industrialized countries puberty now occurs much earlier (Largo and Prader, 1983). The average age of menarche has decreased by about 2–3 months per decade for the past 150 years, from ages 17–18 to about 12–13 years. The average age at menarche is now 12.8 years (Wyshak and Frisch, 1982). This maturational advancement is, like the growth acceleration, largely the result of improved nutrition and health and better socioeconomic conditions. In point of fact, moderate obesity up to 30 percent above normal weight is associated with earlier menarche, whereas pathologic obesity leads to delayed puberty (Hartz, Barboriak, and Wong, 1979). Under optimal conditions of nutrition and child care, genetic factors largely determine the onset of puberty (Zacharias, Rand, and Wurtman, 1976).

An interesting phenomenon that was first documented by McClintock (1971) and contested by Wilson (1992), the convergence of menstrual onset dates, or menstrual synchrony, among girls and women who are friends or living together is still not well understood. Recent work by Weller (Weller, Weller, and Avinir, 1995) suggests that the critical factor may not be the physical contact through close living conditions but emotional synchronization through close friendships and intensive social contact.

9

Psychological growth

Adolescence is a time of intense emotional experiences, and sometimes eccentric behavior, but not necessarily a time of turmoil (Offer, Ostrov, and Howard, 1981). Larson and co-workers (Larson, Csikszentmihalyi, and Graef, 1980) found that adolescents of both sexes, who were paged throughout the day at random intervals and requested to record their mood, reported more rapid and more marked positive and negative mood swings than adults. Continuous turmoil might actually be a sign of psychopathology. Masterson Jr. (1968) observed that many of the tumultuous teenagers displayed symptoms of an affective disorder by late adolescence. Relationships between plasma concentrations of sexual hormones and depression, aggression, or happiness in adolescence are weak and inconsistent (Buchanan, Eccles, and Becker, 1992). So far, it has been difficult to determine even how influences of plasma estrogens or androgens are transmitted to the brain to produce mood changes, because in the male testosterone is extensively converted to estradiol and in smaller amounts to dihydrotestosterone in the brain. Very likely, estrogen receptors also modulate brain neurons in the male (McEwen, 1981).

Preexisting depression has been reported to be more strongly related to depression than coexisting plasma estrogen values (Susman, Dorn, and Chrousos, 1991). Several studies have shown that adolescent girls more frequently report depressed mood and anxiety than adolescent boys (Kandel and Davies, 1982; Petersen, Sarigiani, and Kennedy, 1991; Casper, Belanoff, and Offer, 1996), although no relationship between mood and pubertal status has been observed. One hypothesis that has undergone testing is that girls become oversocialized. Girls tend to be more concerned with expectations and moral issues, to depend more on external approval, and in consequence to develop more easily a negative self-image (Gjerde and Block, 1991). In most cultures, girls are socialized into inhibiting the expression of anger in adverse situations and into internalizing their feelings. Other factors that may account for the higher incidence of depression in women are discussed in Chapter Four.

Body and self-image

Body image in our appearance-conscious society has become a fashionable topic of conversation, mistakenly assumed to reflect a morbid preoccupation with an ideal body shape. Indeed, fear of fatness and of being overweight were expressed by 30 percent of 9-year-old girls in California (Casper, 1995a). Such expression of body dissatisfaction in the young has become a source of concern for parents and teachers. In girls, the preoccupation with weight seems to increase with increasing age, whereas boys tend to interpret weight gain as a sign of strength (Richards, Casper, and Larson, 1990). Studies on the body image in relation to the timing of the onset of puberty have consistently found that in girls early pubertal development is associated with a negative body and self-image (Gargiulo et al., 1987), whereas in boys early puberty affects the body image positively. Early-maturing girls report more conflict with their parents and have been found to describe more depressed affect in 12th grade than late-maturing girls (Petersen, Sarigiani, and Kennedy, 1991). The fact that early maturers are generally shorter than late maturers, but usually weigh more (Garn et al., 1986), might contribute to the negative effects of early menarche, defined as menarche before age 11.

Body image is actually a neutral term (Schilder, 1935). It indicates simply that the brain retains a schematic representation of the body, which under normal conditions rarely, if ever, reaches awareness. For instance, the transformation of the child's into a woman's body, although it occurs gradually, brings with it dramatic changes, yet most of the time these pubertal changes are integrated smoothly into the body image and comfortably accepted into the self-concept. Similarly, most women adapt easily to the changed bodily contours of pregnancy.

Self-concept and self-esteem

Self-esteem, defined in Webster's dictionary as "holding a good opinion of one-self and one of self-respect," develops early in life. Self-regard forms part of the self-concept and draws its substance from the individual's physical and psychological attributes – from the person's genetic disposition, temperament, personality, intelligence, special talents, and attractiveness – and not least from environmental influences. In classical analytic theory the infant moves from being the center of attention and from a position of control (primary narcissism) to the realization of his or her limits and dependence on others (Freud, 1914). The infant learns that despite unavoidable frustrations inherent in any relationship, he or she will be cared for and loved. Such early aquired confident expectations underlie the concept of basic trust (Erikson, 1963). Under optimal conditions, a certain amount of neglect and disappointment leading to anxiety and angry protest will be expected and processed without shattering the individual's sense of worth and confidence.

Most subsequent theories have elaborated on these early relational foundations of self-esteem and their implications for separation and individuation (Mahler, 1963). In a recent study (Roy, Neale, and Kendler, 1995) based on the

Virginia Twin Registry that asked monozygotic and dizygotic twins to complete the Rosenberg self-esteem questionnaire, individual experiences were found to account for about half of the variance contributing to self-esteem. The other half was found to be inherited, with neuroticism and depression contributing most to heritability. Self-esteem was also noted to be fairly stable. Over and above self-esteem, family norms, societal and cultural codes, and the girl's own expectations and conscience subtly mold and negotiate the self-concept in childhood and adolescence and throughout adult life.

Adolescence is a time of increased self-evaluation and at the same time of internal disengagement from family values. Self-consciousness increases with exposure to peer group and societal values as the adolescent begins to realize that social roles and social positions in adult life are fundamental sources of identity. Comparisons and competition create continous conflicts that can affirm or threaten the self-image and self-concept. For girls who grew up in a healthy family and who were accustomed to a matrix of relationships outside the family, autonomy will include reliance on others, whereas for girls who grew up in emotional isolation in dysfunctional families, independence might come to connote self-sufficiency. If female adolescents have been raised with, and as a consequence have developed, an ideal of perfection, there is a constant threat of failure. If their ideal has grown out of a realistic assessment of their innate abilities, their expectations and performance will be in tune with their abilities, and their activities will increase their self-confidence.

Female adolescents for the most part are and feel physically healthy (Casper, Belanoff, and Offer, 1996), but adolescence is a time when minor psychiatric morbidity and more serious disorders rise in frequency, with many of these disturbances showing a female preponderance. Anorexia nervosa typically has its onset in early adolescence, and bulimia nervosa is observed in the late teens (see Chapter Seven). More dramatic is the increased incidence of affective disorders and anxiety disorders and the rise in attempted suicides. Even though only 15–20 percent of female adolescents may be affected (Graham and Rutter, 1973; Leslie, 1974; Hawton and Goldacre, 1982; Angold and Costello, 1995), it is important to recognize these disturbances so that treatment can be initiated.

Conclusions

In industrialized countries, and increasingly all over the world, female adolescents grow up better educated and with more freedom and more choices than their grandmothers had, even if the independent woman may still be considered a contradiction in terms. Greater opportunities, as diverse as they might be, entail greater aspirations and efforts and more responsibilities. It remains a fact of life that women alone can bear children. The debate about how women who are fulfilling several roles will fare in this changing environment has led to many investigations. To give one example, Elliot and Huppert (1991), who surveyed a large British sample of married women under the age of 45, observed that paid employment, particularly full-time work, was beneficial for middle-class women but detrimental for working-class women. Women with one or more preschool children showed the highest prevalence of psychiatric symptoms; surprisingly, the study observed no association between mental health and social class. Women's greater readiness for symptom recognition (Kessler, Brown, and Boman, 1981) might be fortuitous and protective in times of limited access to health care, and so might be the increase in the number of female physicians, who have been found to be more attuned to preventive care for women than male physicians (Lurie et al., 1993). Health and disease are multifaceted. The chapters in this volume describe factors contributing to the disorders for which women are uniquely at risk and present evidence for hormonal and environmental influences on women's health. The last two chapters consider issues in psychopharmacology pertinent to women and present an overview of ongoing intervention trials with a hormonal or a behavioral component in female populations. We hope that greater awareness of the close connections among social, psychological, endocrine, and constitutional factors in disease states will improve treatment options and raise fresh hypotheses for research in women and in men.

CHAPTER TWO

REPRODUCTION AND ITS PSYCHOPATHOLOGY

KATHERINE E. WILLIAMS

AND REGINA C. CASPER

Early writers, such as Hippocrates, saw the womb as the seat of emotions and invoked the image of the "wandering womb" as stirring up emotions in women (Veith, 1965). Women's cookery books and physicians' casebooks from the 17th century abound with prescriptions for "how to put the womb back in her place" with foul-smelling herbs such as asafoetida (Williams, 1990). The notion that the reproductive organs produced substances that could alter mentation was bolstered by reports in the late 19th century which asserted that the "juice" of guinea pig ovaries could cure the symptoms of hysteria (Corner, 1965).

A century later, there is no longer any doubt about the neuropharmacologic effects of the gonadal hormones. Moreover, fluctuations of gonadal steroids premenstrually, during pregnancy and postpartum and in the perimenopausal years, seem to increase the risk of emotional disturbances in certain women. It has become apparent that the ups and downs of hormonal secretion perturb neurotransmitter sites, which regulate emotions and cognition, and not the absolute hormone levels, which show little correspondence. This chapter first briefly reviews the psycho- and neurotropic effects of the gonadal hormones and examines their relationship to psychopathology. It then describes the clinical characteristics of reproductive cycle–related psychiatric syndromes, which can undermine a woman's self-confidence and raise doubts about her ability to function as a partner and a mother.

Neurotropic effects of gonadal hormones

Estrogen and progesterone are lipophilic steroid hormones that directly and indirectly affect central nervous system neurons involved in the regulation of mood and cognition. Neurochemical mapping of rat brain reveals receptors for both hormones distributed thoughout the brain. High densities of estrogen receptors are found in the limbic forebrain, hypothalamus, and pituitary, and high densities of progesterone receptors are found in the hypothalamus, hippocampus, and cerebral cortex; only unbound estradiol and progesterone enter the brain, about 1–3 percent of plasma concentrations (McEwen, 1981). Mean follicular phase preovulatory peak plasma estradiol concentrations range from 139 to 290 pg/ml, and mean luteal phase plasma progesterone concentrations range from 2 to 33 ng/ml (Longcope, 1986). The hormones can enter nerve cells and exert their psychotropic effects in a number of ways. Presynaptically, hormones influence the production of neurotransmitters and receptor modulation, and postsynaptically they can modulate the affinity of receptors for substrates (McEwen, 1981).

Studies suggest that estradiol acts as a weak neuroleptic in both humans and animals (Van Hartesveldt and Joyce, 1986), yet its mechanism of action remains controversial. The effects of estrogen on dopaminergic transmission appear to be dose, time, and region specific. Estradiol inhibits dopaminergic activity in the anterior pituitary and striatum both in vivo and in vitro in rats (Bedard et al., 1979). Chronic estrogen treatment appears to upregulate the number of striatal dopamine receptors (DiPaolo, Poyet, and Labrie, 1981), a mechanism of action similar to neuroleptics in humans. In humans, estrogen can worsen movement disorders associated with dopamine blockade, such as neuroleptic-induced Parkinson's disease (Villeneuve, Langelier, and Bedard, 1980). However, clinically in both animals and humans, estrogen also appears to have some dopamine agonist properties with long-term, high-dose exposure, which has been shown to increase behavioral stereotypies in rats and induce movement disorders such as chorea gravidarum in humans (Lewis and Parsons, 1966).

There is increasing evidence in a variety of studies in both animals and humans that estrogen affects serotonin function. Estrogen effects are dose specific, region specific, and affected by length of exposure and presence or absence of progesterone (Biegon, 1990). Estrogen appears to increase the bioavailability of the serotonin precursor tryptophan by displacing it from its binding sites on plasma albumin, leading to increased free tryptophan available for conversion via tyrosine hydroxylase to serotonin (Aylward, 1973). Estradiol has also been shown to decrease monoamine oxidase (MAO) activity in the basomedial hypothalamus and medial amygdala in rats (Luine, Khylchevskay, and McEwen, 1975) and humans (Klaiber et al., 1979). Thus, estrogen may lead to increased available presynaptic serotonin via inhibition of MAO.

These findings are consistent with observations of significantly increased hypothalamic 5-HT uptake on pre-estrus days in rats when estrogen levels are highest (Biegon, 1990). Similarly, serotonin receptor densities appear to be modulated by estrogen levels in naturally cycling rats. $5-HT_1$-receptor density is lowest during pre-estrus and estrus, when estrogen levels are highest, and receptor density is highest during diestrus, when estrogen levels are lowest (Biegon, 1990). Similarly, acute estrogen administration appears to lead to downregulation of $5-HT_1$ receptors, which persists with chronic administration of estradiol and is unaffected by the presence of progesterone, whereas $5-HT_2$-receptor upregulation with chronic exposure to estradiol can be reversed with progesterone (Biegon et al., 1983; Biegon, 1990). High chronic doses of estradiol affect uptake of serotonin into platelets (Rehavi, Sepcuti, and Weizman, 1987).

Estrogen also promotes norepinephrine release via reduction of tonic presynaptic inhibition of alpha-2-autoreceptors (Etgen and Karkanias, 1994) and modulates norepinephrine receptor density and function. Ovariectomy leads to upregulation of adrenergic recepors in the hypothalamus, corpus callosum, and anterior pituitarty (Petrovic et al., 1983), whereas long-term estrogen exposure leads to noradrengeric downregulation (Biegon et al., 1983) similar to that seen after antidepressant drug treatment in humans. By contrast, progesterone has no effect on adrenergic receptors in rats (Biegon et al., 1983).

Premenstrual dysphoric disorder

In light of the findings from animal studies, investigators set out with much optimism to identify hormonal changes in blood, and rarely in cerebrospinal fluid (CSF), to establish relationships to the symptoms reported in premenstrual dysphoric disorder (PDD). A wealth of studies on the endocrinology of PDD have been conducted, so far with modest results. We review the clinical picture of PDD first and then discuss theories of etiology and treatment.

Premenstrual psychological and somatic complaints are common in women; however, rarely are complaints distressing enough to interfere with activities or relationships. Dysfunction distinguishes premenstrual complaints from premenstrual dysphoric disorder. Technically, at least two cycles of prospective daily ratings that show 30 percent worsening of symptoms during 2 weeks before menses and a clear remission with menses onset are necessary to make the diagnosis (American Psychiatric Association, 1994). Menstrual rating forms include the 21-item Daily Rating Form (Endicott and Halbreich, 1982) and the Moos Menstrual Questionnaire (Moos, 1968). Only 30–40 percent of women who appear to have PDD based upon retrospective reports actually demonstrate these symptoms prospectively (Morse and Dennerstein, 1988; Severino and Moline, 1989), and only 4 percent of this group will ultimately meet the criteria for PDD (Rivera-Tovar and Frank, 1990).

Prospective daily ratings are critical for differentiating PDD from an underlying mood or anxiety disorder. Between 20 and 40 percent of women referred for symptoms of PDD are actually found to be suffering a current mood or anxiety disorder (Pearlstein et al., 1991) rather than PDD. Women with PDD are at increased risk for depression, as 40 to 78 percent of women with prospectively confirmed PDD have a history of anxiety or mood disorders (Hurt et al., 1992).

In order to qualify for the diagnosis of PDD, a woman must have at least five symptoms, and at least one must be an affective symptom, such as depressed mood, anxiety, irritability, or affective lability. Other PDD symptoms include difficulty concentrating, lack of energy, poor appetite, and sleep changes and physical symptoms such as breast tenderness, headaches, and feelings of being overwhelmed (American Psychiatric Association, 1994).

Ever since Frank's original description of "premenstrual tension" in the 1930s, treatments have focused on correcting hormonal imbalances through the use of diuretics, cathartics, venipuncture, and irradiation of the ovaries (Severino and Moline, 1989). The belief that premenstrual dysphoric disorder is due to hormonal imbalance remains very much alive today. Progesterone replacement therapy continues to be widely used as a treatment, despite the many double blind, placebo-controlled studies in prospectively diagnosed PDD patients that have demonstrated its ineffectiveness (Gold and Severino, 1994).

Review of the literature examining hormonal imbalances in premenstrual dysphoric disorder reveals potential methodologic flaws and conflicting results. Major methodologic problems are lack of diagnostic validity due to failure to confirm the presence of symptoms in the luteal phase of the menstrual cycle only, failure to select patients whose symptoms are severe enough to interfere with daily activities and relationships, and failure to confirm the presence or timing of ovulation. Timing of ovulation is important when hormonal values are compared at different stages of the menstrual cycle in symptomatic women and in controls.

Another important variable difficult to control is the apparent pulsatile nature and circadian rhythm of estrogen production. Although hormones that control estrogen production, the gonadotropin-releasing hormones (GnRHs), luteinizing hormone (LH), and follicule-stimulating hormone (FSH) are typically secreted in a pulsatile pattern in humans (Backstrom et al., 1982), the control of estrogen release is not well understood. Animal studies suggest that LH pulses are followed by a transient rise in estrogen and that the frequency of LH pulses determines the amount of estradiol secreted by the ovary (Baird, 1978). A similar pulsatile secretion pattern that leads to significant variability in estrogen levels during the day (Korenman and Sherman, 1973; Lenton et al., 1978) has been observed in humans. Moreover, estrogen levels demonstrate a circadian rhythm, as morning levels have consistently been found to be highest (Backstrom et al., 1982). Thus, the mean estrogen levels reported in studies that do not control for this morning rise in estrogen levels are not as reliable as those that control for the time of day at sampling.

Methodologically sound studies of the relationship between premenstrual symptoms and serum hormone levels can be divided into matched control studies and prospective, intraindividual comparison studies. Three controlled studies fulfill the criteria of prospective confirmation of PDD, and all three reveal no difference in mean concentrations of estrogen and progesterone across the cycle in subjects versus controls (Watts et al., 1985; Rubinow et al., 1988; Dennerstein et al., 1993). No studies exist comparing CSF hormone levels in PDD patients and controls. Parry et al. (1991) has reported no significant differences between follicular and luteal phase CSF estrogen and progesterone levels in a small sample of PDD patients.

Studies of intraindividual differences suggest that some women are more sensitive to changes in hormones and that sensitivity to these changes may lead to psychological symptoms seen in PDD. Hammarback, Damber, and Backstrom (1989) followed 18 women with prospectively confirmed premenstrual syndrome (PMS) for 2 months using daily ratings of visual analog scales during the luteal phase. Sixteen of the 18 women differed in plasma estrogen levels, 13 differed in progesterone levels, and 6 differed in estrogen:progesterone ratios between the two cycles. Six symptoms were associated with high versus low estrogen luteal phase cycles: increased breast swelling and tenderness, less friendliness and more irritability, fatigue, and depression. High luteal phase levels of progesterone also correlated with more PDD symptoms, including anxiety, breast tenderness, irritability, and depression (Hammarback, Damber, and Backstrom, 1989).

Further support for the finding that higher luteal-phase levels of estrogen may predispose to more mental and physical symptoms in women with a history of PDD comes from a study of 11 patients with PDD prospectively confirmed who were randomly assigned either Premarin 0.625 mg or placebo starting 15 days before the expected date of onset of menstruation. Luteal-phase exogenous estrogen was found to be associated with increased mental and physical symptoms of PDD; no serum levels were drawn to determine the correlation between symptoms and change in estradiol levels (Dhar and Murphy, 1990).

The dynamics of hormone change also appear to be important in triggering premenstrual complaints. A faster rate of progesterone decline with a time lag of 4–7 days between hormonal change and onset of symptoms was reported by Halbreich et al. (1986) in a prospectively confirmed group of women with PDD. The dynamics of the fluctuation in hormone levels and their effects on neurotransmitter systems involved in mood regulation in a vulnerable group of women appears to be the most promising area of research in PDD.

Several studies have pointed to abnormalities in the serotonin system in women with PDD. Whole blood serotonin (Rapkin et al., 1987), serotonin platelet reuptake (Taylor et al., 1984; Ashby et al., 1988), and platelet-tritiated imipramine binding (Rojansky et al., 1991) are lower during the luteal phase of the menstrual cycle in women with PDD than in controls. Reduced platelet uptake of serotonin has also been reported throughout the entire cycle in PDD patients as compared to controls (Ashby et al., 1990, Steege et al., 1992). Challenge tests also suggest abnormal serotonergic function in women with PDD, including subsensitivity of 5-HT_{1a} receptors (Yatham, 1994). Acute tryptophan depletion has been shown to aggravate symptoms in women with prospectively confirmed PDD (Menkes, Coates, and Fawcett, 1994), whereas tryptophan has been shown to alleviate symptoms in a pilot study of PDD (Steinberg et al., 1994).

Further support for the findings of serotonin dysregulation in PDD patients comes from reports of the effectiveness of selective serotonin reuptake inhibitors in the treatment of PDD in several double blind placebo-controlled studies (Stone, Pearlstein, and Brown, 1991; Menkes et al., 1992; Wood et al., 1992; Steiner et al., 1995).

The long-term treatment of PDD with SSRIs remains controversial. Anecdotal reports of luteal phase-only dosing and "as needed" dosing of SSRIs in PDD have prompted clinicians and researchers to investigate the possibility of lower doses for shorter time periods, but to date no controlled studies have been published. Thus, a major treatment issue in PDD is "how much SSRI for how long?" The limited number of studies in the literature that have followed patients for 3–47 months suggest that the efficacy of the SSRIs is maintained for the duration of the study. However, once the medication has been discontinued, symptoms return (Pearlstein and Stone, 1994; Elks, 1993; Freeman et al., 1994).

Gonadal steroid effects on circadian rhythms may also underlie PDD. Gonadal steroids, especially estrogen, have been found to affect circadian

Table 2.1. *Current treatments for premenstrual dysphoric disorder: Results of placebo-controlled trials*

Medication	Authors	Conclusion
Alprazolam	Harrison, Endicott, and Rabkin, 1987 Smith et al., 1987 Harrison, Endicott, and Nee, 1990 Schmidt, Gore, and Rubinow, 1993 Berger and Presser, 1994 Freeman et al., 1995	Alprazolam superior to placebo in 5/6 studies
Buspirone	Rickels et al., 1989	Buspirone superior to placebo
Clomipramine	Eriksson et al., 1990 Sunblad et al., 1992	Clomipramine superior to placebo in 2/2 studies
Danazol	Gilmore, Hawthorne, and Hart, 1985 Sarno, Miller, and Sunblad, 1987 Watts, Edwards, and Butt, 1985 Watts, Butt, and Edwards, 1987 Hahn, Van Vugt, and Reid, 1995	Danazol superior to placebo in 5/5 studies. Side effects include nausea, drowsiness. Hot flashes at high doses.
Fluoxetine	Rickels et al., 1990 Stone, Pearlstein, and Brown, 1991 Menkes et al., 1992 Wood et al., 1992 Steiner et al., 1995	Fluoxetine superior to placebo in 5/5 studies
GnRH agonists	Muse et al., 1984 Bancroft et al., 1987 Hammarback and Backstrom, 1988 Helvacioglu et al., 1993 Brown et al., 1994 West and Hillier, 1994	GnRH superior to placebo in 4/6 studies for emotional symptoms Superior in 2/6 studies for physical symptoms only Side effects include hot flushes, mood lability, loss of energy.
Paroxetine	Eriksson et al., 1995	Paroxetine superior to placebo and maprotiline
Sertraline	Yonkers et al., 1996	Sertraline superior to placebo

GnRH, gonadotropin-releasing hormone.

rhythms in animals, perhaps through effects on the suprachiasmic nucleus (Leibenluft, 1993); however, evidence for this relationship in humans is indirect. Just as in depressive disorder, partial early- and late-night sleep deprivation have both been found to be effective in decreasing Hamilton and Beck depression scores in women with PDD, and Parry et al. (1995) suggest that this treatment resets an underlying circadian rhythm disturbance. Women with PDD have been found to have blunted melatonin circadian rhythms compared to normal subjects (Parry et al., 1990). Further studies will need to be done to evaluate the effectiveness of sleep deprivation in PDD and the underlying mechanism of action.

In summary, a diverse array of treatments have been proposed for the treatment of premenstrual dysphoric disorder. Initial therapy includes a thorough psychiatric evaluation to rule out comorbid psychiatric disorders and a careful diet and exercise history. Many women will improve during the 2-month evaluation phase because as they begin to see a pattern to their symptoms, they begin to feel more in control. Aerobic exercise at least three times a week, a well-balanced, low-salt diet, and B vitamin supplementation are recommended initial treatments for premenstrual symptoms (Severino and Moline, 1989). Women who do not improve with these changes in lifestyle may benefit from medications (Table 2.1). Currently, serotonergic agents, such as Fluoxetine, are the most promising interventions, as they lack the addictive potential of the benzodiazepines, which have also been shown to be useful in several placebo-controlled studies (Harrison et al., 1987; Smith et al., 1987; Harrison, Endicott, and Nee, 1990; Schmidt, Grover, and Rubinow, 1993; Berger and Presser, 1994; Freeman et al., 1995).

Pregnancy

Depressive disorders

Several studies have reported that prevalence rates for depressive disorders during pregnancy are similar to those in nonpregnant women (O'Hara et al., 1990). However, psychosocial stressors such as lack of social support, including lack of a partner (O'Hara, 1986), and financial and housing problems are associated with increased rates of depression ranging from 25 to 40 percent of pregnant women in some studies (Hobfoll et al., 1995; Seguin et al., 1995).

Some of the physiologic changes associated with pregnancy, including sleep and appetite disturbances, and low libido and energy, may be difficult to distinguish from the somatic symptoms of depression. Symptoms such as anhedonia, marked memory and concentration disturbances, hopelessness, and suicidality are not normal features of pregnancy and signify a major depressive disorder. Cognitive behavioral therapy and interpersonal therapy offering support and conflict resolution are treatments of choice in pregnant women with a major depressive disorder. Pharmacotherapy and occasionally hospitalization should be reserved for women with severe depressive or psychotic symptoms or suicidality.

Anxiety disorders

The effect of pregnancy upon anxiety disorders appears to vary from individual to individual. Many researchers have postulated that anxiety disorders should improve during pregnancy because progesterone metabolites act similarly to barbiturates to modulate GABA-receptor complexes and have sedative effects (Majewska et al., 1986; Morrow, Suzdak, and Paul, 1987). However, increased levels of estradiol during pregnancy may potentiate noradrenergic functioning, leading to increased anxiety symptoms in some women, especially during the second and third trimesters when estrogen levels are higher than progesterone levels (Verburg, Griez, and Meijer, 1994). New-onset panic attacks have been reported in women initiating hormone replacement therapy (Price and Heil, 1988). Retrospective studies indicate that the majority of women with panic disorder stay the same or improve during pregnancy. The postpartum period is a time of increased risk for new onset or exacerbation of panic disorder (George, Ladenheim, and Nutt, 1987; Metz, Sichel, and Goff, 1988; Cowley and Roy-Byrne, 1989; Villeponteaux et al., 1992; Sholomskas, Wickamaratne, and Dogolo, 1993; Cohen, Sichel, Dimmock, and Rosenbaum, 1994; Northcott and Stein, 1994). Cognitive behavior therapy is the treatment of choice for pregnant women with panic disorder. Pharmacotherapy should be used cautiously. If medication is necessary, tricyclic antidepressants or benzodiazepines should be initiated after the first trimester, if possible, and gradually tapered prior to delivery in order to avoid neonatal withdrawal syndromes (Miller, 1994; Altshuler et al., 1996; see also Chapter Ten in this volume).

In retrospective studies, onset of obsessive compulsive disorder (OCD) occurred during pregnancy in 13–39 percent of women (Buttolph and Holland, 1990; Neziroglu, Anemone, and Yaryura-Tobias, 1992; Williams and Koran, in press). Retrospective studies suggest that OCD symptoms stay the same or improve during pregnancy in the majority of women with preexisting disease (Buttolph and Holland, 1990; Williams and Koran, in press). As in panic disorder, cognitive behavioral therapy is the treatment of choice for obsessive compulsive disorder during pregnancy. The postpartum period appears to be a time of increased risk for exacerbation of OCD and the onset of depression in OCD patients (Williams and Koran, in press).

Psychosis

Several authors report that psychotic disorders such as schizophrenia improve during pregnancy (McNeil, Kaij, and Malmquist-Larsson, 1984; Chang and Renshaw, 1986). It is presumed that this protection from relapse during pregnancy is due to enhanced dopaminergic blockade with increased estradiol levels (Seeman and Lang, 1990). Treatment of a psychotic relapse during pregnancy includes neuroleptics and hospitalization in order to ensure safety for both the mother and fetus. Untreated psychotic pregnant women are at considerable risk for medical complications, in particular lack of prenatal care and substance abuse (Rudolph et al., 1990).

Postpartum blues

The postpartum blues are experienced by 39–85 percent of women (O'Hara, 1987). Classically, the blues begin between 3–5 days after delivery with mood lability, sleep disturbances, fatigue, and problems with memory and concentration. Commonly, these symptoms are mild and self-limited, except, of course, for sleep disruption due to feeding the infant at night. Women are usually back to their usual selves in 2–3 weeks. Presence of a thought disorder, such as ideas of reference or thought broadcasting, or hallucinations differentiates the blues from postpartum psychosis, and persistence of depression beyond 2 weeks differentiates the blues from postpartum depression (O'Hara et al., 1991)

The timing of the onset of the blues coincides with the rapid drop in estrogen and progesterone immediately postpartum, suggesting that postpartum blues might be an endocrine epiphenomenon (Harris et al., 1989; Wieck, 1989). Absolute levels of estrogen or progesterone do not differ on particular days between blues sufferers and controls. O'Hara et al. (1991) reported that women who met criteria for the blues had higher levels of free estriol at week 38 of gestation and on days 2 and 3 postpartum, as well as a greater overall decrease from mean prepartum estriol levels to postpartum levels. Absolute estradiol, progesterone, and prolactin levels were not different (O'Hara, 1991). Feski et al. (1984) observed higher salivary estrogen levels in blues sufferers during the first 5 days postpartum; however, Heidrich et al. (1994) did not find any difference in free plasma hormone levels in postpartum blues patients compared to controls.

By contrast, Harris et al. (1994) found in women with the blues higher prepartum progesterone levels and lower postpartum levels than in women without the blues, and an earlier study by Nott et al. (1976) reported a correlation between decline in progesterone levels after delivery and severity of depression in women during the first 10 days postpartum.

Another correlate is a history of vulnerability to depression during other times of hormonal changes, in particular premenstrually. In a prospective study of 180 women, O'Hara (1991) found women with the blues report more often a history of premenstrual dysphoria and a family history and personal history of depression, including depressive symptoms during the index pregnancy.

Treatment of the blues includes supportive psychotherapy focusing upon educating the family and patient about the "normalcy" of the condition and the need for psychosocial support. Psychiatric follow-up of presenting blues patients is necessary to rule out the emergence of postpartum psychosis or depression.

Postpartum depression

Postpartum blues bear a relationship to postpartum and prepartum depression. In some studies, half the women depressed at 6 weeks reported prepartum depressive symptoms and postpartum blues (Glover, 1992; Hannah et al., 1992). A history of premenstrual dysphoria appears to increase the risk for both postpartum blues and postpartum depression (O'Hara, 1991). Hypomania during the first 5 days postpartum has also been correlated with later development of postpartum depression (Glover et al., 1994), suggesting that some women may have a bipolar diathesis.

Is breast-feeding a risk factor for postpartum depression? Increased prolactin has been associated with irritability, depression, and decreased libido (Koppelman et al., 1987), and it has been hypothesized that in lactating women this hormonal milieu may lead to postpartum depressive symptoms. Alder and Cox (1983) reported that women who breast-fed exclusively had higher depressive symptoms than women who partially breast-fed and supplemented with formula. However, a later study found no relationship between breast-feeding, estradiol or prolactin levels, and mood or sexuality (Alder et al., 1986). In fact, Hannah et al. (1992) reported that depression at 6 weeks postpartum was correlated with bottle feeding and cesarean section; thus, current research does not support a connection between breast-feeding and postpartum depression, and women should not be advised to avoid nursing.

Other risk factors for postpartum depression are similar to risk factors for depression in women in general and include a previous history of depression, a family history of depression, a history of premenstrual dysphoria, and stressful life events (Stowe and Nemeroff, 1995), including a history of severe medical complications during pregnancy such as preeclampsia (Burger et al., 1993) and emergency cesarean section (Boyce and Todd, 1992). Overall, prevalence rates of postpartum depression in a population of mothers with newborns appear to be no higher than depressive disorders in a population of women who are not pregnant (O'Hara et al., 1990).

The risk of relapse for postpartum depression is 10–35 percent (Pitt, 1975) and seems to depend upon the previous psychiatric history. Cooper and Murray (1995) found that women for whom postpartum depression was the index episode had an increased risk for the development of a depressive disorder, but were not at higher risk for postpartum depression. More studies will be needed to determine whether major depression with postpartum onset has the high rates of recurrence seen in postpartum psychosis.

The etiology of postpartum depression remains unknown (Wieck, 1989), and as in premenstrual dysphoria, no studies have found differences between mean gonadal hormone levels when women with postpartum depression were compared to women who did not develop a depression.

In summary, postpartum depression appears to be phenomenologically similar to depressions at other times in a woman's life. Although changes in circulating gonadal hormones postpartum play a role, a history of PDD, undesirable life events, and lack of social support, including marital problems, appear to be equally important in triggering postpartum depression (Braverman and Roux, 1978; Paykel et al., 1980; Kumar and Robson, 1984). Consequently, prevention strategies for PDD include increased prenatal social support and education (Collins et al., 1993; Midmer, Wilson, and Cummings, 1995). Currently, there are no randomized placebo-controlled studies to support the use of progesterone supplementation for treatment of postpartum depression despite its widespread use (Dalton, 1964). One open clinical trial has reported that antidepressant prophylaxis begun during the first week postpartum reduced the recurrence of postpartum depression in a high-risk group (Wisner and Wheeler, 1994). Gregoire et al. (1996) reported that transdermal estradiol for 6 months was more effective than placebo in the treatment of postpartum depression in a double blind study. Forty-seven percent of women in the active treatment group had already been on antidepressants for at least 6 weeks without significant benefit before study entry, and these women subsequently improved with the addition of estradiol, 200 µg per day.

Stuart and O'Hara (1995) have described successful treatment of postpartum depression with interpersonally oriented psychotherapy. One matched control study of new fathers found that men whose wives developed postpartum depression had increased rates of depression themselves (Harvey and McGrath, 1988). Consequently, individual therapy for the postpartum depressed patient's partner and marital therapy may be important in the treatment of women with postpartum depression.

Postpartum psychosis

A woman is at her greatest lifetime risk for psychosis in the weeks immediately following childbirth (Kendell, Chalmers, and Platz, 1987). Fortunately, postpartum psychosis has a low incidence of 1–2:1,000 births (O'Hara, 1987; Videbech and Gouliaev, 1995), but the high rates of maternal and infant morbidity and mortality are alarming. Infanticide is associated with 4 percent of postpartum psychoses (Garvey et al., 1983). As in other psychoses, postpartum psychosis is manifested by disorders of thought content, such as delusions, and disorders of thought pattern, such as looseness of association and tangentiality. The disorder has also been noted to have a "delirium quality," with marked impairment in attention, memory, and concentration (Hamilton, 1989). Thus, in one of the earliest treatises on postpartum psychosis, Marce (1958) spoke of "marked intellectual enfeeblement."

Unlike the risk factors for postpartum blues and depression, which have been found to be closely related to psychosocial variables and life events, risk factors for postpartum psychosis appear to be influenced less by nurture and more by nature (Dowlatshahi and Paykel, 1990; Marks et al., 1991). Women with a history of bipolar disorder appear to be at greatest risk for the development of postpartum psychosis: 25–50 percent (Braftos and Haug, 1966; Reich and Winokur, 1970; McNeil, 1987; Schopf and Rust, 1994). Similarly, postpartum psychosis may constitute the first episode of a bipolar disorder in women, in that 32–40 percent of women in follow-up studies who first experience a psychosis postpartum later on have nonpostpartum episodes. The risk for postpartum relapse in these women can be as high as 30–60 percent (Brockington et al., 1988; Videbech and Gouliaev, 1995).

Support for the finding that women with bipolar or schizoaffective disorder may be especially vulnerable to estrogen-induced changes in dopaminergic function comes from reports that women with a history of postpartum psychosis relapse premenstrually (Brockington et al., 1988). Furthermore, challenge tests with apomorphine, a dopamine agonist, have shown enhanced growth hormone secretion in women with a history of bipolar or schizoaffective disorder who later become ill, as compared to women at risk for psychosis who do not become ill or controls (Wieck and Kumar, 1991; Kumar et al., 1993). However, Meakin et al. (1995) failed to confirm this finding and in fact reported subsensitivity of growth hormone responsiveness on day 4 postpartum in a high-risk group.

Finally, prophylactic estrogen replacement has been found to decrease the incidence of postpartum psychosis in a high-risk group in a small pilot study (Sichel et al., 1995). Eleven women with a history of postpartum affective illness (7 with a history of postpartum psychosis and 4 with a history of major depression) received a 1-month taper of estrogen (tapered from 5 mg BID to 0.625 mg) following delivery. The 9 percent rate of postpartum relapse was significantly lower than the expected 35–60 percent rate without estrogen prophylaxis.

At present, owing to the high correlation between postpartum psychosis and bipolar disorder, lithium prophylaxis beginning 24 hours after delivery is the recommended treatment because lithium in ovariectomized rats prevents apomorphine supersensitivity associated with long-term estrogen exposure (Dorce and Palermo-Neto, 1992). Lithium begun within the first few days postpartum does decrease relapse rates to 10 percent in a high-risk group (Stewart et al., 1991; Cohen et al., 1995). Since valproic acid is now an acceptable and widely used first-time treatment for acute mania (Pope et al., 1991; Keck et al., 1993; McElroy et al., 1993), it may be used in the treatment of postpartum psychosis as well. It is also extremely important to minimize sleep-deprivation postpartum in women because it may induce or exacerbate mania (Strouse, Szuba, and Baxter, 1992).

Further neuroendocrine tests may lead to clarification of which bipolar women are at greatest risk for psychosis. To allow women who do not appear to be supersensitive to estrogen withdrawal to continue to breast-feed, neurendocrine tests need to be developed to clarify which bipolar women are at greatest risk for psychosis because lithium is contraindicated in breast-feeding mothers (Buist, Norman, and Dennerstein, 1990).

Menopause

Menopause reflects ovarian shutdown, which is said to have occurred following cessation of menstrual cycles for 1 year and a rise in FSH to greater than 25 IU/L. This transition to menopause is called perimenopause when cycle length varies due to frequent anovulatory periods and circulating gonadal hormone levels fluctuate. Estrogen levels decrease from a premenopausal mean of 126 pg/ml to a postmenopausal mean of 38 pg/ml, originating in the adrenal gland

(Longcope, 1990) Progesterone levels decrease from a premenopausal mean of 15 nmol/l to 2 nmol/l (Ballinger, Browning, and Smith, 1987). LH and FSH secretion dramatically increase in response to the hypoestrogenic state (Ballinger, Browning, and Smith, 1987).

The involution of the ovaries has long been thought to alter a woman's temper. Schmidt and Rubinow (1991) quote Farnham, who in 1897 wrote, "The ovaries, after long years of service, have not the ability of retiring in graceful old age, but become irritated, and transmit their irritation to the abdominal ganglia, which in turn transmit the irritation to the brain, producing disturbances in the cerebral tissue exhibiting themselves in extreme nervousness or in an outburst of actual insanity."

Kraeplin termed the onset of major depression in midlife Involutional Melancholia due to its symptom profile – hypochondriasis, nihilistic delusions, and agitation – and distinguished the disorder from depressions occurring at other times. Interestingly, Kraeplin believed that Involutional Melancholia affected both men and women; however, during this century the term became synonymous with menopausal depression (Schmidt and Rubinow, 1991).

The existence of Involutional Melancholia has not been confirmed by research. Midlife depressions do not appear to differ in clinical course, severity, or prognosis from depressions arising at other times in a woman's life (Schmidt and Rubinow, 1991). Contrary to common belief, the prevalence of major depression during the menopausal years is not increased (Ballinger, 1990). In fact, women seem to be at their greatest risk for depressive disorders during their childbearing years (Myers et al., 1984).

Multiple cross-sectional surveys of mood complaints during the menopause reveal an increase in minor complaints of psychological distress, but no increase in the prevalence of major psychiatric disorders (Ballinger, 1990). Some studies suggest that clinically significant psychiatric symptoms may increase at the time of perimenopause, when women are menstruating erratically, a time when gonadal hormones show the greatest fluctuation (Jaszmann, van Lith, and Zaat, 1969; Bungay, Vessey, and McPherson, 1980). Women with a history of PDD, postpartum depression, or oral birth control–associated mood changes appear to be at greater risk for perimenopausal mood changes (Stewart and Boydell, 1993).

Hormone replacement and mood

Although over 30 studies have investigated the effects of estrogen and progesterone on mood in perimenopausal and postmenopausal women, only a few have attempted to correlate actual plasma hormone levels with mood (Table 2.2). Low estrogen levels are clearly associated with increased somatic symptoms such as hot flashes and sleep disturbances, especially in younger perimenopausal women (Abe et al., 1976), but not with affective disorders. Ballinger, Browning, and Smith (1987) reported that in early postmenopausal women with higher general health questionnaire scores, plasma estrogen levels were higher than in less symptomatic women. Depression in the menopausal women correlated with higher thyroid-stimulating hormone (TSH) levels but

Table 2.2. *Hormone levels and psychiatric symptoms in perimenopausal and menopausal women*

Author	n	Study population	Measures	Results
Abe et al., 1976	191	Outpatients pre- and post-menopausal	1. Serum: E_2; P_4; FSH; LH 2. Kupperman Index	Kupperman Index correlated with low E_2 and high LH in pre-menopausal women aged 35–39 years
Chakravarti et al., 1979	82	Outpatients pre- and peri-menopausal	1. Serum: FSH; LH; E_2 2. Self-reports of somatic and psychological symptoms	Similar E_2, FSH, and LH regardless of symptoms
Ballinger, Browning, and Smith, 1987	85	Outpatients 45–55 years	1. Serum: FSH; LH; prolactin; cortisol, androstenedione; thyroxine	1. High GHQ scores in early postmenopausal group with significantly higher E_2 2. Depressed late premenopausal subjects had higher TSH and T_3 3. Increased androstenedione levels in early premenopausal group with decreased sexual interest
Pansini et al., 1994	1,161	Outpatients pre-, peri-, and post-menopausal	1. Serum: E_2; P_4; FSH 2. Kupperman Index	No correlation between psychological symptoms and estrogen levels

GHQ, General Health Questionnaire; FSH, follicle-stimulating hormone; LH, luteinizing hormone; TSH, thyroid-stimulating hormone; E_2, estradiol; P_4, progesterone; T_3, triiodothyronine.

not with a reduction in triiodothyronine levels, suggesting subtle dysfunction of the hypothalamic pituitary thyroid axis as is seen in other affective disorders (Ballinger, Browning, and Smith, 1987). In studies of women undergoing oophorectomy, depression scores have been reported to covary inversely with circulating levels of both estradiol and testosterone (Sherwin and Gelfand, 1985; Sherwin, 1988).

Most of the studies investigating the effects of estrogen replacement on mood in menopausal women have failed to use validated, sensitive measures of anxiety and depression. For instance, the Kupperman Index (Kupperman et al., 1959), includes 18 somatic symptoms and only 3 psychiatric symptoms: anxiety, irritability, and depression. Furthermore, hormonal treatment studies are especially difficult to interpret because many of them fail to distinguish between women in early versus late menopause. Baseline estrogen and progesterone levels are not compared to treatment levels or correlated with changes in psychiatric symptoms using validated psychiatric rating instruments. Often, varying dosages of estrogen and progesterone are used without placebo control, which is problematic because perimenopausal complaints are highly responsive to placebo (Coope, Thompson, and Poller, 1975).

Review of estrogen replacement studies that have used validated instruments suggest that estrogen given alone without progesterone may be helpful for improving mood in naturally menopausal women with minor psychological complaints; that is, women who do not meet criteria for a major depression (Table 2.3). Schneider, Brotherton, and Hailes (1977) found that Premarin in doses of 0.3–0.625 mg improved depression scores in patients who were not depressed, but had no effect in depressed patients with a mean Beck Depression Inventory score of 24.5. Best et al. (1992) reported in an open trial a decrease in Hamilton scores from 13.5 to 3.9 after 6 weeks with a 100-mg estradiol implant. In a double blind placebo-controlled trial of 8 weeks of Piperazine estrone sulfate 1.5 mg BID in women with mean pretreatment Hamilton scores of 16–18, suggesting mild to moderate depression, both the estrogen and placebo groups improved (Thompson and Oswald, 1977). An early placebo-controlled study by Klaiber et al. (1979) reported that 25 mg/day of Premarin improved depression in severely depressed women who had failed multiple antidepressant trials (Klaiber et al., 1979), but their mean scores remained at 22, that is, in the depressed range, after estradiol administration. Saletu et al. (1995) reported that placebo and estrogen therapy were both effective in significantly decreasing Hamilton depression scores in a group of depressed menopausal women.

The addition of progesterone to the estrogen leads to cyclical changes in mood similar to those seen in naturally occurring cycles, with increased depression, ten-

Table 2.3. *Placebo-controlled studies of the effect of estrogen on mood in depressed and nondepressed women*

Author	n	Estrogen	Measures	Results
Schneider, Brotherton, and Hailes, 1977	22	Premarin 0.3–0.625 mg/day	BDI	Decrease in depression in non-depressed patients Nonimprovement in depressed patients
Thompson and Oswald, 1977	34	Oral estrone 2 mg/day	HAM-D HAM-A	Decrease in depression and anxiety with both estrogen and placebo in mildly depressed patients
Klaiber et al., 1979	23	Premarin 5–25 mg/day	HAM-D	Improvement in depression with estrogen but not placebo in severely depressed patients Patients remained depressed despite treatment
Coope, 1981	55	Piperazine estrone sulfate 1.5 mg BID	BDI	Decrease in depression with both estrogen and placebo in mildly depressed patients
Ditkoff et al., 1991	36	Premarin 0.625–1.25 mg/day	MMPI BDI POAL WAIS	Decrease in BDI with both doses of estrogen but not with placebo in non-depressed patients
Saletu et al., 1995 placebo	64	Estraderm TTS 50 µg patch twice weekly (0.05 mg/day)	HAM-D	Decrease in depression in depressed patients with both estrogen and placebo

BDI, Beck Depression Inventory; HAM-A, Hamilton Anxiety Scale; HAM-D, Hamilton Depression Scale; MMPI, Minnesota Multiphasic Personality Inventory; POAL, Profile of Adaption to Life; WAIS, Wechsler Adult Intelligence Scale; E, estrogen.

sion, fatigue, and somatic symptoms (Hammarback et al., 1985). Nevertheless, several studies have reported beneficial effects of estrogen on mood with progesterone cycling, and response to progesterone appears to have significant intersubject variability (Dennerstein and Burrows, 1986; von Schoultz, 1986).

In summary, a recent review reported that estrogen replacement therapy is effective for improving mood in naturally menopausal women who are not clinically depressed (Peace, Hawton, and Blake, 1995). Hormone replacement therapy appears to have the clearest and most profound effects on mood in surgically menopausal women (Sherwin and Gelfand, 1985a; Pearce and Hawton, 1996).

Addition of progesterone led to decreases in estrogen's efficacy, whereas addition of testosterone led to further improvement in mood (Sweifel and O'Brien, personal communication). Even when given alone, in dosages ranging from 150 to 200 mg, testosterone appears to be especially helpful for mood in surgically menopausal women (Sherwin and Gelfand, 1985b).

A new direction for research is the investigation of estrogen as an augmentation therapy. Halbreich et al. (1994) reported that estrogen augmented serotonergic activity in postmenopausal women. The serotonin agonist meta-chlorophenyl-piperazine (*m*-CPP) was given to 18 healthy postmenopausal women not on estrogen replacement and 15 healthy menstruating women. Compared with normally menstruating women, postmenopausal women had a significantly blunted prolactin peak after *m*-CPP and a somewhat diminished cortisol peak prior to treatment with estrogen. After 1 month of estrogen (estraderm 0.1 mg) treatment, cortisol and prolactin response to *m*-CPP levels significantly increased.

Thus, theoretically, estrogen augmentation may be a useful adjunctive therapy in postmenopausal depressed women, but few systematic studies have been completed. Prange (1972) reported that the addition of high doses of estradiol, 25 mg, in women already on imipramine led to decreased Hamilton depression scores and improved sleep. Even higher doses (50 mg estradiol) led to toxicity. Similarly, Schneider et al. (1997) reported that in a 6-week trial of Fluoxetine (20 mg/day) for major depression, elderly women (mean age 67 years) maintained on hormone-replacement therapy had a three times greater decrease in their Hamilton scores than did those maintained with placebo.

Estrogen replacement therapy and memory

Memory complaints are frequent in menopausal women; however, the specific changes and their relationship to gonadal hormone levels remain to be clarified. It has been hypothesized that menopausal memory complaints are due to hypoestrogenic states, because animal studies have suggested that estrogen affects cholinergic neurotransmission. Estrogen increases choline acetyl transferase, which is involved in the synthesis of acetylcholine, the neurotransmitter believed to be associated with memory function in humans (Luine, Khylchevskaya, and McEwen, 1975). Estrogen has also been shown to have effects on hippocampal dendrites, the presumed site of memory storage. Ovariectomy in adult female rats resulted in profound decreases in pyramidal cells in the hippocampus, and estrogen replacement prevented this decrease in dendritic spine density. Progesterone augmented the estrogen effect (Gould et al., 1990).

Current studies of the effects of estrogen on memory function in women are difficult to interpret because of the variety of memory tests and differences in age of the women, menopausal status, and estrogen dosages. No studies have prospectively evaluated changes in memory over time, then correlated memory function with changes in estrogen levels and demonstrated improvement with replacement therapy. Available studies are extremely mixed regarding the efficacy of estrogen treatment for memory in naturally menopausal women. Some have reported improvement in various memory tasks (Kampen and Sherwin, 1994; Robinson et al., 1994); others have found no effect on memory (van Hulle and Demol, 1976; Barret-Conner and Dritz-Silverstein, 1993). Studies in surgically menopausal women are more consistent: Estrogen treatment postsurgically appears to prevent decline in some memory tasks such as immediate and delayed recall (Hackman and Gallbraith, 1977; Phillips and Sherwin, 1992).

Similarly, epidemiologic and treatment studies suggest that estrogen replacement therapy may be beneficial in women with Alzheimer's disease. Case control studies show that Alzheimer's disease patients are less likely than control subjects to have used estrogen replacement therapy (Henderson et al., 1994; Pagdnini-Hill and Henderson, 1994), and several case reports (Fillet et al., 1986; Honjo et al., 1995; Ohkura et al., 1995) and one placebo-controlled study (Ohkura et al., 1994) demonstrated that 0.625–1.25 mg estradiol is more effective than placebo in improving psychometric tests of memory and cognition in dementia patients.

Hormone replacement therapy and sleep

Many menopausal women complain of sleep changes that are common with aging in both men and women, such as increased frequency of sleep interruptions and longer latency to sleep onset (Jaszmann et al., 1969; Ballinger, 1976; Stone and Pearlstein, 1994). Frequent awakenings in menopausal women may be due to vasomotor symptoms, but even women who do not complain of night sweats complain of frequent interruptions, suggesting changes in sleep architecture with declining estrogen levels. In a double blind placebo-controlled randomized study of piperazine estrone sulfate 1.5 mg BID, sleep duration significantly increased over the 2 treatment months in both groups. The estrone group had significantly less intervening wakefulness than the placebo group after treatment and significantly increased REM sleep (Thompson and Oswald, 1977).

In a randomized, double blind crossover study, Schiff et al. (1979) investigated sleep in 16 women who had oophorectomies and found that 0.625 mg estrogen was associated with shortened mean sleep latency, longer rapid eye movement (REM) sleep, and a greater percentage of REM sleep. Schiff et al. (1979) also reported a significant disparity between perceived and actual sleep latency. Shaver, Giblin, and Paulsen (1991) confirmed this finding and reported that women who complained of poor sleep but had good sleep as measured by polysomnography had significantly more psychological complaints as measured by the Symptom Checklist (SCL-90). Women with both perceived and documented poor sleep had significantly more hot flashes.

Hormone replacement therapy and sexuality

Many women complain of decreased libido during the menopause; however, in most studies, this decrease in libido is not correlated with estradiol levels but with sexual problems prior to menopause, lack of an available partner, dyspareunia, and psychiatric problems such as major depression (Ballinger et al., 1987; Bachman et al., 1993). Estrogen replacement therapy improves vaginal health and leads to improved sexual satisfaction in women with atrophic vaginitis and dyspareunia (Studd, Chakravarti, and Oram, 1977), but the majority of studies have failed to show a beneficial effect of estrogen replacement on perceived sexual pleasure and sexual behavior in naturally occurring menopause (Myers et al., 1990). Meta-analysis suggests that women with surgical menopause derive greater benefit from hormone replacement therapy than women with naturally occurring menopause (Myers, 1995). The addition of androgens to HRT confers the greatest benefit to sexual functioning in both surgically and naturally menopausal women (Sherwin and Gelfand, 1985, 1987; Myers, 1995; Sherwin, 1995). In 30–40 percent of patients, androgen replacement therapy at physiologic serum levels is associated with downy hair growth, which disappears after cessation of therapy. Supraphysiologic levels of androgens are associated with classic signs of masculinization such as hirsuitism, clitoromegaly, change in voice, weight gain, and increased blood pressure. The effects of exogenous androgens on lipid profiles remain controversial (Sands and Studd, 1995).

Conclusions

Gonadal hormones are potent modulators of the neurotransmitters involved in mood, memory, and sexuality; however, all reproductive cycle–related events except postpartum psychosis are also strongly influenced by psychosocial factors. As reviewed by Wilbush (1980), as early as 1857 Tilt recognized the biopsychosocial nature of symptoms during such events as the menopause when he questioned "how so many phenomena of health and disease can be determined by two little oval bodies." He concluded that symptoms are due not only to involution of the ovaries but also to events such as the loss of one's identity or parents: "One by one snap the cords which anchor a woman's life. At 50, parents may have been gathered to the dust, children may have deserted their roof . . . she must cast aside habits to which she has been wed for so many years and remodel herself on a new plan" (Wilbush, 1980). Future research should focus upon elucidating the complex interplay between hormones and psychosocial events in the etiology and treatment of reproductive cycle–related psychiatric syndromes.

CHAPTER THREE

WOMEN'S SEXUAL FUNCTION AND DYSFUNCTION

DOMEENA C. RENSHAW

Introduction

Before the scientific era produced equipment capable of microscopic scrutiny of semen and ova, human sexuality was shrouded in myth. Female sexuality was hidden in mystique even from women, who were educated by husbands who usually knew less than they did. Infertility was blamed on the wife, and several queens of England lost their lives because there was no male baby.

History

Although sexual enjoyment is not necessarily associated with parity, the early researchers into sexual problems were male gynecologists in the field of infertility. Robert Dickinson, M.D., of Cleveland Clinic, a remarkable gynecologist pioneer, was the first to do couples' counseling when he noted how great a role sexual ignorance played in infertility. He molded wax into models of the genitals with a sagittal section of the female pelvis to educate both husband and wife in internal, as well as external, anatomy and in coital techniques. Dr. Dickinson inspired and advised Alfred Kinsey, Ph.D., whose marathon sociologic sex research team interviewed 8,000 men in the 1940s, and then 12,000 women in the 1950s. By 1950, Joseph Wolpe, a psychiatrist from Philadelphia, had evolved "reciprocal inhibition," a systematic relaxation technique to desensitize women who were anorgasmic, which was then called frigidity (now considered an outmoded and pejorative term because emotional warmth was present).

Building upon the scientific shoulders of the researchers before him, William Masters, M.D., a gynecologist from St. Louis, was also impressed by the many sexual problems of infertile couples (Masters and Johnson, 1966). He first studied his own sexual theories about the cause of sexual symptoms by careful laboratory observations; then, over 5 years, he documented on film the sexual performance of 135 couples (men and women from 19 to 50 years) in solo and coital sexual activity (Masters and Johnson, 1966). Next, Dr. Masters blended these findings into a technique of successful, brief (2-week) treatment of sexual dysfunctions of both men and women (Masters and Johnson, 1970). This was conservative yet revolutionary treatment and a breakthrough in 1970. Subsequently many modifications of the Masters and Johnson 14-day sex therapy have been satisfactorily applied in office practice (Rosensweig and Pearsall, 1978; Lief, 1981; Renshaw, 1983b, 1995; King, Camp, and Downey, 1991).

Child and teen sexuality

How widespread are women's sexual doubts or symptoms? Sexual problems perplex every developing boy, girl, teen, and adult. "Am I sexually normal?" is perhaps the commonest concern about the sexual self, feelings, fantasies, and behaviors. Few youngsters find answers to these questions in the home. Most learn from peers in a haphazard way. Due to sexual abuse concerns and AIDS prevention, public school programs and textbooks of the 1990s usually provide an accurate sex education. Many sexual inaccuracies and modern myths, however, are learned from peers, soap operas, X-rated magazines, cable TV, or videocassettes. A new set of concerns may result: "What's wrong with me?" (I am celibate or not an Olympic sexual athlete as portrayed on the screen.) The infant with a birth defect of the genitals poses a special challenge to pediatrician and parents, who must work together at each growth stage with surgery or hormonal supplements so that needless secrecy and shame are prevented. An approach such as "nature did not quite complete this part of the body so we are helping" can assist parent and patient. Tell the parents it is not their fault.

The sensitive physician has a vital supportive role in giving accurate medical information in clear lay language to gain perspective. This helps the child or teen patient to sort out fact, fears, and fantasy, and to prevent identity confusion. Puberty passions, hormonal peaks, and teen pregnancy have through all ages and cultures combined to evoke intense parental and social protection, particularly for disabled girls, who are also vulnerable to sexual exploitation. Girls with juvenile diabetes, cystic fibrosis, Turner's syndrome, and so on also daydream of boyfriends and romance. They often feel left out and may present with depression. Linkage with a peer group at a community center, church, or library may be of benefit.

Adult sexuality

Sexual dysfunctions may exist (by estimate) in about 50 percent of marriages. What are they? Sexual dysfunctions are impaired, incomplete, or absent expressions of normally recurrent sexual desires and responses. When difficulties with pleasurable climactic resolution of appropriate sexual arousal occur, they may be accepted as transient or become problematic (if they recur or when there is subjective concern or discomfort). In some cases partner dissatisfaction may for the first time precipitate awareness of a dysfunction in a previously accepting individual (e.g., premature ejaculation, anorgasmia, or sexual apathy or lack of interest).

At any age, from in utero to the senium, a definition of orgasm is "a buildup of vasoneuromuscular general and genital tensions." Temperature, heart rate, breathing, and blood pressure all increase to a peak, the penis or clitoris becomes erect, the vagina lubricates, and then there is a discharge of tensions with a few tonic–clonic muscle contractions of all the large and small muscles of the body (including the pubococcygeus encircling the lower vagina). In some women contraction and elevation of the uterus is felt. A return to the preexcitement state follows, with lowered heart rate, breathing, and blood pressure, and total muscle relaxation plus a sense of relaxed well-being. The stimulus for orgasm may be self (masturbation or fantasy), another person (same or opposite sex), or another species (animal).

It must be emphasized that for male and female, the phases or stages of the sexual responses are similar, but the average timing of the cycle is much longer for women (see Fig. 3.1). This information allows the anorgasmic woman and her partner to be relaxed and accepting of their normal differences. The timing difference of male and female sexual response explains why only 20–30 percent of women attain a coital climax. Women have been mislabeled as frigid due to this natural physiologic difference. This basic knowledge can bring relief to many couples because at times a man blames himself for being a poor lover or for having a penis that he thinks is too small if his partner does not have a climax during intercourse.

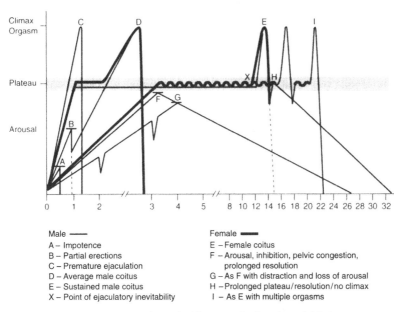

Male ——
A – Impotence
B – Partial erections
C – Premature ejaculation
D – Average male coitus
E – Sustained male coitus
X – Point of ejaculatory inevitability

Female ▬
E – Female coitus
F – Arousal, inhibition, pelvic congestion,
  prolonged resolution
G – As F with distraction and loss of arousal
H – Prolonged plateau/resolution/no climax
I – As E with multiple orgasms

Figure 3.1. Coital graph. (Courtesy D. Renshaw, M.D.)

The clitoris is the analogue of the penis and has lateral crural roots attached to the pelvic arch, where the periosteum is rich in vibratory end organs. These respond well to a pulsating shower or a vibrator and may give an intense orgasm. Unlike the penis, the clitoris has neither reproductive nor urinary function. It is uniquely there for sexual arousal only. A woman needs to realize this basic fact. A climax always involves both clitoris and vagina, whether the stimulus is directly on the clitoris or indirectly by a "pulley" action of the labial attachments, stimulating the clitoris and crura during the thrusting move-ments of coitus. The subjective sensations will, of course, differ. With coitus and partner closeness, the emotional satisfaction may be optimal. Some women fantasize more freely and "let go" more intensely and even more rapidly when alone. Nonetheless, the objective physiologic end result of a climax is total relaxation whatever the mode: coitus, oral, manual, or vibrator. A climax is a climax! One is not better or worse; they may be different. Exploring and under-standing her sexual responses are normal learning and release for every woman. However, thousands of women still need both permission and direction from the physician to overcome anorgasmia. The medical chart should reflect the fol-lowing: CC: lifelong anorgasmia. Diagnosis: 302.73 Female Orgasmic Disor-der. Rx: relaxed masturbation with fantasy on alternate days. Return in

2 weeks. Reading, suggested _____ (Masters and Johnson, 1983; Renshaw, 1983a; Maltz, 1991; Renshaw, 1995).

All persons may be born with similar genital apparatus, but capacities to be aroused and to respond differ. The latter capacity depends on intact brain, spinal cord, peripheral, and autonomic nerves, plus muscles, blood vessels, and end organs. Each woman's personality and early and current life experiences, as well as her response to internal and external erotic stimuli (pleasurable, painful, or conflictual), will influence her response to her partner each day.

Menopause

Sexual changes range from great relief to be free of menses to shock at a late-age pregnancy due to persistent ovulation. Sexual desire and orgasms do not "age," although there may be changes in vaginal and clitoral tissues, with a need for added lubrication and somewhat more intense manual or vibratory simulation. Coitus is very rarely precluded in sexually active seniors.

Some women in midlife grow apprehensive about looks and aging. Continued activity and self-care physically and mentally can prevent anxiety and cosmetic surgery, but some will seek psychiatric support and focus on wrinkle removal to restore confidence.

Is it possible that a woman in the 1990s is unsure whether she is orgasmic? Yes, especially if she expects a different or excessive body response. Her sex education may be marginal. The physician's explicit questions can be educative: During love play or foreplay what happens to your breathing? your heart rate? your body muscles? Do you feel a change in the clitoris? and the vagina? Do you feel small contractions involuntarily in the whole body and lower vagina, then total body relaxation? If she is uncertain, then suggest she check at home and read one of the self-help books listed at the end of the chapter. (1, 7, 14) Ask, "Do you think you can?" Follow up within 2 weeks to ensure cooperation. If there is a belief or moral conflict, suggest she take the materials and talk to her religious adviser. This gives dignity to her question and respects her values as well as providing accurate medical information.

Do women have orgasms during sleep? Yes, during the stage of rapid eye movement (REM) sleep, both sexes from infancy to late age may have normal sexual arousal and sexual dreams, accompanied by rapid breathing, increased heart rate, clitoral engorgement, vaginal lubrication (erections and occasional nocturnal emissions for men), raised blood pressure, an orgasm, and total muscle relaxation. Sometimes an individual may remember a sexual dream or orgasm. Sleep is unconscious and uninhibited, unlike the controls exerted during the day. The woman who asks a question about sleep orgasms can be reassured that she is quite normal and her prognosis is good for waking orgasms: "If you could (in sleep) you can and will again (awake)."

For the woman of the 1990s, delayed childbearing may bring intense pregnancy pursuit when she decides to have a baby. For this lucrative market, fertility clinics have sprung up everywhere. The incidence of endometriosis has increased. Can sexual dysfunctions result? Certainly, and in both partners as they struggle anxiously with baby making and forget the lovemaking. He may suddenly develop impotence, she may have pain or anorgasmia, and the bedroom may become a source of conflict and disappointment

A number of other sexual questions and concerns may be brought to a physician: (1) "I think I had a climax during delivery." This is possible and quite normal. (2) "Is sexual arousal or climax during breast-feeding OK?" This is a normal undifferentiated nipple reflex orgasm response, which may even occur with a breast pump. (3) "What about having intercourse or orgasms during pregnancy?" These are normal and healthy unless there is vaginal bleeding or other complications. (4) "When should I resume intercourse after delivery?" When the genitals have healed, a pelvic exam should be done before answering the question. (5) "Where is the sensationalized G-spot?" This is as yet histologically unsubstantiated as a separate organ or area of prostatelike tissue. Grafenberg wrote that the area at the trigone of the bladder was erogenous and when stimulated digitally caused copious vaginal secretions and orgasms. It remains controversial. (6) "I am feeling depressed and apathetic sexually." A clinical depression causes insomnia, crying, sadness, and lowering of appetites for food, for sex, and for life. If this continues for 6 weeks or more, it may require psychotherapy and/or medication. A single bedtime dose of antidepressants can be used for at least 6 weeks or until the depression lifts (Lief, 1981). Hypnotics are unnecessary because these have a potential for creating dependency; also, hypnotics chemically aggravate a depression. (7) "Will there be sexual changes after a hysterectomy?" If the ovaries remain, then her presurgery sexual pattern should resume after healing. In fact, her satisfaction might even improve if previously there were pregnancy fears. Most patients benefit from reassurance that femininity and desirability will not be altered by a hysterectomy. Her vagina remains receptive and elastic. She will gain weight only if she overeats or does not exercise. There are persistent magazine-perpetuated myths that women become fat and sexless after the uterus is removed. (8) "I have painful orgasms with an IUD." A minority of women have complained of this, which is the result of uterine contractions upon the IUD during a climax. Removal of the

IUD relieves the symptom. (9) "I am bothered by disinterest or sexual apathy." If no physical cause exists such as hypothyroidism or prolactinemia, then check for anorgasmia. If "there's nothing in sex for me," then there may be avoidance. Also ask about masturbatory frequency and if there are other partners (selective sexual apathy). Is fantasy used during loveplay? If the patient replies "No," there will be slow or zero arousal. Fantasy is to arousal what an ignition key is to an engine warmup—essential. If there is moral conflict about thinking of another man, suggest she use memories of their own courtship.

Sexual expression is the only instinct in which deliberate, sustained control or even complete suppression does not result in a threat to the life of the individual, as would cutting off breathing, eating, sleeping, elimination, or circulation. Celibacy is a normal choice. However, if that person marries, sexual avoidance may not be tolerated by the partner. Where "loss of desire" (Hypoactive Sexual Desire 625.8) is the presenting complaint, the question must be raised whether the patient prefers celibacy or if there is selective nonfunction – with one partner but not with another partner or when alone (masturbation). If the sexual disinterest is global, then physical or psychological causes must be excluded. A clinical depression or early sexual trauma or abuse must be sought for and treated.

Mortality

This is rare for sexual dysfunctions. However, a woman may feel desperate about satisfying her partner, who may have threatened divorce. She may attempt or complete suicide. Therefore, the question about suicidal feelings must always be asked and not be trivialized. A suicidal woman will need psychiatric consultation and care.

Etiology

Physical causes such as an intact hymen, vaginitis, endometriosis, congenital abnormalities, and endocrine abnormalities must always be excluded as possible causes of sexual dysfunction; especially dyspareunia (625.0). If all is well physically, then factors such as sexual ignorance; faulty sexual learning; inhibition; shame about the body; religious orthodoxy; guilt or anxiety about normal sexual fantasy or expression; fears (about pregnancy, venereal diseases, AIDS, discovery of an affair, pain, or anticipated pain), chemical factors (alcohol, marijuana, street drugs, needed medications); interpersonal problems; feeling "used," marked conflict, feeling blamed; resentment, unclear communication patterns; another lover; a clinical depression (reduction of all appetites, for food, for sleep, for sex, and for life); deliberate control of her sexual feelings and responses; dissociation (not conscious) of sexual feelings due to early sexual trauma – any or all may combine to interfere with pleasurable sexual expression. It is difficult for a faithful wife of an impotent man. She may doubt her sexual adequacy or his faithfulness and avoid sex to protect herself from perceived rejection. The *Diagnostic and Statistical Manual,* 4th edition (DSM-IV; American Psychiatric Association, 1994) lists

Sexual Desire Disorders

302.71 *Hypoactive Sexual Desire Disorder*

A. Persistently or recurrently deficient or absent sexual fantasies and desire for sexual activity. The judgment of deficiency or absence is made by the clinician, taking into account factors that affect sexual functioning, such as age, sex, and the context of the person's life.

302.79 *Sexual Aversion Disorder*

A. Persistent or recurrent extreme aversion to, and avoidance of all, or almost all, genital sexual contact with a sexual partner.

Sexual Arousal Disorders

302.72 *Female Sexual Arousal Disorder*

A. Either (1) or (2):
  (a) Persistent or recurrent inability to attain or to maintain until completion of the sexual activity an adequate lubrication-swelling response of sexual excitement.
  (b) The disturbances cause marked distress or interpersonal difficulty.
  (c) The sexual dysfunction is not better accounted for by another Axis I disorder (except another Sexual Dysfunction) and is not due exclusively to the direct physiological effects of a substance (e.g., a drug of abuse, a medication) or a general medical condition.

302.73 *Female Orgasmic Disorder*

A. Persistent or recurrent delay in, or absence of, orgasm following a normal sexual excitement phase. Women experience wide variability in the type of intensity of stimulation that triggers orgasm. The diagnosis of Female Orgasmic Disorder should be based on the clinician's judgment that the woman's orgasmic capacity is less than would be reasonable for her age, sexual experience, and the adequacy of sexual stimulation she receives.

B. The disturbance causes marked distress or interpersonal difficulty.

Sexual Pain Disorders

302.76 *Dyspareunia*

A. Recurrent or persistent genital pain in either a male or a female.

B. The disturbance causes marked distress or interpersonal difficulty.

C. The disturbance is not caused exclusively by Vaginismus or lack of lubrication, is not better accounted for by another Axis I disorder (except another Sexual Dysfunction), and is not due exclusively to the direct physiological effects of a substance (e.g., a drug of abuse, a medication) or a general medical condition.

306.51 *Vaginismus*

A. Recurrent or persistent involuntary spasm of the musculature of the outer third of the vagina that interferes with sexual intercourse.

B. The disturbance causes marked distress or interpersonal difficulty.

C. Is not due to the direct physiological effects of a general medical condition.

Some disorders are lifelong, others acquired. They may be situational or generalized (global), due to physical, psychological, or combined factors. Whether they cause or result from a sexual dysfunction, there may be marked feelings of inadequacy concerning body habitus, size and shape of sex organs, sexual performance, or other traits related to self-imposed standards of masculinity or femininity – even persistent and marked distress about sexual orientation. Other terms widely in use follow.

Primary anorgasmia is never ever (by hand, mouth, vibrator, or coitus) having experienced an orgasm or climax.

Secondary or situational anorgasmia is not global, as in some circumstances orgasm can be attained.

Hypoactive Sexual Desire Disorder may present as a variety of statements, such as "I'm not interested in sex," "I hate sex," "Sex is a hassle," "I'm sick of sex, it's boring. I get nothing out of sex, it hurts," or "I'm too exhausted for sex, by the time I've done my office job and housework, it's just one more job." For the clinician it is vital to "scratch" a desire disorder because there's often a dysfunction underneath it. Under some of the comments there may be dyspareunia, anorgasmia, or withdrawal from interpersonal conflicts. Fatigue is real. Advice to sleep for 1 ½ hours, set the alarm, wake, make love for 30 minutes, then complete the night's rest, may be practical. Medical conditions to rule out are hypothyroidism and hyperprolactinemia.

Dyspareunia describes genital pain on intercourse. It is very common in gynecologic practice but is usually transient and due to an acute local infection that will heal with local medication. However, if it is unrelated to vaginal infection, intact hymen, or vestibulitis, then lack of lubrication or other physical factors must be sought.

Vaginismus is defined as involuntary spasms of the outer third of the vagina (pubococcygeus muscle) in response to attempts at vaginal penetration. This prevents not only intercourse but also the physician's examining finger.

For this diagnosis there must be no physical pathology to account for the vaginal contraction. It is estimated that 2 percent of women have the condition, which can be diagnosed only after physical and pelvic examinations have been done. The muscle is not hypertrophied but is hyperresponsive, even in anticipation of pain (anxiety). Reassurance, relaxed slow exhalation, finger insertion daily, even brief use of local anesthetic jelly for not more than one tube can be a turning point.

Some women with vaginismus admit to being fearful of pregnancy, childbirth, and penetration pain. Many have shame, conflict, and guilt about their genitals, due to early learning. Others insist they yearn for a child and present seeking conception. A few will say sex seems dirty or abhorrent; some will tell of early sex abuse or an attempted rape. This may represent an underlying sexual aversion beneath the hypoactive desire. Marriage may have been contracted "for companionship only" in a few.

Several other women with vaginismus have admitted to being sexually aroused on a regular basis, lubricated well, and accepted, enjoyed, and reciprocated with oral and manual contact to orgasm for the partner, who corroborated the history.

The presence of a tight intact hymen on the pelvic exam may explain the difficulty in penetration and the pain. Hymenotomy and healing together with encouragement and reassurance will facilitate final entry and consummation of the marriage.

Deliberate contraction of the pubococcygeus muscle for her own or her partner's sexual enhancement has been practiced for centuries in various cultures. Arnold Kegel in 1952 reported that regular exercises of this muscle assisted women patients to control mild urinary incontinence and also enhanced their orgasmic responses. These Kegel exercises (about 60 successive contractions several times daily) are now part of standard sex therapy to increase vaginal awareness by constricting and relaxing the muscle voluntarily (as if to stop urine flow midstream). This reassures the woman that the control is hers, locally at the lower vagina. Through thinking of these muscles she can self-instruct to relax or contract them.

Occasionally there may be a noninflammatory cause of focal coital pain in the vaginal area, such as at the site of a healed episiotomy or a hymenal remnant that requires excision with good results. Due to pain or in anticipation of pain, the circular muscles of the outer or lower third of the vagina (pubococcygeus or sphincter vaginae) may contract protectively to prevent penetration. This is usually a transient response related to the actual physical problem and is not considered to be psychogenic vaginismus.

Unconsummated marriage has not found its way into the International Classification of Diseases (ICD) or the DSM-IV, but it does present for treatment (Renshaw, 1989). Men may be virginal, may be unable to penetrate, or may ejaculate vaginally. There are women virgins with dyspareunia, vaginismus, or other genital problems that preclude coitus. Sometimes both partners have a dysfunction. They may be otherwise compatible and faithful for up to 21 years before sex therapy is sought (Renshaw, 1989).

Sex therapy

Brief office counseling to manage sexual dysfunctions consists of

1. *General and sexual history from each partner* (Table 3.1).

2. *Physical examination of each partner.* This is extended into an educational sexologic examination, using a mirror for the woman to view her own genitals, in the presence of the husband. Both should be guided by the physician to see and feel the clitoris and vaginal contractions. This experience is of inestimable therapeutic benefit to the couple. It tells them that the condition is known and understood by the physician. Also, with the lights on, the doctor authoritatively gives them permission to look at, learn about, touch, and understand their own genitals. The medical chart must state "Routine sexologic exam done with spouse and nurse X."

Table 3.1. *Explicit sexual history*

How is your sexual functioning? _____
Do you have sexual questions/concerns/worries? _____
Does your partner have a sexual problem? _____
Does your partner blame you or pressure you sexually? _____
How frequently per month do you try intercourse? _____
How frequently per month do you have intercourse? _____

How frequently per month do you have vaginal pain/spasm? _____

Where? (at entrance/mid-vagina/deep inside) _____

Do you use tampons? _____

How frequently per month do you have sexual desire? _____

How frequently per month do you have sexual fantasy? _____

How frequently per month do you have sleep orgasms? _____

How frequently per month do you have waking orgasms? _____

  How? _____

How frequently per month do you have oral-genital contact? _____

If uncertain whether orgasmic, answer the following:

What happens to your heart rate? _____

What happens to your breathing? _____

What happens to your clitoris? _____

  Throbbing? _____

What happens to your vagina? _____

  Lubrication/Contractions? _____

What happens to your body muscles? _____

  Tension? _____

  Contractions? _____

Relaxation afterward? _____

How frequently per month do you masturbate each other? _____

How frequently per month do you masturbate alone? _____

How frequently per month do you use a vibrator? _____

How frequently per month do you handshower on the genitals? _____

How have you been best able to climax? _____

Have you had any sexual experiences that were negative or upsetting? _____

  Details: _____

Does your partner know? _____

How do you feel about being pregnant? _____

  Your partner? _____

Do you have worries about pregnancy? _____About pain? _____

Have you ever been pregnant? _____

Had a miscarriage? _____Discussed adoption? _____

Have you been for an infertility work-up? _____

Last pelvic examination? _____

  Details? _____

Date of last menstrual period? _____

  Any nonmenstrual bleeding? _____

Any vaginal discharge? _____

What books have you read about sex? _____

Do you regard yourself as sexually inhibited? _____Open? _____

Do you regard your partner as sexually inhibited? _____Open? _____

What do you see as your greatest sexual problem? _____

Anything else? _____

How can the physician best be of help to you? _____

Further comments? _____

3. *Sex education:* The physician shows and names each aspect of the genitals; for example, "This is a normal-sized soft penis, which is circumcised. These testes are normal and hang asymmetrically (and so on). This lower outer vaginal muscle is circular, called the pubococcygeus muscle. As you can tell your circular muscles in the eye, mouth, and rectum to contract and relax voluntarily, you can do the same here. Tighten it. Good. Now loosen or relax it." This is done by the doctor before a digital examination. Point out the labia. Take the woman's index finger and place it on her clitoris. When she identifies it, take the husband's index finger to place on her index finger, which she is then asked to remove and guide husband's finger to roll the clitoris from side to side. Many couples are not in touch with their genitals and benefit greatly from the instruction. (In non-vaginismus cases the pelvic exam and Pap smear follow in husband's presence.) At *no* time is it appropriate to sexually stimulate the patient in the office or on the exam table. This is considered sexual misconduct and may have severe legal repercussions (often beyond coverage of malpractice insurance).

4. *Clarify possible causes of the sex symptom if possible.* Clearly connect for the couple perceived antecedent factors (for example, shame, guilt, inhibitions, trauma, abuse, painful intercourse, or anticipatory pregnancy or delivery fear) with the symptom (Masters and Johnson, 1966, 1970; Lief, 1981). This statement initiates patient understanding preliminary to taking individual responsibility to resolve whatever the conflict (Renshaw, 1981, 1983a, 1989). A detached helpless reply of "I don't know why" perpetuates the problem. Invite and answer questions, and suggest selected home reading (1–14).

5. *Reassurance from the physician must be given when all is healthy.* Then tell the couple that if they have motivation to change, through assigned exercises at home all sex symptoms, even vaginismus, are highly reversible. Such therapeutic optimism is well founded. The muscle spasm can indeed be voluntarily relaxed away. For an older woman with atrophic vaginitis and dyspareunia, replacement hormones under a gynecologist's supervision may be indicated.

6. *Relaxation exercises for dyspareunia or vaginismus:* With the woman still on the examining table, in the presence of her husband, instruct her in open-mouth, slow, deep breathing, first in to the count of 4, then out and hold out to the count of 4, to relax herself and the vaginal introitus. The physician should insert a single, well-lubricated, gloved examining fingertip as she begins to exhale: "Relax . . . in to 4 and out to 4 again." The patient is also requested to contract the pubococcygeus very tightly against the examining finger, then to relax and repeat the contraction. This, of course, is a simple illustration of the Kegel exercises. Say so, and tell her to practice herself at home, using her own fingers in preference to mental dilators, because this provides double sensory

value (both fingers and vagina) plus there is not only permission but prescription to touch her genital herself (11). In the pelvic exam guide her own finger (lubricated) into the vagina (Renshaw, 1989). Comfortable insertion of a child-size or nasal speculum is possible after a gentle one-finger pelvic examination as she slowly breathes out with an open mouth. On a tense and resistant patient, this relaxed pelvic examination with both partners present must occasionally be repeated on later visits. Patience, time, and encouragement do help.

7. *Lab studies:* Routine urinalysis and blood tests can be done as medically indicated when pathology is noted or discovered. A routine Pap smear is done if needed.

8. *Brief sex therapy for psychiatric women patients* when requested by them differs very little from that of women without a psychiatric diagnosis.

Because a clinical depression may cause sexual apathy, the diagnostic test would be a course of antidepressant medication, which by about the fourth week usually restores all of the appetites for food, sleep, life, and sex. Another consideration is the patient's use of psychotropic medications because some of these (like some antihypertensive medications) may reversibly cause delayed orgasms or frustration at having no orgasms. "Muted" or "anemic" orgasms, lessened sensations, and feeble muscle contractions are all complaints reported with the use of anxiolytics or serotonin blockers (SSRIs).

In the manic phase a woman with bipolar depressive illness may manifest intense pursuit of sexual outlet that may lack discrimination, appropriateness, or regard for consequences. Also, there may be a quality of insatiable sexual urgency in that despite orgasm she immediately repeats the stimulus but this may fail to provide relief in spite of the sexual release. Lithium alone or combined with antipsychotics can reduce this hypersexuality.

9. *Differential diagnosis:* Physical factors (e.g., side effects of medications), hormonal changes (e.g., hyper- or hypothyroid), prolactinemia, menopausal atrophic vaginitis, concurrent illness, fear of pain, pregnancy avoidance, and so on must be ruled out.

10. *Home exercises for all sexual symptoms:* The couple is asked to make the time (30 minutes daily) for loveplay, kissing, and body massage, but no breast or genital touching for the first 2 weeks (Masters and Johnson, 1970; Renshaw, 1995).

For dyspareunia or vaginismus the patient is also to spend 5 to 15 minutes solo, twice daily. The door is to be locked and the phone off the hook, so she will not be disturbed. Sexual fantasy is essential. Relaxed, open-mouthed breathing with simultaneous vaginal insertion of (a) for 2 days, one finger, and (b) for the next 2 days, two fingers. She must continue this daily for 2 weeks. In week 3 her husband's lubricated index finger can be guided into the vagina by her after plenty of general and genital foreplay. In week 4, the same exercises with foreplay and finger insertion can precede the husband, who lies supine, with wife on top. She then stuffs into the vagina his soft penis lubricated with saliva, KY jelly, or baby oil (which must also be placed on her vaginal opening). She must breathe slowly out to the count of 4. If the penis is erect or semierect, this may be uncomfortable for her. Therefore, it is to be emphasized that insertion or stuffing is of the soft penis. When a husband says he cannot be soft due to a reflex erection in proximity to his wife's vagina, tell both that this arousal is positive and a compliment. However, prescribe (in the presence of both) that he masturbate and ejaculate first to ensure flaccidity for an hour. Then she can mount and insert the soft penis.

In all of these graded tasks, she is told to relax as well as contract the vaginal muscles so that she may get in touch with this voluntary muscle of her body and know how it works. For all these steps, she is active and the husband passive. The trap of "you are hurting me" is thus avoided. She is now to be the active partner, assertive and responsible for finding comfortable, relaxed insertion without blaming him. Suggest they read a sex manual, such as those listed at the end of this chapter, together or taking turns. This reinforces the office counseling. These home instructions can effectively reverse the vaginismus of many years' duration if the patient is motivated to change. Treatment may require a total of five or six 30-minute office visits spaced over 12 weeks. Victims of sexual or other trauma can also obtain relief from the listed home reading.

Masturbatory exercises solo or side by side can help the anorgasmic woman to attain orgasm. Some patients and their husbands were highly pleased at the relief of the dyspareunia and/or vaginismus and attained pain-free coitus. This was "sufficient pleasure for now" one couple said. Neither wished to pursue her orgasmic attainment.

Fear of loss of self-control by having an orgasm may be for some women a stressful thought. The clinician can leave an open door for them to return for further therapy, if and when they are ready.

Clinicians assist persons to attain their optimal sexual pleasure. We cannot take them further or faster than they are willing or able to go. It is their index of sexual satisfaction and not ours that must always be respected.

Fashions and fads

The search for aphrodisiacs has waxed and waned through the centuries. Some are more dangerous than others. In this time-starved era the quick fix of a "sex pill" keeps health food stores in business. Again on the horizon for women is testosterone. No matter how minute the dose, the side effects may include facial hair growth with thinning of hair on the head, thickening of the vocal cords with a bass voice, and unknown tumor possibilities. Hyperplasia of the clitoris with resultant suicide occurred in Illinois in the 1970s. The physician lost his license and spent 4 years in jail. Hormones must be regarded with respect.

Prognosis

For the first time in centuries the outlook is optimistic for sexual symptom reversal. Accurate sex education and the application at home of sex therapy exercises can lead to relaxed pleasuring. It is a conservative, noninvasive treatment that achieves much. Self-help paperbacks (bibliotherapy) can extend the help and are at libraries or inexpensively available (see suggested reading list).

Conclusions

Because sex clinics are few and often overloaded, front-line sex therapy by the practicing physician merits a diagnostic trial. It can be provided for women patients – solo, in a group therapy instructional setting, or as a couple. There is no subspecialty of sexology, yet the knowledge has been available for over two decades and is waiting for a much wider application in the 1990s.

Suggested self-help reading

1. Barbach, L. G. (1975 and 1991). *For Yourself (Women)*. New York: Doubleday.
2. Bloomfield, H. (1983). *Making Peace with Your Parents*. New York: Random House.
3. Donovan, M. E., and Ryan, W. P. (1989). *Love Blocks*. New York: Penguin Books.
4. Goldberg, H. (1976). *The Hazards of Being Male*. New York: Signet Publications.
5. Hendriks, H. (1988). *How to Get the Love You Want*. New York: Harper & Row.
6. Maltz, W. (1991). *The Sexual Healing Journey*. New York: HarperCollins.
7. Mason, T., and Green-Norman, V. (1988). *Making Love Again*. Chicago: Contemporary Publications.
8. Masters, W., Johnson, V., and Kolodny, R. (1986). *Sex and Human Loving*. Boston: Little, Brown.
9. Renshaw, D. C. (1984). *Incest: Understanding and Treatment*. Boston: Little, Brown.
10. Renshaw, D. C. (1984). *Sex Talk for a Safe Child*. Milwaukee, WI: AMA.
11. Renshaw, D. C. (1995). *Seven Weeks to Better Sex*. New York: Random House.
12. Visher, J., and Visher, E. (1979). *Stepfamilies: Myths and Realities*. Secaucus, NJ: Citadel.

13. Zilbergeld, B. (1978). *Male Sexuality.* Boston: Little, Brown.
14. *Our Bodies Ourselves* – A Book by and for Women. (1975 and 1985). New York: Simon & Schuster.

Note: Try your library or local bookstore.

There are normal differences in how each individual reacts to the same materials. Tell patients to respect these differences and to try to understand how each family, religion, childhood experience, and so on may affect adult sexual feelings.

CHAPTER FOUR

GENDER DIFFERENCES IN BRAIN MORPHOLOGY AND IN PSYCHIATRIC DISORDERS

LAURA MARSH AND REGINA CASPER

Epidemiologic and clinical studies in psychiatry consistently reveal gender-based differences in the prevalence and manifestations of certain psychiatric disorders. In particular, women may be more vulnerable to developing depressive or anxiety disorders, whereas men may be more prone to substance-related disorders. Other conditions, such as schizophrenia or bipolar disorder, occur with a relatively similar frequency in men and women, yet differ in age of illness onset, symptomatology, illness course, and treatment response. These dissimilarities have implications in terms of clinical management as well as in our heuristic understanding of the etiologies of various psychiatric conditions. Sex differences in brain anatomy and function may underlie certain gender biases in psychiatric disorders or possibly confer protective or predisposing influences in the development of psychiatric illness. However, other factors are also important, such as genetic predisposition, endocrine status, and sociocultural issues. Part I of this chapter discusses the fundamental processes underlying sexual differentiation of the brain and the ramifications on brain structure and function. Part II consolidates the literature on gender differences in psychiatric illnesses and provides an overview of gender differences in the prevalence, clinical features, proposed mechanisms, and nonpharmacologic treatments of six major psychiatric conditions – major depression, bipolar affective disorder, alcoholism, anxiety disorders, somatization disorder, and schizophrenia. Given the range of subject matter covered in this chapter, references to more extensive reviews on each topic are provided. Psychopharmacologic issues are discussed in Chapter Ten.

Part I
GENDER DIFFERENCES IN
BRAIN MORPHOLOGY

In the context of normal variability and overlap among individuals of either sex, the brains of men and women demonstrate relatively consistent structural and functional differences. These differences present as variations in neuronal number, morphology, and connectivity, which are associated with differences in brain physiology, cognitive development, and behavior. Gonadal hormones exert the greatest influence on sexual differentiation in terms of early neuronal organization and the later activation of sex-related behaviors. However, numerous environmental factors and experiences, present during fetal development, subsequent to birth, and throughout the adult life span, further interact with hormonal levels and anatomic templates to contribute to gender differences in brain morphology and function.

Sexual differentiation of the brain

Sexual differentiation and organization of the brain begin early in fetal development in response to gonadal hormones. Detailed reviews of the hormonal influences on sexual differentiation of the nervous system and the behavioral consequences are available (MacLusky and Naftolin, 1981; Seeman and Lang, 1990; Hines and Green, 1991; Breedlove, 1994; Lewine and Seeman, 1995). Initially, the nervous system and gonads are undifferentiated, and neurons contain intracellular estradiol receptors in both sexes. In males, genes linked to the Y chromosome result in conversion of the embryologic gonads to testes, which secrete testosterone. Testosterone crosses the blood–brain barrier, where it is converted to estradiol, which binds to brain estrogen receptors that subsequently regulate gene transcription. These estradiol-dependent gene products permanently organize the developing brain through a cascade of mechanisms that promote different maturational rates and different patterns of neuronal formation, programmed cell death, and synaptic connectivity in the male brain relative to the developing female brain. Absence of testosterone and its related gene products during critical periods of development will result in brain structures and gonads with the female somatic phenotype (regardless of genotype). However, in females, ovarian secretions influence brain development, although the mechanisms and gene products facilitating female patterns of brain organization are less established (Bardoni et al., 1994).

Gender differences in brain structure

Many gross neuroanatomic structures demonstrate sexual dimorphism in the adult human brain (Table 4.1); microscopic differences are less established and seem to vary with age. At birth, the only gender difference consistently detected is a modest increase in brain weight in males (Breedlove, 1994), suggesting that subsequent events, hormonal and otherwise, influence development of the gross structural differences apparent in adults. In adult men, the increase in brain weight and volume is not wholly accounted for by their increased height and weight (Dekaban

Table 4.1. *Anatomic dimorphisms in the adult human brain*

Region	Differences (women relative to men)
Whole brain	
Weight	Smaller
Volume	Smaller
Hemispheric asymmetries	
Sylvian fissure and planum temporale	Smaller; reduced left-right differences
Cortex	
Superior temporal gyrus	Greater neuronal density and percentage of gray matter
Prefrontal	Greater percentage of gray matter
Interhemispheric commissures	
Corpus callosum	Larger
Anterior commissure	Larger
Massa intermedia	More frequently present
Hypothalamus	
Sexually dimorphic nucleus of the preoptic area (SDN-POA)	Fewer neurons and smaller size
Bed nucleus of the stria terminalis	Smaller volume
Suprachiasmatic nucleus	Elongated in females, spherical in males

and Sadowsky, 1978). Thus, gender differences in total brain size may be related to sex-specific patterns of neuronal differentiation and not just body size.

In addition to nonspecific differences such as brain weight, certain brain regions consistently demonstrate sexual dimorphisms. Sex-related differences in the magnitude of hemispheric asymmetry are particularly noted for the planum temporale (the posterior region of the superior temporal gyrus, which consists of the auditory association cortex). In men, the left planum temporale and its associated structures tend to be larger than the right hemisphere. Women are less likely to show this pattern of leftward asymmetry, as are non-right-handed men (Witelson and Kigar, 1992). It is hypothesized that the leftward asymmetry in males results from inhibited neuronal loss in left hemisphere structures in the presence of testosterone and relatively more left hemisphere cortical estrogen receptors (Craft et al., 1992). This theory is partially supported by animal studies in which male rats show greater asymmetry in patterns of cortical thickness and cell numbers than females. However, the patterns vary over the age span and in response to concentrations of both gonadal and nongonadal steroids, such as from the adrenal gland. Thus, sex-specific genetic factors as well as nongenetic and non-gender-related factors (e.g., stress) influence brain development and patterns of cortical asymmetry (Diamond, 1991). Structures connecting the two hemispheres also manifest gender differences, with evidence for enhanced hemispheric connectivity in women. This is supported by a recent meta-analysis of data from 43 postmortem and neuroimaging morphologic studies on the corpus callosum (the major fiber tract connecting the right and left cerebral hemispheres), which found a larger corpus callosum in women, provided that overall brain size was taken into account (Driesen and Raz, 1995). Another discrete example of male–female structural differences is the sexually dimorphic nucleus. This structure in the anterior hypothalamus/preoptic area has a larger neuronal size and number in males beginning in late childhood, but the magnitude of the gender discrepancy wanes with age (Allen et al., 1989).

Gender differences in brain function

The neuroanatomic sexual dimorphisms and asymmetries complement gender differences in physiologic and cognitive function. Several studies have shown higher cortical blood flow in women relative to men (e.g., Gur et al., 1982) and sex differences in regional cerebral metabolic activity (Gur et al., 1995). Sex-linked differences are also apparent in biogenic amine neurotransmitter distribution (Heller, 1993), including the magnitude of hemispheric asymmetries

(Craft et al., 1992). For both sexes, cognitive functions are typically lateralized, with the left hemisphere subserving verbal processes and the right hemisphere nonverbal processes. However, certain cognitive sex differences are consistently recognized (Maccoby and Jacklin, 1974; Heller, 1993). Men tend to show greater lateralization of brain function than women, and this may account for better performance by men on tasks requiring spatial reasoning. Conversely, relatively less hemispheric specialization and greater interhemispheric connectivity in women is thought to confer better performance on tasks requiring verbal abilities and processing of emotional information. Of course, there is considerable variation among individuals of either sex, and social factors may enhance such gender differences in cognitive attributes. For example, better visual-spatial skills in boys may be nurtured through encouragement to partake in nonverbal physical activity, whereas relatively better verbal skills in girls are amplified by their increased verbal social interactions. However, the essential basis for such cognitive sex differences is thought to rest in prenatal gender-specific patterns of neuroanatomic organization in response to gonadal hormones. Outcomes of natural experiments support this position. For example, women exposed in utero to androgenic steroids prescribed to prevent miscarriage (e.g., diethylstilbestrol) showed greater lateralization of cognitive function on dichotic listening tasks relative to their unexposed sisters (Hines, 1982). Furthermore, women are less likely than men to manifest developmental disabilities, such as dyslexia, or to suffer the same extent of language dysfunction after cerebrovascular accidents, indicating that language functions in men are relatively more lateralized (Halbreich and Lumley, 1993).

Hormonal influences on the sexually differentiated brain

The extent to which neuroanatomic dimorphisms interact with sex hormones to modulate gender differences in adult behavior or psychopathology has not been established. The presence of structural dimorphisms in brain regions integral to mood and behavioral regulation (e.g., the hypothalamus) certainly suggests that the dimorphisms have functional consequences. Inherent gender-based differences in neurotransmitter function, receptor distribution, and neuronal connectivity may modulate the clinical expression of a given psychiatric illness or the predisposition to developing psychiatric illnesses in men and women. Different thresholds in male and female brains for vulnerability to injury or genetic errors during neurodevelopment may modify the risks for developing psychiatric illnesses more strongly in one gender than the other because neural ontogeny and neuronal ultrastructure are not the same across the genders. Likewise, innate cognitive differences, with women better able than men to process emotional stimuli and express themselves verbally, could influence clinical presentation in terms of symptom awareness, help-seeking behavior, and coping strategies in response to emotional distress.

With the onset of puberty, activational effects of gonadal hormones and, in females, gonadal hormone cyclicity exert further effects on neurotransmitter functioning in the sexually differentiated brain. These differential effects may be related to gender differences in psychiatric disorders. Testosterone, estradiol, estrogen, progesterone, and related metabolites influence both genomic and direct nongenomic effects on transmitter function, including regulation of receptor number, modulation of receptor binding affinity, neurotransmitter synthesis and metabolism, and synaptogenesis (McEwen, 1991). For example, in rats, estradiol induces an acute reduction in serotonin receptor numbers and a delayed increase in serotonin receptors in specific brain regions containing estrogen receptors (i.e., the amygdala, the preoptic area, and the hypothalamus), areas thought to be involved in affective regulation in humans (Biegon and McEwen, 1982). In another animal study (Häfner et al., 1993), neonatal and adult rats treated with estradiol showed attenuation of dopamine-mediated behaviors relative to untreated rats, but only the treated neonatal rats showed reduced dopamine receptor affinity. Together with their differential organizing effects during brain maturation, these gonadal hormones in the adult continue to exert gender-related influences on neural functioning. Thus, in some psychiatric illnesses, such as schizophrenia and mood disorders, sex-related variations in gonadal hormones potentially modulate the prevalence, expression, and response to treatment of psychiatric illness.

Part II
GENDER DIFFERENCES IN
PSYCHIATRIC DISORDERS

The study of gender differences in psychiatric illnesses is in its nascent stages. A better understanding of the epidemiologic and clinical characteristics distinguishing men and women with similar psychiatric conditions will help identify predisposing factors and appropriate treatment methods for each sex. It is possible further that gender differences will point to separate sex-linked pathogenetic mechanisms. Alternatively, gender differences may represent different expressions of a single etiology affected by neurohormonal, psychological, or cultural issues.

After all, male and female patients with the same disorder have many more clinical characteristics in common than they have differences, suggesting that the central pathogenetic mechanisms are similar between affected individuals.

Recognition of gender differences in psychiatric illness has been greatly advanced by relatively recent large-scale epidemiologic studies that used operationalized diagnostic criteria, reliable diagnostic assessment instruments, and research designs enabling estimation of both lifetime and cross-sectional prevalence rates. One important study was the National Epidemiologic Catchment Area (ECA) Survey Program (Regier et al., 1984), a federally funded program that provided prevalence and incidence data on psychiatric illness occurring in a large cohort of subjects (over 20,000) from five different community samples in the United States. In follow-up, the National Comorbidity Study (NCS) performed diagnostic interviews using DSM-IIIR criteria in 8,098 participants aged 15 to 54 years who resided throughout the continental United States (Kessler et al., 1994). These two studies showed that psychiatric disorders are more prevalent than previously believed, that they occur more frequently in women for certain conditions, and that a substantial number of probands (>15%) have a history of three or more comorbid illnesses. Comorbidity was particularly evident in women. As shown in Table 4.2, lifetime prevalence rates for psychiatric disorders in men and women from epidemiologic studies conducted in other nations support the general findings of the NCS, although prevalence rates vary with geographic location (Canino et al., 1987; Bland, Orn, and Newman, 1988; Lee et al., 1990; Wittchen et al., 1992).

Major depression

Prevalence

Major depression affects women two to three times more often than men (Weissman and Klerman, 1977; Paykel, 1991; Weissman et al., 1993). These different prevalence rates emerge in adolescence and prevail in most industrialized cultures. Prior to adolescence, rates of depression among boys and girls are about equal, or possibly higher in prepubertal boys (Angold and Worthman, 1993). Multiple explanations are proposed for these findings, including biologic, genetic, environmental, and psychosocial determinants. To the extent that these factors interact, interpreting the results of the collective studies on gender differences in depression is confounded by methodologic differences in terms of depressive symptom assessment (such as the use of self-report inventories vs. diagnostic interviews) and definitions of mental illness (e.g., presence of

Table 4.2. *Lifetime prevalence rates (in percentages) of psychiatric disorders[a] in adult women and men*

Psychiatric disorder	United States[c] F (n = 4,251)	United States[c] M (n = 3,847)	Canada[d] (Edmonton) F (n = 1,928)	Canada[d] (Edmonton) M (n = 1,330)	Korea[e] (Seoul) F (n = 1,644)	Korea[e] (Seoul) M (n = 1,490)	Germany[f] (Munich) F (n = 251)	Germany[f] (Munich) M (n = 232)	Puerto Rico[g] F (n = 859)	Puerto Rico[g] M (n = 654)
Affective disorders	23.9	14.7	13.2	7.1	6.6	4.3	18.7	6.4	10.9	4.7
Major depressive episode	21.3	12.7	11.4	5.9	4.1	2.4	13.6	4.0	5.5	3.5
Dysthymia	8.0	4.8	5.2	2.2	3.0	1.8	5.4	2.5	7.6	1.6
Manic episode	1.7	1.6	0.4	0.7	0.3	0.6	0.5	0.0	0.4	0.7
Alcohol abuse and dependence	—	—	—	—	—	—	—	—	1.3	13.4
Abuse	6.4	12.5	—	—	1.6	25.6	—	—	0.3	9.0
Dependence	8.2	20.1	—	—	1.0	17.2	—	—	0.4	2.1
Abuse/dependence	—	—	6.7	29.3	—	—	5.1	21.0	2.0	24.6

	F	M	F	M	F	M	F	M	F	M
Anxiety disorders	30.5	19.2	–	–	12.7	5.3	18.1	9.1	15.7	11.2
Generalized anxiety disorder	6.6	3.6	–	–	4.3	2.4	–	–	–	–
Panic disorder	5.0	2.0	1.7	0.8	1.8	0.3	2.9	1.7	1.9	1.6
Phobias	–	–	11.7	6.1	8.6	2.9	–	–	14.3	9.9
Agoraphobia	7.0	3.5	4.3	1.5	3.3	0.7	8.3	2.8	8.7	4.9
Simple phobia	15.7	6.7	9.8	4.6	7.9	2.6	10.3	5.5	9.6	7.6
Social phobia	15.5	11.1	2.0	1.4	1.0	0.0	(simple and social phobia)		1.6	1.5
Obsessive-compulsive disorder	–	–	3.1	2.8	2.4	2.2	2.3	1.8	3.1	3.3
Somatization disorder	–	–	0.1	0.0	0.1	0.0	1.6	0.0	0.7	0.7
Schizophrenia	–	–	0.6	0.5	0.2	0.4	–	–	1.2	1.9
Nonaffective psychoses[b]	0.8	0.6	–	–	–	–	–	–	–	–

F = female, M = male.

[a]According to DSM-III diagnostic criteria, except Kessler, et al., 1994 (DSM-IIIR).

[b]Includes schizophrenia, schizoaffective, and delusional disorders and atypical psychosis.

[c]Kessler, et al., 1994 (sample derived from across the continental United States).

[d]Bland, Orn, and Newman, 1988.

[e]Lee et al., 1990.

[f]Wittchen et al., 1992.

[g]Canino et al., 1987.

psychological distress vs. clearly defined psychiatric syndromes). However, more recent epidemiologic studies using standardized assessment instruments and diagnostic criteria report similar prevalence figures (Table 4.2).

Some schools of thought contest the validity of data suggesting higher prevalence rates for depressive illness in women (reviewed by Paykel, 1991). One theory suggests that the excessive rate for depressive illness in women is an artifact resulting from women's greater tendency to seek medical help, report symptoms of distress, and receive treatment. Indeed, a recent study showed that primary care physicians, regardless of their gender, were more likely to prescribe antidepressants for their women patients with depression than for men with similar diagnoses (Williams et al., 1995). Inherent differences in men and women with respect to affective expression may invoke different manifestations of illness behavior, that is, the response to physical or emotional discomfort (Briscoe, 1982, 1987), and thereby alter prevalence rates of reported depressive illness. Even among adolescents, irrespective of their ethnic background, girls tend to report more depressive symptoms than boys (Casper, Belanoff, and Offer, 1996). These different styles of expression may develop from biologic determinants and/or differential socialization of boys and girls, as discussed in Part I. However, prevalence rates from community surveys (which do not necessarily involve cases receiving treatment) refute the artifact hypothesis, and the magnitude of the effect of different styles of affective expression is felt to be relatively small. Thus, the increased reporting of depressive symptoms by women seems to be because women are simply more often affected by depressive illnesses.

A second alternative view maintains that social influences and social conditions, and not biologic factors, account for divergent prevalence rates among men and women (Jenkins and Clare, 1985; Wilhelm and Parker, 1994). Evidence cited includes (1) studies of depression in nonindustrialized nations, which show equal prevalence rates among men and women, if not lower rates in women; (2) a lack of sex differences in prevalence rates in studies of homogenous populations in which the variance attributable to social status is minimized (e.g., college students or civil servants of the same employment grade); and (3) the peak incidence of depression in married women 20–40 years old who also have children. The factors that might contribute to females experiencing greater social burdens, which lead to stress, and, ultimately, depression are described next.

Clinical manifestations

There are relatively few gender differences in the clinical features of unipolar depression (reviewed by Weissman and Klerman, 1977; Pajer, 1995; Shaw, Kennedy, and Joffe, 1995). Increased frequency of comorbid anxiety disorders in women is one of the more salient clinical differences that may partially explain the higher rate of depression in women. This is supported by evidence from a longitudinal epidemiologic study (n = 1,007), which showed that gender differences in the prevalence of major depression were largely attributed to concomitant anxiety disorders and that an increased rate of prior anxiety disorders in women contributed to their greater risk for developing depression (Breslau, Schultz, and Peterson, 1995). A study of gender differences in patients from a university research clinic reported similar findings of increased comorbid anxiety in women (Rapaport et al., 1995). A second notable clinical difference is the greater frequency of suicide attempts in younger women and completed suicides in older men. A third difference is that women with depression are more likely to have certain medical illnesses, including thyroid disease, autoimmune conditions, and migraine headaches. Whereas both sexes tend to have an equal predisposition toward recurring episodes or chronicity (Kessler et al., 1993; Weissman et al., 1993), some evidence suggests that women might become ill at an earlier age and experience more recurrent and longer episodes (Ernst and Angst, 1992).

Biologic influences – neurotransmitter and neurohormonal regulation

Neurotransmitter and neurohormonal dysfunction are both invoked in the etiology and pathophysiology of depression, regardless of gender. However, gender differences in these biologic systems may generate sex-related variance in the prevalence of depression (reviewed by Halbreich and Lumley, 1993). As described earlier, gender-based differences in neurodevelopment yield inherent differences in neurotransmitter systems. Presumably, in the context of these normal gender differences, abnormalities in the noradrenergic and serotonergic systems are implicated in affective modulation, pathologic mood states, and antidepressant activity. These abnormal systems are further influenced by gonadal hormones, which modulate receptor-binding affinity, receptor density, and neurotransmitter metabolism. In addition, sex-related differences in cortisol secretion and regulation, with cortisol levels increasing with age and fluctuating with hormonal cyclicity in premenopausal women, may also affect synthesis of biogenic amines. Functional neuroimaging studies of major depression suggest frontal–subcortical dysfunction (reviewed by Marsh et al., 1996), although it is not established how gonadal hormones or other gender differences might facilitate disruption in regional connectivity. Often cited are effects of cycling female sex steroids on the hypothalamic-pituitary-adrenal (HPA) axis and cortisol release, although evidence for this mechanism is limited (reviewed by Blehar and Oren, 1995). Gender differences in the neuropsychological concomitants of major depression have received little attention, although further research in this area may provide insight into the role of inherent gender differences in cognitive function on the expression of depressive illness and on brain structure–function relationships in depression (reviewed by Heller, 1993). For example, enhanced performance by women on cognitive tasks requiring emotional processing may represent greater specialization of right hemisphere functioning, which also renders women more vulnerable to dysfunction involving such cognitive processes. At the same time, heightened verbal skills and a lesser degree of hemispheric specialization for language may facilitate the use of verbal strategies by women in response to emotional distress and the increased diagnosis of depressive disorders.

The differential effect of hormonal cyclicity on neurotransmitter function is another side of the biologic hypotheses explaining gender differences in the development of depression. These theories hypothesize that hormonal shifts induce depressive symptomatology in women who are vulnerable to affective disorder for either genetic or psychosocial reasons. Although some women develop depressive symptoms when hormones are fluctuating, studies linking depressive episodes directly to hormonal changes are inconclusive. An increased rate of depression is particularly evident during the postpartum period, although other determinants, such as social supports, are relevant (O'Hara, 1987). It also appears that affective state in a subset of women with depression is exquisitely sensitive to changes in hormonal levels during the menstrual cycle, but premenstrual depression in most women patients is not correlated with hormonal changes (Endicott, 1993). Similarly, studies have not substantiated increased rates of depression with menopause (reviewed by Paykel, 1991) or, despite the established female predominance of depression in adolescence, higher rates of depression in girls in association with the hormonal changes at puberty relative to pubertal boys (Angold and Worthman, 1993). However, it is worth noting that many investigations of these hormonal correlates involved small sample sizes and may not have employed comprehensive approaches for detecting hormonal levels.

Biologic influences – genetic factors

Genetic factors appear important to the transmission of depression, as demonstrated by a greater risk for affective disorders in first-degree relatives of patients diagnosed with depression and by higher concordance rates for mood disorders in monozygotic compared to dizygotic twins (reviewed by Weissman and Klerman, 1977; Kendler et al., 1993). Whether genetic factors account for women being more prone to depression is unclear. Genetic studies indicate evidence for X-linked transmission in bipolar disorder, but not unipolar disorders. A polygenic mode of inheritance may confer increased susceptibility to depression in the context of other interpersonal and environmental variables. There are also theories that women tend to develop depression, whereas male relatives develop alcoholism and sociopathy when there is a family history of these conditions (Winokur, 1979).

Interpersonal influences

The contribution of personality differences between men and women has been explored in theories on gender differences in depression, but there is little consensus among investigations (reviewed by Blehar and Oren, 1995; Nolan-Hoeksema, 1995; Pajer, 1995). The essence of such theories is that women tend to place a greater value than men on interpersonal relationships and have increased psychological dependency on others, which may lead to lower self-esteem, stress, internal conflicts, and depression when relationships are disrupted. It has also been suggested that women tend to ruminate over their problems, blame themselves for stress, and show greater passivity. One problem with such studies is that the psychological constructs under examination (e.g., passivity, dependency, and assertiveness) are variably defined and difficult to measure with validity given the complexity of human relationships and individual behavior. Sampling issues (e.g., college students vs. homemakers with small children) also influence the results of such studies. In general, however, there is no evidence that increased depression in women can be attributed to women's increased dependency or passivity or decreased assertiveness. In fact, demonstration of competence and intelligence in women who defy female social stereotypes may increase their risk of depression (reviewed by Nolan-Hoeksema, 1995). Although some studies show decreased rates of depression in married versus unmarried men, the effects of marriage on the development of depression in women is not established. However, a supportive social network appears to be a protective factor against developing depression for some women (Nolan-Hoeksema, 1995). Thus, psychological tendencies in women may influence the individual expression of depression, but their effects cannot, as yet, be extended to explain the excessive prevalence of unipolar depression in women than men.

Social factors

Social factors contributing to depression in women have been studied extensively (reviewed by Briscoe, 1982; Paykel, 1991; Nolan-Hoeksema, 1995). These investigations tend to focus on those gender-related aspects of socialization that result in increased stress and vulnerability to depression for women.

Such gender-specific consequences include greater tolerance for women in the sick role, the differential demands of marriage on men and women, occupational factors such as the demands of housewives with small children versus women employed outside the home (who may also have children), the lower social status attributed to women in their work roles, whether as a housewife or in the work force, and discrimination suffered by women when they attempt to achieve greater independence. Although these issues affect the quality of life for women, the effects of these various factors are also modified by the social value imparted by a given culture or social class for different roles served by women, making it difficult to draw broad conclusions. An additional problem is that few studies have examined these factors in comparable groups of men. Differential effects of stress on men and women are also not established, although stressful life events are known risk factors for developing depression. Whereas women report greater symptom intensity in relation to stress, women, compared with men, do not have more stressful life events or consider their life events more stressful (Uhlenhuth and Paykel, 1973). More general and concrete influences on rates of depression in women, and no doubt chronic stress, are poverty and sexual abuse. Both conditions affect women more often and are associated with increased rates of depression.

Treatment

As with men, comprehensive treatment of women should take into account the various social, psychological, and biologic influences on the depressive syndrome and integrate these into the individual treatment plan (reviewed by Pajer, 1995). Initial assessment of women with depression must especially consider the greater likelihood of other psychiatric and medical conditions, some of which can be treated in concert with depression (e.g., antidepressants are also prescribed for chronic pain). Psychotherapeutic approaches should examine social issues (including gender role and related expectations), personality vulnerabilities, and past traumata, which increase the risk of depression. Some women may particularly benefit from group and cognitively oriented therapies, which enhance problem-solving skills and a sense of mastery while discouraging rumination.

Bipolar disorder

The topic of gender differences in bipolar disorder and their basis has received little attention in the psychiatric literature. Although many clinical features of bipolar disorder are similar in affected men and women, gender differences in the course of the illness are consistently reported. The findings from two extensive reviews (Bardenstein and McGlashan, 1990; Leibenluft, 1996) are summarized here.

The course of bipolar disorder tends to involve more episodes of depression in women than men. Several clinical studies indicate that women are up to three times more likely than men to experience rapid-cycling bipolar disorder (i.e., occurrence of four or more affective episodes annually). Less established are findings that women with bipolar disorder seem predisposed to developing depressive syndromes, with more frequent depressive episodes or mixed states of concomitant depression and mania relative to men affected with bipolar disorder. Further, the initial affective episode is more often depressive in women relative to men, although the difference is modest (75 vs. 67 percent). Despite the relatively greater prevalence of depressive syndromes in bipolar women, which may be associated with their greater suicide risk, men are more likely to have comorbid substance abuse and a poorer global outcome. Otherwise, the prevalence of bipolar disorder, the age of symptom onset and of initial hospitalization, the presence of schizophrenia-like symptoms, family history variables, and response to lithium treatment are not distinguishable among affected men and women. Some data suggest that women are overrepresented in groups of late-onset bipolar disorder (after age 45 years), although this is controversial. The nature of greater affective cyclicity and frequency of depressive episodes in bipolar women is unclear; thyroid hormone abnormalities, hormonal fluctuations inherent to menstrual cyclicity, and antidepressant treatment approaches have been implicated.

Alcohol dependence

Prevalence

Over the last two decades, many investigations have distinguished men and women on a number of differences in the characteristics, complications, and potential etiologies of alcohol dependence. It is well established in clinical and epidemiologic studies that men start drinking at an earlier age, consume more alcohol, and have a greater rate of alcohol dependence (reviewed by Lex, 1995). Thus, the different prevalence rates could reflect decreased reporting of female alcoholism because the criteria used for dependence are mostly based on consumption patterns and related complications in men. For example, studies that define heavy alcohol consumption at lower levels for women than for men (Whitehead and Layne, 1987) or correct for differences in amount of body fluid

(Mercer and Khavari, 1990) find similar rates of heavy alcohol use for each sex. Similarly, application of symptom criteria based only on the physiologic or psychosocial consequences of excessive alcohol use can affect prevalence rates; men may be more likely to experience alcohol-related social consequences because they have more full-time employment or show behavioral disturbances when intoxicated. However, they may be less likely to endorse symptoms suggesting powerlessness or physical effects of alcohol (Dawson and Grant, 1993). Cultural factors affecting societal tolerance or pressure for increased drinking among women also influence gender ratios in prevalence rates (Dawson and Grant, 1993; Hill, 1995b).

Clinical features

Consumption patterns vary greatly between men and women and with age (Gomberg, 1993a, 1993b). In general, men consume larger amounts of alcohol in a single setting and over the duration of their drinking life. Women begin drinking at a later age, consume less in a single setting, binge less often, and have more periods of abstinence. In both men and women, younger age is associated with higher rates of heavy episodic drinking, intoxication, alcohol dependence, and drinking problems. Women over 65 years old drink less than younger women and men in general. Although women, like men, drink more often in social settings, women drink alone or surreptitiously with a greater frequency. Consumption among younger women has increased over the last few decades, but use patterns over the life span also change with marital status, employment, parenthood, and whether or not these life changes are perceived as desirable (Wilsnack and Wilsnack, 1995). It is therefore difficult to make broad generalizations about the effect of these factors on drinking patterns and problem drinking.

Greater psychiatric comorbidity in female alcoholism is one of the most salient gender differences and has substantial effects on treatment outcome. The ECA data showed that 65 percent of alcoholic women met lifetime criteria for another psychiatric diagnosis, whereas 44 percent of alcoholic men had other lifetime diagnoses (Helzer, Burnam, and McEvoy, 1991). In particular, depressive disorders frequently accompany alcoholism in women, appear to precede their onset of problem drinking, and may be associated with relapse and a higher risk for suicide (reviewed by Davidson and Ritson, 1993; Gomberg, 1993a). Men also develop depressive disorders, but they are less common, and they tend to develop secondary to alcoholism and with continuous drinking (Shuckit, Irwin, and Smith, 1994). One study showed that a lifetime diagnosis of depression conferred a better prognosis in women but was associated with a poorer outcome in men (Rounsaville et al., 1987). However, Davidson and Ritson (1993) caution that evidence for gender differences remains preliminary because few comparison studies have examined the issue of comorbidity in mixed gender groups. By contrast, antisocial personality disorder (when present) typically predates alcoholism in men but develops in the context of substance abuse in women. Both men and women with alcoholism have an increased risk for abusing psychoactive drugs, but men typically use illicit substances, whereas women more often abuse prescribed medications. Anxiety disorders, especially panic and phobic disorders, are also often seen in women alcoholics, as are eating disorders, especially in younger patients. Sexual dysfunction or sex-related problems occur commonly in women with alcoholism, including evidence for higher rates of sexual abuse and incest as children or adults (reviewed by Wilsnack and Wilsnack, 1995).

Alcohol-related complications

Compared to men, women with alcoholism develop medical complications within a shorter interval since the onset of drinking and at an increased rate relative to the amount of alcohol consumed, suggesting that alcohol in excess is more harmful to women than men (reviewed by Hill, 1995a; Lex, 1995). Several studies showed higher rates of alcohol-related hepatitis and cirrhosis in women, but cardiovascular, neurologic, gastrointestinal, and reproductive dysfunction also occur commonly. It is not clear why women should be more susceptible to alcohol-related damage inasmuch as their consumption is less than men. One explanation may be that women have lower gastric alcohol dehydrogenase activity and first-pass metabolism in the liver, which result in higher acetaldehyde levels (Frezza et al., 1990). Women also have a greater average percentage of body fat than men, which results in higher blood alcohol levels at equal consumption levels.

Psychosocial complications associated with alcohol abuse and dependence differ between men and women. Prevailing societal attitudes confer a greater stigma and disapproval toward women who drink. In addition, women report more marital discord and divorce in the context of their drinking, even when both spouses drink. However, men have more frequent contact with the legal system, although younger women show more arrests than older women, which may be related to their different social contexts for drinking. Differences between men and women in the relationship between occupational disturbances and drinking are difficult to assess in the presence of increasing numbers of women employed outside the home. However, traditionally, drinking-related problems in employed men were more overt relative to women homemakers who drank. Excessive alcohol use in women may also be associated with greater risk of exposure to sexually transmitted diseases while intoxicated or to domestic violence by others who also drink, thereby indirectly creating additional health-related problems (Hill, 1995a).

Biologic influences

The mechanisms underlying gender differences in the development of alcoholism are not known. Interestingly, drinking patterns in rodents are opposite to those of humans, with female rats tending to consume more alcohol than males. These opposing patterns suggest that gonadal hormones influence alcohol intake in the rat, but that a variety of other nonbiologic factors play a role in human drinking patterns. Gender-related biologic phenomena are increasingly being considered as the subject of animal research on alcoholism and by inclusion of women subjects in study populations. Of relevance to the development of alcoholism are differential effects of the neuroendocrine system in response to alcohol on gene expression and its pharmacokinetics in the brain (Lancaster, 1995). For instance, compared to females, alcohol has been found to induce less activation of the HPA axis in both men and male rats, an effect thought to be related to activational effects of testosterone rather than organizational effects of neonatal androgens (Ogilvie and Rivier, 1996). It is likely that chronic hypercortisolemia in alcoholic women may contribute to the increased medical and psychiatric complications, but it does not explain the gender disparity in prevalence rates. Sex-related differences in the mesolimbic dopamine system, with female rats showing greater dopamine release in specific brain regions in response to lower doses of alcohol, indicate that there may be differential neurotransmitter-mediated patterns of reinforcement and sensitivity to alcohol effects that influence the development of alcoholism (Blanchard and Glick, 1995).

Genetic factors are common to both male and female alcoholism; whether the extent of genetic mediation differs between the sexes is unclear (reviewed by Hill, 1995b). Adoption and twin studies indicate a substantial genetic influence on male alcoholism. However, the heterogeneity of data from studies on the heritability of alcoholism indicate that some subgroups are more likely to have a genetic liability (Pickens et al., 1991). For example, in men, Type II alcoholism is described as a more severe early onset form of alcoholism with a greater genetic transmission, whereas Type I alcoholism is later onset, less severe, and related to environmental stressors. There is some evidence for this pattern in women, in that family histories of alcoholism and psychiatric illness in first-degree relatives occur more commonly in female probands. In the Virginia Twin Study, consisting of 1,030 female twin pairs of known zygosity, Kendler et al., (1995) reported greater heritability for alcoholism, which was not shared by the other psychiatric conditions (affective, anxiety, and eating disorders). Even though comorbidity is common, these data suggest that the vulnerability to alcoholism is unrelated to those genetic factors that predispose to other psychiatric disorders. Comparable data are not available for men.

Psychosocial influences

The profile of psychosocial risk factors for alcohol-related problems in women varies over the life span, whereas the role of personality variables is relatively unclear (reviewed by Gomberg, 1993a, 1994). Impulsivity in adolescence seems consistently reported as a direct risk factor, and factors related to development of depression or loss in middle age are also relevant. Claims about personality features predisposing to alcoholism are often anecdotal. For instance, alcohol abuse is said to be associated with feelings of low self-esteem and inadequacy, but these qualities may precede the onset of alcoholism for many years.

Treatment

In general, treatment programs for women involve the same practices as for men – detoxification, treatment of comorbid conditions, education, and relapse prevention. However, gender-specific treatment approaches are particularly relevant given that alcohol-related problems occur in different contexts for each gender and referral patterns are different (reviewed by Beckman, 1994). The need for alcoholism treatment in women may be overlooked for a variety of reasons (e.g., their excessive use is more often covert, singular treatment of a primary affective illness may take precedence, or alcohol use may be viewed as an appropriate coping mechanism). Barriers to treatment and risks of treatment noncompliance in women are largely personal, including denial, fears of stigmatization, and feelings of guilt, shame, or low self-esteem. Lack of financial resources, discouragement by a using partner from entering treatment, and beliefs by therapists that treatment of women alcoholics has a poor prognosis present additional deterrents. By contrast, the tendency in men to greater psychosocial disruption, such as impaired school or work performance and more legal infractions, increases referrals for treatment and improves compliance.

Anxiety disorders

Prevalence

The anxiety disorders include generalized anxiety disorder (GAD), panic disorder, agoraphobia, social phobia, specific phobia, posttraumatic stress disorder (PTSD), and obsessive-compulsive disorder (OCD). As a group, the anxiety disorders constitute the most prevalent psychiatric conditions among both men and women, with estimated lifetime prevalence rates of 25–44 percent (Lindal and Stefansson, 1993; Kessler et al., 1994). The character and basis of gender differences in anxiety disorders have not been researched to the same extent as in depression, schizophrenia, and alcoholism, despite the greater prevalence of most anxiety disorders in women (Yonkers et al., 1992; Zerbe, 1995). As seen in Table 4.2, gender ratios vary with the type of anxiety disorder, but lifetime and cross-sectional prevalence rates are often two to three times higher in women. The exception to female predominance is OCD, which occurs about equally in adult men and women, but has a greater prevalence in boys and earlier age of onset in boys and men (Rasmussen and Eisen, 1992). Likewise, for panic disorder, results from studies in the United States, Canada, Germany, and Taiwan show an increased prevalence rate in women compared to men, but the difference is often not significant (reviewed by Wittchen and Essau, 1993). Prevalence rates for PTSD are highly variable, from 1 percent in the ECA study to 9 percent in a community sample, with women affected more often (Yonkers et al., 1992).

Comorbidity

In most populations studied, anxiety disorders are frequently accompanied by comorbid psychiatric illnesses, including other anxiety disorders, substance abuse, and depression (e.g., Scheibe and Albus, 1992; Lindal and Stefansson, 1993; Dick, Bland, and Newman, 1994; Kessler et al., 1994). The rate of comorbidity is disproportionately higher in women (Kessler et al., 1994), although only a few studies examined whether certain patterns of comorbidity are specific to women or distinguished between comorbidity within the anxiety disorders or with other psychiatric conditions. Among the anxiety disorders, agoraphobia and specific phobia occur together most commonly, although panic disorder frequently accompanies either (Wittchen and Essau, 1993). The common co-occurrence of anxiety and depression has led to the proposition of a "mixed anxiety–depression" subcategory to include patients (typically women) who do not meet full current diagnostic criteria for either condition but nonetheless suffer substantial psychiatric morbidity (Zerbe, 1995). The basis for such a diagnostic subcategory is supported by data from a large clinical sample (n = 1,051) in which the ratio of women to men affected with comorbid anxiety and depression was nearly 2:1, but 1:1 when there was only one disorder (Ochoa, Beck, and Steer, 1992). In OCD, women may be more likely to develop concomitant depression and eating disorders (Noshirvani et al., 1991). Generalized anxiety disorder is often accompanied by dysthymia. Clinical studies suggest that panic disorder and somatization are more often seen together in females, although few studies have addressed whether somatization disorder has increased comorbidity with panic disorder (reviewed by Wittchen and Essau, 1993). The impact of increased comorbidity in women is substantial, creating an overall increase in the degree of personal distress, disability, chronicity, risk for treatment unresponsiveness in any of the comorbid psychiatric conditions, and risk for other complications such as suicide (Weissman et al., 1989; Schweizer, 1995).

Clinical features

Few investigations have studied whether specific clinical features of anxiety disorders differ among men and women. Most anxiety disorders tend to be chronic and unremitting, with the onset of symptoms fairly early in life, such as in adolescence or young adulthood. This is especially true for women with agoraphobia or post-traumatic stress disorder. In contrast, women with OCD have an older age of onset and less morbidity than men (Yonkers et al., 1992). Phobias, for example, of animals, environmental conditions, and specific situations such as elevators, predominate among women, but the blood-injection-injury subtype is less gender specific (American Psychiatric Association, 1994, p. 408). In OCD, men tend to have checking compulsions (e.g., develop rituals around the need to check whether a door is locked), whereas women tend to have compulsive washing (Noshirvani et al., 1991; Khanna and Mukherjee, 1992), raising the possibility of sex-linked expressions of phenomenologic subtypes (Rasmussen and Eisen, 1992). The clinical phenomena of panic disorder are the same for men and women, although several studies report an exacerbation of panic symptoms in the premenstrual period and more frequent associations with hyperthyroidism and mitral valve prolapse in women (reviewed by Yonkers et al., 1992). The risk of suicide attempts in patients with panic disorder was three times higher in women than in men, an effect that was independent of coexisting psychiatric illnesses (Weissman et al., 1989).

Biologic factors

Genetic and familial influences appear to be substantial factors in the development of the various anxiety disorders. In the Virginia Twin Study, contributions of genetic and environmental factors to psychiatric disorders were examined in a large sample of female twin pairs (Kendler et al., 1992a, 1992c, 1992d, 1995). Although these data cannot delineate gender differences, they indicate a higher concordance rate for monozygotic versus dizygotic twins for most anxiety disorders. Thus, genetic factors increase the risk of developing these conditions; however, the degree of heritability is generally modest, with variation among anxiety disorder subtypes. The genetic predisposition is relatively strongest for OCD, which has 20–25 percent heritability and 60 percent concordance rates in monozygotic twins. Other family and twin studies indicate four to ten times higher lifetime rates of panic disorder among first-degree relatives of patients with panic disorder (Weissman, 1993). Panic disorder and depression are often comorbid illnesses, but the two conditions are transmitted independently. Despite the greater prevalence of anxiety syndromes in women, their familial nature, and modest heritability, there is no evidence for sex-linked transmission.

Other biologic factors predisposing to gender differences in anxiety syndromes have been difficult to establish (Zerbe, 1995). One hypothesis maintains that anxiety is an adaptive survival mechanism in which women are rendered more sensitive to environmental stimuli and thereby have a lower threshold for expressing fear or anxiety. Hormonal influences acting on neurotransmitter systems are implicated in the development of puerperal anxiety disorders as well as fluctuations in panic and PTSD symptoms over the menstrual cycle. In structural neuroimaging studies of panic disorder and PTSD that implicate the limbic system (Ontiveros et al., 1989; Bremner et al., 1995), or in functional imaging studies of social phobias (Davidson et al., 1993), gender differences are either not apparent or were not examined. Neuroimaging studies of OCD are suggestive of hypermetabolism in the orbitofrontal cortex and caudate nuclei, but consistent neuroanatomic abnormalities or gender differences are not evident (reviewed by Marsh et al., 1996).

Psychosocial factors

Psychosocial influences clearly affect the occurrence of anxiety, although the incidence of anxiety syndromes in women in relation to such factors is not established (reviewed by Yonkers and Gurguis, 1995; Zerbe, 1995). For women, adjustments to changes in gender roles and professional opportunities may generate anxiety and conflicts regarding personal and societal expectations.

The impact of past trauma, including abuse, may confer an increased predisposition to anxiety disorders, notably PTSD. Developmental issues and social learning, in which women are encouraged to seek protection by others, have been suggested as relevant to the genesis of phobias. Early parental loss seems clearly associated with the later development of anxiety disorders and depression (Kendler et al., 1992b), although many other factors, such as the presence of another secure attachment figure may mitigate against adverse effects. Suggestions of an association between panic disorder and separation anxiety, however, are not substantiated (Wittchen and Essau, 1993).

Treatment

Treatment of the various anxiety disorders in women is confounded by the tendency toward greater comorbidity, a longer duration of illness, and a worse prognosis than in men. As with all conditions, a comprehensive and individualized approach is indicated. For GAD, some treatment approaches that focus on specific worries may generate gender-based approaches to treatment, after accounting for individual nuances.

Somatization disorder

Prevalence

Somatization disorder, once referred to as hysteria, is regarded as typically affecting women. In Table 4.2, somatization disorder is exclusively female in three of the reported studies, whereas the gender ratio is equal for the Puerto Rican sample. It is not clear whether this discrepancy is related to cultural factors in Puerto Rico that enhance the endorsement of somatic symptoms in men (Canino et al., 1987). A recent literature review (Wool and Barsky, 1994) examined the contribution of gender differences in patterns of somatization to the prevalence of somatization disorder. This review indicated that somatization and somatization disorder occur in men, but that women are predominantly affected by both, with the increased prevalence rates persisting even after controlling for increased visits to the doctor for gynecologic care.

Clinical features

Somatization disorder is characterized by help-seeking behavior for multiple somatic complaints for which there is not an adequate physiologic basis. It tends to begin in young adulthood, has a chronic disabling course, and is more likely to occur in lower socioeconomic groups, the less educated, and the previously married. There have been few investigations of gender differences in somatization disorder. Women are more likely to be referred for psychiatric evaluation, but direct comparisons show no differences in symptomatology, impairment, psychiatric comorbidity, or demographic features between men and women (Slavney and Teitelbaum, 1985; Golding, Smith, and Kashner, 1991). The high rate of comorbidity with other psychiatric illnesses, namely, depressive and anxiety disorders, is seen in both men and women with somatization disorder. One study indicated that referrals for men with somatization disorder hinged upon greater disruption in life functioning (Smith, Monson, and Livingston, 1985), whereas women are more inclined to seek medical help earlier.

Biologic influences

Certain features of somatization disorder implicate biologic factors in its underlying pathogenesis, which are further modulated by gender-specific and cultural factors that affect the expression of somatic complaints. First, there is increased comorbidity with psychiatric illnesses that have obvious biologic underpinnings and an increased prevalence in women. Second, there is a genetic component to somatization disorder with evidence for increased concordance among monozygotic twins relative to dizygotic twins and an increased occurrence of psychiatric illness, including somatization disorder, in first-degree relatives of patients with somatization disorder (Golding et al., 1992; Kaplan, Sadock, and Grebb, 1994). Third, innate gender differences in perception, with women being more likely to incorporate extrasomatic cues and emotional stimuli when interpreting bodily sensations, may render women more vulnerable to expressing concern over otherwise benign bodily sensations (reviewed by Wool and Barsky, 1994). Immune system dysfunction and its effects on central nervous system function have also been proposed as potential mediators of some of the symptoms seen in somatization disorder, although these data are controversial (Manu, Lane, and Mathews, 1992).

Psychosocial influences

Psychosocial explanations for the development of somatization disorder have been proposed. A large body of literature has examined the phenomenon that women seek medical attention more than men and the multiple social and interpersonal influences that mediate the easier expression of physical complaints by women relative to men (e.g., Cleary, Mechanic, and Greenley, 1982). It is difficult to delineate the manner in which these general social and cultural factors increase the risk for somatization disorder in women. However, it seems that illness behavior is more readily manifested by women, including abnormal illness behavior. Although not necessarily gender specific, psychological explanations are also proposed, including some evidence that histories of early childhood emotional trauma are overrepresented in women with somatization disorder and predispose toward somatization (Morrison, 1989). An accompanying view is that such early stressors modify brain function in response to stimuli (Bell, 1994).

Treatment

Treatment of somatization disorder in men or women involves the same essential principles: maintaining regular contact with a primary care physician to monitor symptoms and plan appropriate diagnostic tests. The frequent coexistence of mood or anxiety disorders, which occur with an increased frequency in women, and the potential history of childhood abuse would indicate a need for careful consideration of these possibilities in treatment approaches.

Schizophrenia

Prevalence

Gender differences in schizophrenia were recognized early in the century by Kraepelin and have subsequently been the subject of extensive epidemiologic and clinical investigations. A prevailing caveat is that men and women have about an equal risk for developing schizophrenia but differ in the clinical manifestations of the illness. However, a recent careful review of all epidemiologic studies since, 1980 showed that the incidence is higher in men in most studies and that male:female prevalence rates vary from 1.0 to 2.1 (Goldstein, 1995b). Whether the reported rates were statistically significant depends upon a variety of factors, such as population sampling, diagnostic criteria, and statistical methodology, as well as the variable expression of schizophrenia by men and women. For example, gender differences in reported rates for schizophrenia are minimized when the schizophrenia spectrum disorders (e.g., delusional and schizoaffective disorders) are included because these conditions tend to predominate in females. Rediagnosis of affective disorders in some women originally thought to have schizophrenia may also account for a relative decrease in the diagnosis of schizophrenia in women. Variation in male:female ratios might be seen when the sampled population is restricted to the community or a younger age range, because men are more likely to reside in hospitals and women are older at symptom onset. Cultural influences may also affect prevalence rates, with higher male:female ratios for the diagnosis of schizophrenia in developing countries as compared to lower ratios for Eastern European regions and middle values for Western Hemisphere nations (Hambrecht, Maurer, and Häfner, 1993).

Clinical differences

Gender exerts a profound pathoplastic effect on the clinical expression of schizophrenia, largely in relation to the onset and course of the illness (reviewed by Lewis, 1992; Goldstein, 1995b; Seeman, 1995). Relative to affected men, most women with schizophrenia have a later age of onset, a more acute course with less insidious onset, better premorbid adjustment, and higher premorbid intellectual abilities. Symptom onset is most frequently between ages 18 and 25 years for men and after age 25 years through the mid-thirties for women (Angermeyer and Kuhn, 1988). However, incidence peaks a second time for women older than 45 years, whereas men rarely develop new onset of illness at this stage of life. Women also have a more favorable treatment outcome, with more affective symptoms, a faster and more superior response to neuroleptics, higher remission rates, fewer relapses and involuntary hospitalizations, less concomitant substance abuse, and fewer symptoms of the deficit state (e.g., social withdrawal, amotivation). Perhaps complementary to their later age of onset and better premorbid functioning, women schizophrenic patients have better social skills and are more often married. These differential clinical patterns have not been attenuated by the rediagnosis of affective disorder in some women initially diagnosed as schizophrenic.

Biologic influences: Neurohormonal factors

Estrogen is implicated as a primary determinant of gender differences in the clinical expression of schizophrenia; its etiologic role remains quite speculative (Seeman and Lang, 1990; Seeman, 1995). The central thesis of the estrogen hypothesis, as it is called, is that high estrogen levels in females exert a protective role that delays the onset of schizophrenia in predisposed women until after puberty. Further, the risk of illness onset or relapse is lower during pregnancy, whereas it is increased when estrogen levels are low, such as premenstrually, during the postpartum period when levels drop precipitously, or after menopause. A potential mechanism for this protective effect is via neuromodulatory effects of estrogen, which downregulate dopaminergic receptor affinity (Häfner et al., 1991). Antidopaminergic properties of estrogen may also contribute partially to the better outcome in women in that they require lower neuroleptic doses. However, refuting this idea, others have found that neuroleptic use does not consistently increase after menopause (Salokangas, 1995), suggesting that increased neuroleptic doses in younger men may be related to other gender-bound issues, such as increased smoking habits or increased body weight in most men.

Biologic influences: Neuroanatomic factors

Biologic theories on the nature of schizophrenia implicate neurodevelopmental, genetic, and environmental factors that affect brain structure and function. Structural brain abnormalities in schizophrenia have been consistently demonstrated since the mid-1970s and provide a solid marker for a neuropathologic process integral to the illness (reviewed by Marsh et al., 1996). These include evidence for widespread reductions in cortical gray matter volumes, especially in prefrontal and temporal regions, enlargement of ventricular and sulcal spaces, and discrete abnormalities in temporal-limbic regions, such as cytoarchitectural disarray in the hippocampus. A prevailing theory proposes that these abnormalities are the result of aberrations occurring early in brain development that interact with subsequent maturational events in the brain to result in clinical expression of the illness. It is not clear whether distinctive neuropathologic processes or sex-related patterns of normal brain development that influence patterns of neuroanatomic abnormalities in schizophrenia account for the aforementioned clinical gender differences. Evidence that men with schizophrenia have a disproportionate number of minor physical anomalies and neurologic soft signs and a disproportionate history of obstetric complications during birth might reflect and/or result in deviations from normal brain structure and function. Although studies on the extent of gender differences in neuroanatomic pathology are somewhat inconsistent in their results, many studies suggest more abnormalities in schizophrenic men (Lewine and Seeman, 1995). Some researchers argue further that left-sided abnormalities are relatively greater in schizophrenia, especially in schizophrenic men, and that these develop out of gender-modulated factors in brain development (Crow et al., 1989). Another hypothesis proposes several subtypes of schizophrenia with different underlying mechanisms, including an early-onset form characterized by male preponderance and neurodevelopmental damage versus a later-onset form that predominates in women and is genetically transmitted (Castle and Murray, 1991).

Biologic influences: Genetic factors

Regardless of gender, genetic factors are evident in the transmission of schizophrenia, with a marked increase in the risk of developing the illness when first-degree relatives are affected (3–15 percent) and in monozygotic twins (15–65 percent) (Torrey, 1992). Although gender effects on the heritability and expression of schizophrenia are apparent, the nature of this effect is unclear (Goldstein, 1995a). Interpretations of the collective data on gender and genetic transmission are affected by the different diagnostic criteria used to define the schizophrenia phenotype. For example, same-sex concordance in monozygotic twins was reported as greater in male twins in some studies and in female twins in other studies. Of particular interest are family transmission studies, which suggest that relatives of women schizophrenics are at greater risk for developing schizophrenia and related psychotic illnesses than are relatives of schizophrenic men. Some researchers argue that maternal or paternal transmission dictates same-sex concordance as well as gender-based differences in the expression of the illness, as in theories implicating homologous schizophrenia susceptibility genes on the X and Y chromosomes (e.g., Crow et al., 1994). A recent series found no gender effect in terms of age of onset in cases of familial schizophrenia (Gorwood et al., 1995).

Psychosocial influences

Reviews of the psychosocial factors related to gender differences in schizophrenia (Seeman and Lang, 1990; Seeman, 1995) stress that social expectations of women influence clinical manifestations of the illness and that different treatment approaches are necessary for affected men and women. Higher cultural expectations of men, versus tolerance of dependency in women, may precipitate the earlier onset of schizophrenia in vulnerable men. More frequent aggression in schizophrenic men may relate to premorbid differences in socialization. Along with their later age of onset and increased marriage rates, women are more likely to have more financial resources, better integration of personal strengths, and a broader and more accommodating social network – all features that contribute to a more positive course.

Treatment

Treatment of schizophrenia centers around neuroleptic treatment and psychosocial rehabilitation, regardless of gender, and there is always a need for individualization of treatment approaches. In keeping with their better prognosis, women tend to respond more positively to lower doses of neuroleptic medications and to psychosocial interventions (reviewed by Seeman, 1995).

Conclusions

This chapter describes gender differences in psychiatric illnesses as they relate to prevalence rates, clinical features, underlying biologic, psychological, and environmental factors, and treatment approaches. A review of sex differences in brain morphology serves to introduce the concept of inherent differences in mental functioning in men and women, and how these might relate to the expression of psychiatric illness.

In this general overview, the most striking gender difference in psychiatric illnesses is the variation in lifetime prevalence rates for different disorders in men and women across multiple nations (Table 4.2). These figures indicate that women are substantially more affected by depressive illnesses, anxiety disorders, and somatization disorder than men, and, compared to men, women are more likely to have comorbid psychiatric conditions, which increases their morbidity and refractoriness to treatment. Men suffer significantly more from alcoholism and might have a greater tendency, albeit modest, to develop schizophrenia or OCD.

In many respects, the various psychiatric illnesses in men and women are more alike than they are different, aside from differences in prevalence. Schizophrenia is the only condition for which the clinical characteristics are not the same, but these differences revolve around the course of the illness and not its basic phenomenology. For both alcoholism and schizophrenia, there is some evidence for discrete neuroanatomic and physiologic differences between affected men and women. By contrast, sociocultural and, possibly, neurocognitive sex differences are more salient factors in the affective and anxiety disorders. Treatment, including psychopharmacologic, psychotherapeutic, and psychosocial approaches, is highly individualized, regardless of gender, although certain themes or caveats apply more to one gender or the other for a given condition.

To the extent that men and women are inherently different organisms on the basis of respective differences in brain development and their varying hormonal milieu over the life span, gender is an important mediating variable in psychiatric illness. More recent research strategies using operationalized diagnostic criteria have facilitated better descriptions of each of these illnesses from the neurobiologic, interpersonal, and sociologic perspectives. Thus, exploration of the role of gender in the context of each of these perspectives should lead to a better understanding of both the nature and management of the different psychiatric illnesses.

Acknowledgments

This work was supported by the Theodore and Vada Stanley Foundation and the National Institute of Health (Grants MH-30854 and AA-05965). The authors are grateful to Teresa Sung and Scott Spears for research assistance.

CHAPTER FIVE

THYROID HORMONES IN MAJOR DEPRESSIVE AND BIPOLAR DISORDERS

NASEEM AHMED SMITH AND

PETER T. LOOSEN

Part I
THYROID GLAND: PHYSIOLOGY, PATHOLOGY, AND EPIDEMIOLOGY

Physiology

The principal hormones of the hypothalamic-pituitary-thyroid (HPT) axis are thyroxine (T_4) and triiodothyronine (T_3), the latter being the more potent biologically (Larsen and Ingbar, 1992). Although both T_4 and T_3 are released from the thyroid gland, about 90 percent of circulating T_3 is derived from T_4 by monodeiodination in (mainly) liver, kidney, and other tissues by the enzyme 5'-deiodinase-I (5'D-I). In serum, more than 99.5 percent of T_4 and T_3 are bound to thyroxine-binding globulin (TBG), albumin, and thyroxine-binding prealbumin (TPBA), leaving less than 0.5 percent of T_4 and T_3 unbound and biologically active (Larsen and Ingbar, 1992). Alterations in deiodination and/or serum protein concentrations can therefore profoundly affect thyroid hormone economy (Israel et al., 1979; Israel and Orrego, 1984).

Biosynthesis and release of T_4 and T_3 from the thyroid gland are primarily controlled by the anterior pituitary hormone thyrotropin (thyroid-stimulating hormone, TSH). In turn, biosynthesis and release of TSH from thyrotroph cells are mediated principally by the tripeptide thyrotropin-releasing hormone (TRH). TRH is released directly into the portal venous system, which connects the hypothalamus and the pituitary gland, from hypothalamic neurons that originate in the paraventricular nucleus. TRH also stimulates the release of prolactin from pituitary lactotroph cells. Homeostatic control within the HPT axis is assured through negative feedback inhibition by T_4 and T_3 at the thyrotroph cell, leading to diminished synthesis and release of TSH. Thyroid hormones have also been shown to selectively reduce TRH biosynthesis in the hypothalamus, which may provide yet another means of regulation (Segerson et al., 1987). Finally, many neurotransmitters and non-HPT-axis hormones affect TRH and TSH release (Morley, 1981).

A wealth of laboratory studies provide evidence for both a neuroregulatory role of thyroid hormones (Table 5.1) and a homeostatic mechanism by which brain intracellular T_3 concentrations are enzymatically maintained within narrow limits (Leonard, 1990). The enzyme 5'-deiodinase-II (5'D-II) – found in the central nervous system, anterior pituitary, brown adipose tissue, and placenta –

Table 5.1. *Evidence for a neuroregulatory role of thyroid hormones*

- Thyroid hormone receptors are widely distributed throughout the brain (Dratman et al., 1982).
- Both T_4[a] and T_3[b] enter the brain by a high-affinity saturable transport mechanism (Dratman et al., 1976, 1982).
- Within the brain T_4 and T_3 are differentially distributed regionally and highly localized in synaptosomes (Dratman et al., 1976, 1982).
- The rate of conversion of T_4 to T_3 is many times greater in brain than in liver (Leonard, 1990).
- There is evidence that T_4 may be converted into T_3 within nerve terminals (Dratman, Crutchfield, 1978).
- Despite extremes of T_4 availability, brain T_4 and T_3 concentrations and brain T_3 production and turnover rates are kept within narrow limits (Dratman et al., 1983; Leonard 1990), suggesting that small changes in brain thyroid hormones may produce significant changes in behavior.
- Hyperthyroidism increases striatal β-adrenoreceptors and striatal dopaminergic activity, whereas hypothyroidism reduces striatal and hypothalamic β-adrenoreceptors (Atterwill et al., 1984).
- Hyperthyroidism increases, and hypothyroidism decreases, presynaptic α_2-adrenoreceptor function (Atterwill et al., 1984).
- Hypothyroidism causes a significant increase in serotonin and substance P levels in rat brain nuclei (Savard et al., 1983).

[a]Thyroxine.

[b]Triiodothyronine.

has been shown to increase three- to fivefold within 24 hours of thyroidectomy, and to decrease by 80–90 percent within 2–4 hours after injection of a saturating dose of T_3 (Leonard, 1990). The thyroid hormone-induced changes in 5′D-II activity in vivo and in cell cultures are due to changes in the half-life of the enzyme (in euthyroid animals the half-life of 5′D-II is about 30 minutes; it increases to 4–6 hours in hypothyroid animals) and do not depend on transcription or translation. Moreover, T_4 and rT_3 are more than 100-fold more effective than T_3 (Leonard, 1990). In contrast, 5′D-I activity is decreased in thyroidectomized rats, and at least 3 to 5 days of hypothyroidism are required to observe this fall in activity (Leonard, 1990).

Pathology

Thyroid structure and function undergo subtle changes during the human life cycle (Table 5.2). As we will discuss later, many of these changes (e.g., increased

Table 5.2. *Changes in thyroid function with age*

Thyroid gland structure	
• Glandular weight	↓
• Microscopic and palpable nodularity	↑
• Cellular infiltrates	↑
• Autoimmune damage	↑
Thyroid disease	
• Hyperthyroidism (Graves' disease)	↓
• Hypothyroidism	↑
• Subclinical hypothyroidism	↑
• T_3[a] toxicosis	↑
• Toxic multinodular goiter	↑
Thyroid hormones in blood and hormone production	
• Renal iodine clearance	↓
• Rate of iodine accumulation in thyroid	↓
• MCR[b] of T_4[c]	↓
• Serum T_3[d]	↓
• TRH-induced TSH response in men	↓

[a] Triiodothyronine.

[b] Metabolic clearance rate.

[c] Thyroxine.

[d] Note that serum T_3 concentrations are lowered in patients undergoing caloric deprivation as well as in a great variety of patients with acute or chronic systemic illnesses (Larsen and Ingbar, 1992).

frequency of palpable nodularity, goiter, autoimmune damage, and overt and subclinical hypothyroidism) are more common in (aging) women than in men. It is not known whether some of these age-related changes (e.g., decreased glandular weight, increased nodularity, decreased renal iodine clearance, reduced serum T_3 concentrations, and attenuated TSH responses to TRH in men) are of any medical or behavioral significance.

Fetal, infantile, and child hypothyroidism

Thyroid hormone deficiency during fetal life does not appear to affect growth and maturation, suggesting that brain development in utero is not significantly thyroid dependent (Fisher, 1986). However, infants with untreated congenital hypothyroidism are likely to show, in addition to the usual thermogenic (e.g., lowered body temperature), metabolic (e.g., constipation, hypotonia), and organ (e.g., enlarged tongue, dry skin) dysfunctions, growth deficiency, delayed bone maturation, and delayed dental development. Brain effects are generally profound in both sexes, with mental retardation and specific motor and sensory dysfunctions being common (Fisher, 1986). Laboratory experiments have shown that the lack of thyroid hormones during infancy, if uncorrected, will lead to significantly diminished brain weight, reduced size of cortical neurons, severely retarded dendritic arborization of Purkinje cells, reduced synaptogenesis, decreased myelinization, and changes in brain enzyme activity and RNA transcription (Adams and DeLong, 1986). Impaired neuronal maturation and connectivity are the net result of these changes.

After age 3, the brain's dependency on thyroid hormones wanes, most likely because its maturation is largely completed by this time. Hypothyroidism occurring after this age is thus not associated with mental retardation, but school performance may be obtunded to a variable degree. Growth retardation, delayed bone maturation, and delayed sexual maturation are common (Fisher, 1986).

Adult hypothyroidism

The earliest sign that patients may develop hypothyroidism is a rise in serum TSH, associated initially with normal thyroid hormone values. As the disease with its insidious nature and multiple presentations progresses, first T_4 and later T_3 levels fall below the normal range. At this time, patients begin to develop signs and symptoms of hypothyroidism (e.g., anemia, bradycardia, brittle hair and cool skin, cold intolerance, fatigue, lethargy, dry skin, hypothermia, slow speech, and weight changes) and benefit from treatment. In general, hypothyroidism is a graded phenomenon, being classified as overt, mild, and subclinical (Table 5.3).

Overt hypothyroidism (Table 5.3) can arise from a variety of causes, including iodine and iodine-containing medications, treatment of primary hyperthyroidism (e.g., radioiodine, surgery, antithyroid drugs), inadequate replacement therapy for overt hypothyroidism, and, most commonly, autoimmune (Hashimoto's) thyroiditis (Ross, 1991; Larsen and Ingbar, 1992). It can also arise during lithium therapy (Calabrese et al., 1895; Myers et al., 1985; Lazarus et al., 1986; Bocchetta et al., 1991; Lombardi et al., 1993).

The behavioral sequelae of hypothyroidism have been noted early. After Gull's (1873) report, "On a cretinoid state supervening in adult life in women," the Clinical Society of London established a committee on myxedema (i.e., primary hypothyroidism) to study the relationship between this condition and behavioral disorders. In 1888, they reported that in 109 patients with myxedema "delusions and hallucinations occurred in nearly half of the cases," and that "insanity" was seen in an equal number of patients (Clinical Society of London, 1888). This "myxedematous insanity" was characterized by "mania," or "dementia melancholia, with a marked preponderance of suspicion and self-accusations." The committee also observed a general slowing of thought processes in their patients. These observations are still valid today. Cognitive changes, with alterations in attention, concentration, and perception are common, as are depression and lethargy (Bauer, Droba, and Whybrow, 1987; Whybrow, 1991). Over the last fifty years, there have been only three studies of unselected hypothyroid patients. Jain (1972) reported that 43 percent of 30 patients presented with depression and 33 percent with anxiety. Crown (1949) found cognitive deficits in each of the 24 patients studied. Whybrow, Prange Jr., and Treadway (1969) found each of the 7 hypothyroid patients to be either

Table 5.3. *Grades of hypothyroidism*

Grade	Clinical features	Serum T$_4$	Serum T$_3$	Serum TSH
Overt	Obvious symptoms and signs of hypothryoidism	Low	Usually low	Very high
Mild	Mild or nonspecific symptoms or signs	Low or normal	Normal	Moderately high
Subclinical	None	Normal	Normal	Slightly elevated

Modified from Ross, 1991.

confused (6), depressed (5), or irritable (1); none was without any psychiatric symptom. The psychiatric problems of hypothyroidism in the adult respond to adequate replacement with thyroid hormone, but endocrine and behavioral remission may not run a parallel course. Improvement is usually greatest among patients whose mental changes were mild and of recent origin (Wilson and Jefferson, 1985; Bauer, Droba, and Whybrow, 1987).

Subclinical hypothyroidism

The diagnostic criteria of subclinical hypothyroidism are listed in Table 5.3; its causes are the same as the causes of overt hypothyroidism (Larsen and Ingbar, 1992). Asymptomatic autoimmune thyroiditis, based on the evidence of circulating thyroid antibodies with normal thyroid function, is common, particularly in older women (Tunbridge and Caldwell, 1991). In the Wickham Survey, overt hypothyroidism developed at the rate of 5 percent per annum in subjects with antibodies and raised TSH level (Tunbridge and Caldwell, 1991). Whether subclinical hypothyroidism should be treated on the basis of preventing such deterioration is a matter of debate. Treatment may be indicated to prevent progression to overt hypothyroidism, especially in patients with TSH levels above 14–20 mU/ml and/or microsomal antibody titers of 1:1,600 or greater.

Primary hyperthyroidism (Graves' disease)

No test predicts the development of Graves' disease. A rise in serum T_3 and a fall in TSH are the earliest signs of thyroid overactivity, followed later by a rise in T_4 (Table 5.3) (Tunbridge and Caldwell, 1991). In the Wickham Survey, the prevalence of newly diagnosed primary hyperthyroidism was 4.7 per 1,000 women and that of previously diagnosed and treated hyperthyroidism was 20 per 1,000 women. The prevalence of established hyperthyroidism was 10 times more common in women than in men, and the mean age at diagnosis was 48 years (range 25–70) (Tunbridge and Caldwell, 1991).

The true incidence of psychiatric symptoms in patients with primary hyperthyroidism is difficult to estimate because of the lack of use of objective diagnostic criteria. Most studies of hyperthyroidism have been concerned with syndromal prevalence of behavioral problems; they reported mild cognitive decline in 20–54 percent of patients (Wilson, Johnson, and Smith, 1962; Whybrow, Prange Jr., and Treadway, 1969), depressive symptoms in 20–58 percent (Wilson, Johnston, and Smith, 1962; Whybrow, Prange Jr., and Treadway, 1969), and nervousness and/or irritability in 71–100 percent (Whybrow, Prange Jr., and Treadway, 1969; Rockey and Griep, 1980; Wallace and McCrimmon, 1980). Kathol, Turner, and Delahunt (1986) studied 26 females and 7 males with newly diagnosed, untreated hyperthyroidism using operational (DSM-III) criteria. Ten patients (30 percent) were found to have depression and 15 (45 percent) anxiety. The number of anxiety symptoms paralleled the number of hyperthyroid symptoms whereas depressive symptoms did not. Prior history of psychiatric disease and family history of psychiatric disease did not predict anxiety or depression. The number of patients with depression and anxiety was felt to be artificially inflated by the concurrent presence of somatic thyroid symptoms. In another report of 29 consecutively studied hyperthyroid patients, the same investigators (Kathol and Delahunt, 1986) found depression in 31 percent and generalized anxiety disorder in 79 percent of patients. All depressed patients and 21 of the 23 with anxiety displayed complete resolution of these symptoms with antithyroid therapy alone. Are these behavioral symptoms the direct result of increased serum thyroid hormone concentrations? This was suggested by the report of Kathol, Turner, and Delahunt (1986), cited earlier, as well as the study by Wilson, Johnson, and Feist (1996), which showed that the experimental administration of T_3 to 11 normal volunteers produced marked changes in interpersonal functioning and caused dysphoria, depression, jitteriness, and decreased friendliness.

However, recent work has clearly demonstrated that behavioral problems are common in subclinical hyperthyroidism, where serum thyroid hormone concentrations are normal (but TSH and TSH response are reduced). Nowotny et al. (1990) investigated two groups of 10 patients each who suffered from subclinical hyper- or hypothyroidism, respectively, and 10 euthyroid controls. Psychological testing was performed by questionnaires concerning subjective somatic symptoms, emotional disturbances, psychomotor performance, cognitive impairment, and personality. Patients with subclinical hyperthyroidism were more subject to somatic symptoms and affective complaints than were those who had subclinical hypothyroidism. As compared with controls, patients were more depressed, anxious, irritable, and emotionally labile. Rockel et al. (1987) demonstrated that behavioral symptoms were equally common in subclinical (n = 20) and overt (n = 20) hyperthyroidism; they included anxiety, emotional lability, a sense of not feeling well, an increased lack of vitality and activity, and a tendency toward depression. Bommer et al. (1990) showed that 43 percent of 45 euthyroid patients who had suffered from hyperthyroidism still complained of "seriously reduced wellbeing," with feelings of fear, hostility, and inability to concentrate.

Pregnancy, postpartum, and menstrual function

Although goiter, hypothyroidism, and hyperthyroidism are not uncommon during pregnancy, thyroid dysfunctions generally occur more frequently in the peripartum or postpartum period than during pregnancy (Emerson, 1991). The two most common forms of postpartum thyroid dysfunction are postpartum Graves' disease and postpartum thyroiditis. It is worthwhile to warn women with a history of thyroid disease that the underlying condition may worsen after delivery. Although postpartum thyroiditis, its incidence ranging from 3 to 8 percent of postpartum women, is not responsible for most cases of postpartum psychosis (Stewart et al., 1996), women who develop depression, lethargy, and emotional lability after delivery should have thyroid function tests.

In adult women, hypothyroidism results in menorrhagia, anovulation, and an increase in fetal wastage (Emerson, 1991). For many years, fertility was thought to be markedly impaired in hypothyroid women, but recent studies appear to be more optimistic in showing that pregnancy in hypothyroid women is less rare, perhaps because mild hypothyroidism can now be detected early. When hypothyroidism is diagnosed during pregnancy, T_4 should be instituted promptly to increase the chances for a normal pregnancy. It is noteworthy that T_4 administration is not useful in treating euthyroid patients for infertility, menstrual irregularity, or premenstrual syndrome (Emerson, 1991).

Part II
THYROID HORMONES
AND MAJOR DEPRESSION

Peripheral thyroid hormones before and during treatment

Peripheral thyroid hormone concentrations were assessed in acutely depressed patients and compared to normal controls, euthymic patients, or both; the results are equivocal. Most depressed patients appear to be euthyroid (Kirkegaard, 1981; Loosen, 1988a, 1988b; Briggs et al., 1993). However, some investigators reported serum T_4 levels in the upper normal range (Dewhurst et al., 1968; Hatotani et al., 1974; Kirkegaard and Faber, 1981; Kjellman et al., 1983; Styra, Joffe, and Singer, 1991) or found increased serum concentrations of reverse T_3 (rT_3) (Linnoila et al., 1979; Kirkegaard and Faber, 1981; Kjellman et al., 1983), the hormonally inactive analogue of T_3 (Larsen and Ingbar, 1992).

Other investigators reported lowered thyroid function in depressed patients, including reduced mean levels of free T_4 index (FT_4I) and free T_4 (FT_4) (Rybakowski and Sowinski, 1973; Rinieris et al., 1978a, 1978b), and T_3 (Linnoila et al., 1979; Joffe et al., 1985; Orsulak et al., 1985; Rupprecht et al., 1989; Wahby et al., 1989).

Are there dynamic changes in thyroid function during treatment of depression? If so, are these changes related to remission of symptoms? Although these questions cannot be answered with certainty, studies that have addressed them have revealed remarkably consistent results. Most (Board, Wadeson, and Persky, 1957; Gibbons, Gibson, and Maxwell, 1960; Whybrow et al., 1972; Ferrari, 1973; Kirkegaard et al., 1975, 1977; Kirkegaard and Faber, 1986; Unden et al., 1986; Joffe and Singer, 1987; Baumgartner et al., 1988; Muller and Boning, 1988; Brady and Anton, 1989; Mason et al., 1989; Southwick et al., 1989; Joffe and Singer, 1990b; Hoeflich et al., 1992; Kusalic, Engelsmann, and Bradwejn, 1993), but not all (Kolakowska and Swigar, 1977; Leichter, Kierstein, and Martin, 1977; Karlberg, Kjellman, and Kagedol, 1978; Shelton et al., 1993) studies reported that significant reductions in serum T_4 concentrations after remission were induced by a wide range of somatic treatments, including various antidepressants, lithium, sleep deprivation, and electroconvulsive therapy (ECT). Four studies (Roy-Byrne et al., 1984; Southwick et al., 1989; Joffe and Singer, 1990b; Kusalic, Engelsmann, and Bradwejn, 1993) documented that the T_4 reduction was greater in treatment responders than in nonresponders, suggesting that increased thyroid function may facilitate treatment response. This was first noted by Whybrow et al. (1972), who showed that heightened thyroid activity before treatment was positively correlated with a prompt clinical response to imipramine.

Thyrotropin/subclinical hypothyroidism/antithyroid antibodies

The following TSH and/or autoimmune dysfunctions are not uncommon in depression: an abnormal circadian TSH rhythm, elevated basal serum TSH concentrations, and elevated titers of antithyroid antibodies. The latter two are frequently seen together in subclinical hypothyroidism.

Abnormal circadian thyrotropin-secreting hormone rhythm

Depression is often associated with disturbances in circadian behavioral (e.g., changes in emotional well-being during the day, commonly with early morning worsening) and biologic (e.g., abnormalities in body temperature and cortisol secretion) rhythms. To these dysfunctions we can add an abnormal diurnal TSH rhythm, often characterized by a lack of the nocturnal TSH surge (Table 5.4). In addition to depression, this abnormality can be found in central hypothyroidism (Adriaanse et al., 1993), in euthyroid patients with suprasellar extensions of pituitary lesions (Adriaanse et al., 1993), and after naloxone administration (Samuels et al., 1994). The latter, of course, suggests that endogenous opioids have significant stimulatory effects on TSH secretion, predominantly during the nocturnal TSH surge.

Subclinical hypothyroidism

Between 1 and 4 percent of patients with a variety of affective illnesses show evidence of overt hypothyroidism, and between 4 and 40 percent show evidence of subclinical hypothyroidism (Table 5.5).

It appears that subtle, but not overt, thyroid dysfunctions are rather common in depressed patients, and that they are not clinically irrelevant. Comorbid subclinical hypothyroidism can lower the threshold for the occurrence of depression (Haggerty Jr. et al., 1993) and for panic disorder (Joffe and Levitt, 1992). It can also be associated with cognitive dysfunction (Haggerty Jr., Evans, and Prange Jr., 1986; Haggerty Jr., Garbutt, Evans et al., 1990) and/or a diminished response to standard psychiatric treatments (Haggerty Jr., Garbutt, Evans et al., 1990; Joffe and Levitt, 1992). That some depressed patients with subclinical hypothyroidism responded behaviorally to thyroid hormone substitution (Gold, Pottash, and Extein, 1981, 1982; Gewirtz et al., 1988) suggests that it may be useful to intervene therapeutically and to broaden the list of index symptoms for initiating thyroid hormone replacement to include depression and memory faults in addition to the somatic symptoms of fatigue, weight gain, and cold intolerance (Haggerty Jr. and Prange Jr., 1995). Haggerty Jr. et al. (1993) demonstrated that the lifetime frequency of depression was significantly higher in depressed patients with subclinical hypothyroidism (56 percent) than in those without (20 percent).

Antithyroid antibodies

In a wide spectrum of depressed patients prevalence of antithyroid antibodies ranged from 9 to 20 percent (Table 5.6), compared to the about 5 percent found in the general population (Tunbridge and Caldwell, 1991).

It is unclear whether high antibody titers are of clinical relevance if they are accompanied by normal serum TSH concentrations (Nemeroff et al., 1985; Joffe, 1987). Summarizing the experience of the Chapel Hill group, Prange Jr. et al. (1990) concluded that (1) in 148 patients with mental disorders, 8 percent of patients with major depression had antithyroid antibodies, none of bipolar/manic patients, 20 percent of bipolar/depressed patients, 33 percent of bipolar/mixed patients, and 7 percent of schizophrenic patients; (2) in 41 bipolar patients (18 had received lithium at some previous time, 23 had never taken lithium), the prevalence of antibodies was slightly, but insignificantly, higher in those patients who had not been exposed to lithium; (3) studying the relationship between FT_4I and clinical response to tricyclic antidepressants (TCAs) in 80 depressed patients, good responders were found to have a significantly higher, albeit within the normal range, FT_4I than poor responders; (4) patients with antithyroid antibodies had a poorer average treatment response than those without antibodies; and (5) in 50 depressed patients receiving ECT, ratings of ECT-induced organicity were inversely correlated with baseline FT_4I concentrations.

Thyroid hormones in cerebrospinal fluid

The studies evaluating concentrations of various hormones of the HPT axis in cerebrospinal fluid (CSF) of affectively ill patients are summarized in Table 5.7. As shown in the table, levels of T_4, rT_3, and FT_3 have been reported to be increased in some depressed patients. Moreover, increased TRH levels have also been reported in some patients, but not all studies agree.

The thyrotropin-releasing hormone test

The TRH test, that is, measurement of serum TSH following TRH administration, has been widely used in psychiatric patients. To date, more than 80 studies, involving more than 2,500 patients, the majority of whom had the diagnosis of major depressive disorder, allow identification of individual patients with TSH blunting, usually defined as a Δ_{max} (i.e., peak minus baseline) TSH response of less than 5.0 or 7.0 μU/ml. Approximately 30 percent of patients had a blunted TSH response during depression (Loosen and Prange, 1982; Loosen, 1986, 1988b; Kirkegaard, 1981), although methodologic issues such as the use of different doses of TRH, the use of different assays, and the lack of controls in some studies make a precise estimate of prevalence uncertain.

TSH blunting also has been demonstrated in some patients with alcoholism,

Table 5.4. *Circadian variation in thyroid function in depression*

Study	n	Diagnosis	Thyroid measure	Comment
Weeke and Weeke (1978)	12	ED	T_4, T_3, FT_4, FT_3, TSH 2 A.M. and midnight	Absence of diurnal TSH variation and free hormones related to symptom severity
Weeke and Weeke (1980)	4	ED	T_3, TSH q1h for 24 hours	No difference from controls
Goldstein et al. (1980)	13 8	ED: 5 BP, UP	TSH q60min/day or q30min/night for 24 hours	Nocturnal TSH peak absent in UP
Kjine et al. (1982)	9	ED	T_4, T_3, TSH q4h	No difference between depression and recovery
Kjellman et al. (1984)	32	MDD	TSH q2h for 24 hours	24h TSH secretion reduced during depression, normalization upon recovery
Unden et al. (1986)	31	MDD	T_4, T_3, TSH q4h, but q2h (midnight–8 A.M.)	TSH reduced in depression. No change in T_3, T_4 between depressed patients and controls
Souetre et al. (1988)	8	BP	TSH q1h for 25 hours, body temperature	Nocturnal body temperature increased and nocturnal TSH surge blunted during depression; both normalized upon recovery
Souetre et al. (1989)	16	ED, 15 recovered	TSH q1h for 25 hours, body temperature	Amplitude reduction during depression significantly correlated with depression scores; normalization of circadian rhythms upon recovery
Bartalena, Placidi, Martino et al. (1990)	15	ED	TSH q1h (midnight–2 A.M.)	Nocturnal TSH surge abolished in 14 patients
Coiro et al. (1994)	7	SAD	TSH q1h (11 P.M.–2 A.M. and 7 A.M.–9 A.M.)	No difference between spring/summer and fall/winter tests. At both periods, patients lacked nocturnal TSH surge.

ED, endogenous depression; MDD, major depressive disorder; UP/BP, unipolar/bipolar depression; SAD, seasonal affective disorder.

Table 5.5 *Subclinical hypothyroidism in affectively ill patients*

Study	n	Diagnosis	Prevalence (%)	Comment
Gold, Pottash, and Extein (1981)	250	Depression and/or anergia	1 (grade 1) 4 (grade 2) 4 (grade 3)	Of the 20 patients with some degree of hypothyroidism, 6 were later discharged after thyroid replacement alone.
Gold, Pottash, and Extein (1982)	100	Depression and/or anergia	15 (grades 1–3)	Of these 15 patients, 60 percent had detectable antimicrosomal antibodies.
Targum et al. (1984)	21	Refractory depression	24 (grade 3)	Five of 7 patients who responded to combined thyroid hormone–antidepressant treatment had grade 3.
Haggerty et al. (1987)	102	Affective disorder	10 (grade 3)	Dexamethasone nonsuppressors were significantly more likely to have elevated TSH levels than suppressors. 20 percent of patients had antithyroid antibodies.
Tappy et al. (1987)	157 104	Psychogeriatric Medical-surgical	4 (grade 1) 2 (grade 1)	There were 157 psychogeriatric and 104 medical-surgical admissions. 15 percent of 27 patients with neurotic depression had grade 1 hypothyroidism.
Joffe and Levitt (1992)	139	Unipolar depression	14 (grade 3)	Depression with grade 3 differed from depression without grade 3 by the presence of a concurrent panic disorder and a poorer antidepressant response.
Gewirtz et al. (1988)	15	Refractory depression	40 (grades 2,3)	The 6 women with hypothyroidism all responded behaviorally to thyroid substitution.

Grade 1, overt hypothyroidism; grade 2, mild hypothyroidism; grade 3, subclinical hypothyroidism.

Table 5.6. *Antithyroid antibodies in affectively ill patients*

Study	n	Diagnosis	Prevalence (%)	Comment
Gold, Portash, and Extein (1982)	100	Depression and/or anergia	9	Of 15 patients with some form of thyroid abnormality, 60 percent had positive antibody titers.
Nemeroff et al. (1985)	45	Affective disorder	20	Each of the 9 patients with symptomless autoimmune thyroiditis had normal baseline serum TSH, T_4, and T_3 uptake, and FT_4I concentrations.
Haggerty et al. (1987)	102	Affective disorder	20	TSH levels were normal in 7 of these patients and elevated in 14. Thyroid antibodies were present in 14 percent of the dexamethasone nonsuppressors and 19 percent of the suppressors.
Haggerty, Evans, Golden et al. (1990)	99	Affective disorder	9	Although the overall frequency of positive antibody titers did not differ in affective and nonaffective disorders, patients with bipolar affective disorder–mixed or bipolar affective disorder–depressed had a higher rate of positive antibody titers than other patients.
	68	Nonaffective disorder	10	
Joffe et al. (1987)	58	Unipolar depression	9	Antimicrosomal and antithyroglobulin antibodies. The presence of detectable antibody titers was not related to abnormal thyroid function tests.

Table 5.7. *Thyroid hormones in cerebrospinal fluid of patients with depression or bipolar illness*

Study	n	Diagnosis	Thyroid measure	Comment
Linnoila et al. (1983)	34 11	MDD BPD	$rT_3 \uparrow$	$rT_3 \uparrow$ in unipolar depression
Kirkegaard and Faber (1991)	12	MDD	$FT_4, FrT_3 \uparrow$	Decrease in both hormones with recovery
Kirkegaard et al. (1979)	15 20	MDD Neurologic disease	TRH $\uparrow$	TRH higher in depressed patients, both before and after recovery, than in neurologic disease
Banki et al. (1988)	14 4 12	MDD Somatization disorder Neurologic disease	TRH $\uparrow$	TRH markedly higher in depressed patients than in the other patient groups
Gjerris et al. (1985)	21 13 8 9	ED Non-ED Mania Schizophrenia	TRH	No significant difference among patient groups
Roy et al (1994)	17	MDD	TRH	No significant difference between patients and controls

MDD, major depressive disorder; BPD, bipolar disorder; ED, endogenous depression.

borderline personality disorder, mania, chronic pain, panic disorder, primary degenerative dementia, and premenstrual syndrome (Loosen, 1986, 1988b). In anorexia nervosa, TSH responses are normal in magnitude, though often delayed in their timing. Such delay may be due to starvation rather than being causally associated with the disease; delayed responses also occur in secondary amenorrhea with simple weight loss, suggesting either hypothalamic dysfunction or altered TSH plasma clearance. Although TSH blunting is not specific for any psychiatric disorder, it does not seem to be the result of mental stress per se. Schizophrenic patients, undoubtedly suffering from severe mental upheaval and "stress," usually do not show TSH blunting, at least not at the level of frequency reported for depression or alcoholism.

Sources of variance

The following factors have been reported to reduce the TRH-induced TSH response: increasing age (in males), being male, acute starvation, chronic renal failure, Klinefelter's syndrome, repetitive administration of TRH, and administration of somatostatin, neurotensin, dopamine, thyroid hormones, and glucocorticoids (Loosen, 1986, 1988b). Most investigators have controlled for these factors. Less well controlled is nutritional state, although profound appetite disturbances often accompany depression.

In depression, such clinical and endocrine factors as the patient's age, height, weight, and body surface; severity of depression; previous intake of antidepressant drugs (i.e., excluding lithium); and increased activity of thyroid hormones, corticosteroids, somatostatin, or dopamine do not appear to be associated with TSH blunting. Nor does the abnormality seem to aid in the distinction between primary and secondary depression, or between unipolar and bipolar subgroups. However, there is preliminary evidence suggesting that a long duration of illness and a history of violent suicidal behavior are associated with TSH blunting. A blunted response during acute illness also seems to point to an increased risk for suicide during follow-up (Loosen, 1986, 1988b), but not all studies agree (Korner, Kierkegaard, and Larsen, 1987).

State-trait considerations

In depression and alcoholism, TSH blunting was observed in both acutely sick and remitted patients (Loosen, 1986, 1988b). In nine studies of remitted depressed patients, 35 percent of 93 patients showed a blunted TSH response (Loosen, 1989). In 43 patients, the rate of normalization of (initially) blunted TSH responses were studied; it ranged from 0 to 71 percent (mean: 32 ± 12; $x \pm SD$).

The data suggest that TSH blunting, when present during depression, may normalize in fewer than half of remitted depressed patients.

Nine studies evaluated the TSH response to TRH during abstinence from ethanol; all but one reported the occurrence of a blunted TSH response to TRH in some patients (Loosen, Sells, Geracioti, Garbutt et al., 1992). In all, 163 patients received TRH; of these, 26 percent showed a blunted TSH response.

The occurrence of TSH blunting in depression and alcoholism deserves special mention. In both conditions, the abnormality was observed during the acute illness and after complete remission, suggesting that it may represent a trait marker, at least in some patients. Whether TSH blunting represents a biologic link that parallels the epidemiologic and genetic similarities between alcoholism and depression (Cloninger, Reich, and Wetzel, 1979; Winokur, 1983) remains to be determined.

Prediction of outcome

Five studies have examined whether the TRH test is useful as a correlate of improvement after treatment with TCAs or ECT, and as a predictor of early relapse after TCA- or ECT-induced remission (Loosen and Prange, 1982; Loosen, 1986, 1988b). The difference in Δ_{max} TSH between the first (initial) and second (posttreatment) testing (i.e., $\Delta\Delta_{max}$ TSH) was used as the endocrine variable. It was shown that (1) a positive trend in $\Delta\Delta_{max}$ TSH (i.e., a Δ_{max} TSH that is bigger on second testing than on first) was correlated with a "good" response to treatment, (2) a persistently low TSH response (i.e., a $\Delta\Delta_{max}$ TSH < 2.0 µU/ml) predicted early relapse, usually within 6 months, and (3) clinical relapse predicted by the TRH test can be prevented by administration of amitriptyline. The outcome data need to be interpreted with caution because different doses of TRH were used and patients were studied with and without continued antidepressant treatment.

The thyrotropin-releasing hormone test and other putative biologic markers

In depression, no clear association between dexamethasone suppression test (DST) abnormalities and TSH blunting has been noted, suggesting that neither abnormality is an (endocrine) epiphenomenon of the other (Kirkegaard, 1981; Loosen and Prange, 1982; Loosen, 1986, 1988b). However, the finding that the corticotropin-releasing hormone (CRH)–induced ACTH response and the TRH-induced TSH response are associated in depressed patients and normal controls suggests that both axes may be regulated, at least in part, by a common mechanism (Holsboer et al., 1985).

When depressed patients were studied with both TRH test and electroencephalograph (EEG) sleep recordings (Rush et al., 1983), 13 (59 percent) of 22 patients were identified by either a reduced rapid eye movement (REM) latency or by a blunted TSH response. All three tests detected 15 patients (68 percent).

Associations between TSH response and measures of serotonergic activity have also been studied. Gold et al. (1977) found a significant negative correlation between TSH response and CSF 5-hydroxyindoleacetic acid (5-HIAA) levels in patients with primary depression. Robertson et al. (1982) reported a significantly reduced uptake of labeled serotonin in blood platelets of euthyroid depressed patients with TSH blunting, as compared to normal controls.

Significance of thyrotropin-stimulating hormone blunting

There is sufficient evidence to posit two preliminary endocrine hypotheses for TSH blunting. The first hypothesis suggests that TSH blunting may be due to chronic hypersecretion of (endogenous) TRH. In this condition, the thyrotroph cells in the anterior pituitary are thought to become hyporesponsive to TRH, possibly because of downregulation of thyrotroph cell TRH receptors. After TRH challenge, these patients would then show TSH blunting. The second hypothesis regards the status of the thyrotroph cells, which may receive increased inhibitory input (the possibility that these cells may be primarily disordered is presently not testable) in patients with TSH blunting. Although, as mentioned earlier, thyroid hormones are unlikely causes of TSH blunting, it is possible that small alterations in the *free* concentration of thyroid hormones are responsible for the TSH response changes reported (Kirkegaard and Faber, 1986).

Triiodothyronine augmentation of antidepressants

There is evidence that a small amount of thyroid hormone accelerates the response to TCA in women and converts TCA nonresponders into responders in both sexes. Augmentation of the therapeutic effect of antidepressants with thyroid hormones appears clinically useful with a variety of antidepressants and, preferably, should utilize T_3 rather than T_4.

Enhancement of treatment response

Delayed onset of action, at times as long as 6 weeks (Prien and Kupfer, 1986), is a significant limiting factor of standard antidepressant therapy. It is thus understandable that means were sought to shorten this delay. Augmentation of TCAs with sleep deprivation (Loosen, Merkel, and Amelung, 1976; Wehr, 1990; Wu and Bunney, 1990; Kuhs and Toelle, 1991), lithium (Garbutt et al., 1986; Joffe, Levitt, Bagby, MacDonald, and Singer, 1993; Stein and Bernadt, 1993), or thyroid hormone (Prange et al., 1969; Goodwin et al., 1982; Joffe and Singer, 1990a; Joffe, Singer, Levitt, and MacDonald, 1993) achieves this goal.

Most (Prange et al., 1969; Wilson et al., 1970; Coppen et al., 1972; Wheathley, 1972), but not all (Feighner et al., 1972; Steiner et al., 1978) studies have shown that when TCAs are given in usual doses and accompanied by as little as 25 μg T_3 per day, the antidepressant effect of the regimen occurs much faster than with TCAs alone. This acceleration of the therapeutic response has been more marked in women than in men. In all six of the above cited double blind, controlled studies patients were euthyroid at the outset and remained euthyroid throughout the course of treatment. T_3 has not increased toxicity; in one study (Coppen et al., 1972) the hormone appeared to reduce toxicity.

Conversion of treatment failures

T_3 augmentation has also been addressed to a related problem – TCA inefficacy. Most (Cavalca, Covezzi, and Boncinelli, 1974; Ogura et al., 1974; Banki, 1975, 1977; Earle, 1979; Tsutsui et al., 1979; Goodwin, Searles, and Tunk, 1982; Hullett and Bidder, 1983; Schwarcz et al., 1984; Targum et al., 1984; Joffe, 1988a, 1988b; Joffe and Singer, 1990a; Browne et al., 1990) but not all (Garbutt et al., 1986; Gitlin et al., 1987; Thase, Kupfer, and Jarrett, 1989) studies have demonstrated that the addition of T_3 will convert TCA nonresponders into responders, even when TCA blood levels are in the therapeutic range (Goodwin, Searles, and Tunk, 1982). The studies have involved a variety of TCAs and other antidepressants in a variety of doses with various amounts of T_3. The conversion rate – therapeutic failure to therapeutic success – is in the order of two thirds; it appears to be about as high in men as in women. Although there are no clear clinical or laboratory indicators that allow separating T_3 responders from nonresponders (Joffe, Levitt, Bagby, MacDonald, and Singer, 1993), several studies found increased TSH responses to TRH in those patients who later responded to T_3 augmentation (Tsutsui et al., 1979; Schwarcz et al., 1984; Gitlin et al., 1987). However, T_3 appears to be significantly more efficacious than T_4 in converting TCA nonresponders into responders (Joffe and Singer, 1990a). The mechanism(s) by which T_3 accelerates the TCA response in pharmacologically naive women and converts TCA failures to success in both sexes are not known.

Part III
THYROID HORMONES AND
BIPOLAR DISORDER

Peripheral thyroid hormones before and during treatment

Several investigators reported increased serum concentrations of T_4 or FT_4I in some acutely ill bipolar adult (Muller and Boning, 1988; Mason et al., 1989; Southwick et al., 1989; Styra et al., 1991) or adolescent (Sokolov, Kutcher, and Joffe, 1994) patients. Other investigators found reduced thyroid hormone concentrations in acutely ill (Rybakowski and Sowinski, 1973; Bartalena, Pellegrini, Meschi et al., 1990) and normal concentrations in euthymic (Kjellman et al., 1985) bipolar patients. In contrast to depression, changes in serum T_4 concentrations are not common during behavioral shifts from mania into depression (Bauer and Whybrow, 1988).

Thyrotropin/subclinical hypothyroidism/antithyroid antibodies

When examining thyroid function in bipolar illness, it is useful to distinguish between rapid-cycling and non-rapid-cycling bipolar disorder. By definition, rapid cyclers experience four or more affective episodes per year (American Psychiatric Association, 1987). Approximately 10–15 percent of bipolar patients experience rapid cycling; although they are similar to other bipolar patients nosologically and demographically, they tend to have a longer duration of illness and a more refractory course (Dunner and Fieve, 1974). Furthermore, women are disproportionately represented, making up 80–95 percent of rapid-cycling patients, compared to about 50 percent of non-rapid-cycling patients (Bauer and Whybrow, 1988). A variety of factors may predispose bipolar illness to a rapid-cycling course, including treatment with TCAs, monoamine oxidase inhibitors (MAOIs), lithium, and antipsychotics (Wehr et al., 1988). To these factors we can now add comorbid hypothyroidism.

In recent years, investigators have increasingly focused on the associations of various states of hypothyroidism with bipolar illness. Wehr and Goodwin (1979) first reported that TCAs induced rapid cycling in 5 female bipolar patients; 3 had a history of thyroid disorder. Cho et al. (1979) demonstrated that 6 percent of lithium-treated women developed hypothyroidism; most (71 percent) were rapid cyclers. They also noted that significantly more rapid-cycling women (31 percent) than non-rapid-cycling women (2 percent) were on postlithium thyroid medication. Cowdry et al. (1983), conducting a retrospective chart review, found evidence of hypothyroidism in half of the 24 rapid-cycling patients and in none of the 19 non-rapid-cycling patients. Moreover, 42 percent of the rapid cyclers and 32 percent of the nonrapid cyclers presented with subclinical hypothyroidism, resulting in an overall prevalence of some variety of hypothyroidism totaling 92 percent in rapid cyclers compared with 32 percent in nonrapid cyclers. Bauer, Whybrow, and Winokur (1990) reported that 23 percent of 30 patients with rapid-cycling bipolar disorder had grade I hypothyroidism, whereas 27 percent had grade II and 10 percent had grade III abnormalities. Other investigators confirmed the high prevalence of hypothyroidism of some sort in bipolar illness, but found similar rates in rapid-cycling and non-rapid-cycling patients (Joffe, Kutcher, and MacDonald, 1988; Wehr et al., 1988; Bartalena, Pellegrini, Meschi et al., 1990). Instead they demonstrated that spontaneous or lithium-induced hypothyroidism was associated with female sex (Joffe, Kutcher, and MacDonald, 1988) or duration of lithium treatment (Joffe, Kutcher, and MacDonald, 1988; Bartalena, Pellegrini, Meschi et al., 1990).

If hypothyroidism during bipolar illness predisposes to a rapid-cycling course, what are the effects of treatment with thyroid hormones? O'Shanick and Ellinwood (1982) first suggested that such treatment may be beneficial. In the most extensive study to date, Bauer, Whybrow, and Winokur (1990) entered 11 rapid-cycling bipolar patients whose symptoms were refractory to their current treatment into an open trial of high-dose T_4. T_4 was added to the baseline medication regimen, and the dosage was increased until clinical response occurred or until side effects precluded further increase. When the patients received T_4, their depressive and manic symptoms decreased significantly compared with baseline. Improvement was due to response of depressive symptoms in 10 of 11 patients, with manic symptoms responding in 5 of the 7 patients who exhibited them at baseline. Four patients then underwent single or double blind placebo substitution; 3 relapsed into either depression or rapid cycling. Treatment response did not depend on thyroid status at intake. In 9 of 10 responsive patients, supranormal levels of serum free T_4 were necessary to induce clinical response; however, side effects were minimal, and there were no signs of T_4-induced hypermetabolism. Baumgartner, Bauer, and Hellweg (1994) treated 6 patients with severe forms of non-rapid-cycling bipolar disorder whose symptoms had previously been refractory to all current antidepressant and/or prophylactic medications with supraphysiologic doses of T_4 (250–500 μg/day) as "art adjuvant" to their previous medications for an average of 28 months. The mean number of relapses declined, and the mean duration of hospitalizations shortened significantly during follow-up. Three patients had no further relapses at all. The side effects were negligible. However, Cowdry et al. (1983) noted that efforts to treat rapid cycling with thyroid hormones have met with inconsistent results.

Part IV
CONCLUSIONS

There are many associations between thyroid hormones and behavior in regard to both clinical relevance and gender specificity. It is noteworthy that, with the possible exception of the profound effects of thyroid hormone deficiency on the developing brain, the exact nature of these associations remains unknown.

Clinical relevance

Disturbances in thyroid function have more to do with affective state than with any other aspect of mentation, except possibly cognition. *First,* thyroid hormone deficiency during infancy (i.e., infantile hypothyroidism), if not corrected within the first 3 months of life, will inevitably result in mental retardation and specific motor and sensory dysfunctions. Because thyroid hormones are vital for normal brain development and maturation, infants are now routinely checked for congenital hypothyroidism and immediately substituted, if necessary. *Second,* depression and cognitive decline are the most frequently observed psychiatric symptoms in patients suffering from adult hypothyroidism. *Third,* a small dose of thyroid hormone, preferably T_3, will accelerate the therapeutic effect of various antidepressants in women, and convert antidepressant nonresponders into responders in both sexes. *Fourth,* administration of TRH may induce an increased sense of well-being and relaxation in normal subjects and patients with neurologic and psychiatric disease, including depression (Prange et al., 1969; Prange, Nemeroff, and Loosen, 1978; Prange, Loosen, and Nemeroff, 1979; Loosen and Prange, 1984; Loosen, 1986). *Fifth,* most longitudinal studies have revealed intriguing dynamic reductions in serum T_4 concentrations in depressed patients during a wide range of somatic treatments, including various antidepressants, lithium, sleep deprivation, and ECT. There is also evidence that the T_4 reduction was greater in treatment responders than in nonresponders. However, despite their consistency, the data need to be viewed with caution. Some acutely ill psychiatric patients with diagnoses other than depression show transient hyperthyroxinemia during acute hospitalization, suggesting that the finding is disease nonspecific, and T_4 levels normally quickly decline even if there is no therapeutic intervention or behavioral change. Moreover, most studies have included only a small number of patients and, more important, did not control for independent effects of such drugs as carbamazepine or lithium on depression and on peripheral thyroid hormone metabolism. There is a clear need for longitudinal studies, ideally without treatment or at least with delayed treatment. *Sixth,* although overt thyroid disease is rare in major depression, more subtle forms of thyroid dysfunction are common. Studies most consistently point to three abnormalities: (1) absence or flattening of the diurnal TSH curve, often caused by a reduction in the nocturnal TSH surge; (2) a blunted TSH response after administration of TRH; and (3) subclinical hypothyroidism and/or positive antithyroid antibodies (subclinical hypothyroidism and positive antibody titers are often seen together in the same patient). Are these findings clinically relevant? We don't know in the case of abnormal diurnal TSH secretion or positive antibody titers (without the clinical picture of subclinical hypothyroidism). However, although the diagnostic utility of the TRH test appears to be compromised due to disease nonspecificity and low sensitivity (Loosen, Garbutt, and Prange Jr., 1987), TSH blunting has shown promising clinical utility in predicting outcome to standard antidepressant treatment and in assessing the risk for violent suicide attempts (though both need replication in larger samples). The possible medical and psychiatric consequences of subclinical hypothyroidism are still a matter of intense debate. Medically, it is not known whether patients with subclinical hypothyroidism are at the same risk for developing cardiovascular disease as are patients with overt hypothyroidism (Ross, 1991). Although there is no uniform improvement in cardiac contractility, a subgroup of patients with prolonged systolic time intervals had reductions to normal values during therapy, and left ventricular function during maximal exercise improved (Cooper et al., 1984). The controversy regarding serum lipid levels is also unsettled. It can be argued that subclinical hypothyroidism carries no significant biologic disadvantage for most and treatment is not without risk of exacerbating ischemic heart disease in older women, who are largely those affected (Tunbridge and Caldwell, 1991). In practice, however, many physicians who identify subclinical hypothyroidism in a patient initiate T_4 replacement therapy (Tunbridge and Caldwell, 1991). The major benefits of treatment, based on two randomized trials, appear to be improvements in clinical symptoms and psychometric test results (Ross, 1991). Psychiatrically, comorbid subclinical hypothyroidism appears to negatively affect the clinical course of depression. *Seventh,* bipolar disorders are often associated with various forms of hypothyroidism, including subclinical hypothyroidism. As in depression, such comorbidity seems to negatively affect the course of the illness (by predisposing the individual patient to a rapid-cycling course). As in depression, substitution with T_4 has proven useful in some patients, but often high doses are necessary to induce clinical response. Conceptually, these findings have led to the hypothesis that a relative central thyroid hormone deficit may predispose to the marked and frequent mood swings that characterize rapid-cycling bipolar disorder. However, as noted by Bauer, Whybrow, and Winokur (1990), there are several confounding issues in studies involving rapid cycling and thyroid function. First, because of their more severe course, rapid-cycling patients are more likely to have received thyroid hormone treatment and may then be erroneously classified as hypothyroid in retrospective studies. Second, the female preponderance in rapid-cycling bipolar disorder may elevate the rate of hypothyroidism, because both disorders are more common in women. Last, the use of lithium and carbamazepine, known goiterogens, is not examined in some studies. Here we also may add that it remains to be determined whether such a central thyroid hormone deficit serves only as a risk factor for the development of rapid cycling in a known bipolar patient, or whether it can predispose most affectively ill patients to any major behavioral change (i.e., the switch from depression into recovery or from depression into mania).

Gender specificity

Thyroid function is similar in *normal* women and men (Gambert, 1991). Although TBG concentrations are slightly higher and TBPA concentrations are slightly lower in women than in men, serum total and free T_4 and T_3 concentrations are similar, as are serum TSH concentrations and T_3-uptake values. However, sex differences have been reported in the TRH-induced TSH response, with young and middle-aged women having slightly greater responses than men of similar age. There are also variations in TSH response during the menstrual cycle: TSH release is greater in the preovulatory phase, and the postovulatory phase response is similar to the response in men (Gambert, 1991). Estrogens do acutely inhibit the rate of hormone release from the thyroid in adults, but any effect appears transient because both men and women taking chronic estrogen therapy have normal serum free T_4, free T_3, and TSH levels (Gambert, 1991).

Whereas thyroid function appears similar in normal women and men, there are marked gender differences in the prevalence of established thyroid gland pathology (Table 5.8). Adult hypothyroidism, subclinical hypothyroidism, primary hyperthyroidism (Graves' disease), sporadic endemic goiter, and comorbid and subclinical hypothyroidism (in depression and bipolar disorder) are all seen with much greater frequency in women than in men. Furthermore, a small amount of T_3 will accelerate the therapeutic effect of various antidepressants, and this effect is more pronounced in women than in men. However, infantile hypothyroidism, if not corrected timely, will inevitably result in mental retardation in both sexes.

Table 5.8. *Thyroid function and gender*

Clinical syndrome	Behavioral findings/significance	Gender effect
Thyroid disease		
Infantile hypothyroidism	Mental retardation, cretinism, specific motor and sensory dysfunctions	No
Adult hypothyroidism	Depression, cognitive decline, mental slowing, lethargy	Yes (F » M)
Subclinical hypothyroidism	Unknown	Yes (F » M)
Primary hyperthyroidism (Graves' disease)	Agitation, increased anxiety, cognitive decline, irritability	Yes (F » M)
Simple goiter	Unknown	Yes (F » M)
Thyroid function in depression		
Serum T_4[a] elevation at intake	May facilitate treatment response	Unknown
Dynamic T_4 change during treatment	Change greater in responders than non-responders	Unknown
TSH blunting	May predict treatment outcome and identify patients at risk for violent suicide	No
Subclinical hypothyroidism	May negatively affect outcome	Yes (F » M)
T_3[b] augmentation of TCA[c]	T_3 accelerates the response to TCA	Yes (F » M)
	T_3 converts TCA nonresponders into responders	No
Thyroid function in rapid-cycling bipolar disorder		
Subclinical hypothyroidism	Likely to affect course and outcome by predisposing to rapid cycling	Yes (F » M)

[a] Thyroxine.

[b] Triiodothyronine.

[c] Tricyclic antidepressants.

F = female; M = male; » = much greater than.

Data from the Wickham Survey indicated a prevalence of established hyperthyroidism of about 2 percent in women, and the established incidence was about 3 cases per 1,000 women annually. The prevalence of established hyperthyroidism was 10 times more common in women than in men (Tunbridge and Caldwell, 1991). The prevalence of established, spontaneous hypothyroidism was 10 per 1,000 women, rising to 15 per 1,000 women when the possible but unproven cases were included (Tunbridge and Caldwell, 1991). Numerous people, particularly older women, have asymptomatic autoimmune thyroiditis on the evidence of thyroid antibodies, with normal thyroid function. In the Wickham Survey, the prevalence of high levels of thyroglobulin antibodies was 4.6 percent in women and 1.1 percent in men. The prevalence of serum TSH elevations in the absence of overt hypothyroidism was 7.5 percent in women and 2.8 percent in men (Tunbridge and Caldwell, 1991). Three percent of the sample (5 percent of women and 1 percent of men) were found to have both thyroid antibodies and high TSH levels. Mean TSH levels were significantly higher in both men and women with antibodies than in those without. When the age and sex distributions of TSH were examined, no significant variation was found in men, but there was a marked rise in TSH in women over age 40 (in women over age 75, the prevalence of subclinical hypothyroidism was 17.4 percent); this rise was almost abolished when women with any marker of thyroid disease, particularly thyroid antibodies, were excluded (Tunbridge and Caldwell, 1991). There is general agreement that the prevalence of endemic sporadic goiter is also increased in women, showing a female:male ratio of at least 4:1 (Tunbridge and Caldwell, 1991). However, the age distribution of "simple" goiter contrasts noticeably with the age distribution of both thyroid antibodies and TSH. Whereas frequency of positive thyroid antibody titers and concentrations of serum TSH increase sharply after age 30 or 40 in women, "simple" goiter is most frequent before the age of 40, declining sharply thereafter (Tunbridge and Caldwell, 1991).

To conclude, thyroid pathology is much more common in women than in men (Table 5.8). Adult hypothyroidism, subclinical hypothyroidism, primary hyperthyroidism (Graves' disease), sporadic endemic goiter, and comorbid hypothyroidism and subclinical hypothyroidism (in depression and bipolar disorder) are all seen with much greater frequency in women than in men. Furthermore, a small amount of T_3 will accelerate the therapeutic effect of various antidepressants, and this effect is more pronounced in women than in men. However, infantile hypothyroidism, if not timely corrected, will inevitably result in mental retardation in both sexes.

CHAPTER SIX

THE HYPOTHALAMIC-PITUITARY-ADRENOCORTICAL SYSTEM

DOMINIQUE L. MUSSELMAN,

GAIL ANDERSON,

MARYFRANCES R. PORTER, AND

CHARLES B. NEMEROFF

Introduction

The hypothalamic-pituitary-adrenal (HPA) axis has undoubtedly received more psychobiologic scrutiny than any other endocrine axis. Historically, one rationale for the intensive study of adrenocortical function in patients with primary psychiatric disorders was the observation that patients with primary endocrine disorders such as Addison's disease (Fava, Sonino, and Murphy, 1987; Lobo et al., 1988) or Cushing's syndrome (Loosen, Chambliss, DeBold, Shelton, Orth et al., 1992; Kling et al., 1993) exhibited a higher than expected psychiatric morbidity. This led to the so-called neuroendocrine window strategy based on a large literature which indicates that the secretion of the target endocrine organs, for example, the adrenal or thyroid, is largely controlled by their respective pituitary trophic hormones. The pituitary tropic hormones, in turn, are controlled primarily by the secretion of their respective hypothalamic release and/or release-inhibiting hormones. There is now considerable evidence that the secretion of these hypothalamic hypophysiotropic hormones is controlled by serotonin, acetylcholine, and norepinephrine, neurotransmitters previously posited to play a preeminent role in the pathophysiology of affective and/or anxiety disorders. This neuroendocrine window strategy remains an impetus for continuing investigation of the major endocrine axes in psychiatric disorders. However, the hypothesis that information about higher central nervous system (CNS) neuronal activity, such as the activity of serotonergic neurons in a particular disease state, may be inferred solely by measuring the activity of a specific endocrine axis is far from proven and is fraught with problems. It is unclear if alterations in peripheral adrenal hormone secretion or altered secretion of pituitary and hypothalamic hormones primarily contribute to the pathogenesis of depression. What the neuroendocrine window strategy has provided, however, is clear evidence for alterations in the activity of the HPA axis in depression and an appreciation of the complexity of the regulation of its activity in women and in men. This chapter briefly reviews the major findings concerning altered HPA-axis activity in unipolar depression, the relationship between HPA-axis and ovarian physiology, HPA-axis morphology in depression, and implications for future research.

Pathophysiology of the HPA axis in major depression and other affective disorders

The most intensive scrutiny of the HPA axis have been conducted in patients with major depression. Corticotropin-releasing factor (CRF), composed of 41 amino acids, is released from the hypothalamus and is the major physiologic mediator of the secretion of adrenocorticotropic hormone (ACTH) and β-endorphin from the anterior pituitary (Vale et al., 1981). Neurons containing CRF project from the hypothalamic paraventricular nucleus to the median eminence (Swanson et al., 1983). Activation of this circuit occurs in response to stress, resulting in an increase in synthesis and release of ACTH, β-endorphin, and other pro-opiomelanocortin (POMC) products. As discussed later, numerous reports document HPA-axis hyperactivity in drug-free patients with major depression, including CNS (i.e., CRF), pituitary (i.e., ACTH), and adrenal (i.e., glucocorticoid) involvement. CRF neurons, both hypothalamic and extrahypothalamic, coordinate the endocrine, behavioral, autonomic, and immune responses to stress.

Evidence for the involvement of CRF in the pathophysiology of depression includes elevated CRF concentrations in cerebrospinal fluid (CSF), which has been documented in multiple studies of drug-free patients with major depression (Nemeroff et al., 1984; Arato et al., 1986; Banki et al., 1987; France et al., 1988; Banki et al., 1992; Risch et al., 1992) as well as in suicide victims (Arato et al., 1989), with the exception of Roy and colleagues, 1987, who found no such relationship. In that study, however, dexamethasone test (DST) nonsuppressors had higher CSF CRF concentrations than DST suppressors. Elevations of CRF concentrations in CSF are believed to be due to central CRF hypersecretion (Post et al., 1982). Reductions in CSF CRF concentrations have been observed following administration of desipramine, a tricyclic antidepressant, in healthy, nondepressed volunteers (Veith et al., 1992) and following treatment of depressed patients with ECT (Nemeroff et al., 1991) or with fluoxetine, a selective serotonin reuptake inhibitor (DeBellis et al., 1993). Thus, CSF CRF concentrations are elevated in major depression, normalize after treatment with antidepressants or ECT in depressed patients, and are reduced by desipramine in normal controls.

There are several methods for assessing the HPA-axis activity, which are outlined later. One particularly sensitive method to assess the activity of the HPA axis is the CRF stimulation test. CRF is administered intravenously (usually in a dose of 1 μg/kg or a fixed 100-μg bolus), and the subsequent ACTH (or β-lipotropin [LPH]/β-endorphin) and cortisol response is measured over a 2- to 3-hour period (Hermus et al., 1984; Watson et al., 1986). In drug-free depressed patients, the ACTH and β-endorphin response to exogenously administered ovine CRF (oCRF) is attenuated compared with that of normal comparison subjects (Gold et al., 1984; Holsboer et al., 1984; Gold et al., 1986; Amsterdam et al., 1988; Kathol et al., 1989; Young et al., 1990). The blunted ACTH response to CRF occurs in depressed DST nonsuppressors but not in DST suppressors (Krishnan et al., 1993). The diminished ACTH response to CRF is likely, at least in part, due to chronic hypersecretion of CRF from the median eminence resulting in downregulation of adenohypophyseal CRF receptor number and decreased pituitary responsivity to CRF, as has previously been demonstrated in laboratory animals (Wynn et al., 1983; Wynn et al., 1984; Aguilera et al., 1986; Holmes, Catt, and Aguilera, 1987; Wynn et al., 1988). Further evidence for hyperactivity of hypothalamic CRF neurons in depression has been provided by Raadsheer et al. (1994, 1995) who reported that postmortem tissue of depressed patients exhibits a fourfold increase in the numbers of CRF-containing paraventricular hypothalamic neurons as well as a marked increase in CRF mRNA expression, as assessed by in situ hybridization. Moreover, decreased CRF receptor numbers in the frontal cortex have been reported in postmortem tissue of suicide victims (Nemeroff et al., 1988), likely due to CRF receptor downregulation secondary to CRF hypersecretion.

The majority of the work in HPA-axis activity in depression has used measures of cortisol hypersecretion, for example, elevated plasma corticosteroid concentrations (Gibbons and McHugh, 1962; Carpenter and Bunney, 1971), and increased levels of cortisol metabolites (Sachar et al., 1970). Elevated 24-hour urinary free cortisol concentrations and nonsuppression of plasma hydroxycorticosteroid levels after the administration of dexamethasone (using the DST) have also been utilized. In the standard DST paradigm, patients ingest 1 mg of dexamethasone, a synthetic glucocorticoid, by mouth at 11 p.m. Blood samples, which were originally utilized to confirm screening measures of hypercortisolemia, are obtained at 4 p.m. and 11 p.m. the following day to measure plasma cortisol concentrations. One half to two thirds of depressed patients exhibit dexamethasone nonsuppression (plasma cortisol concentrations ≥ 5 ng/ml) whereas healthy, nonobese patients will almost always suppress plasma cortisol concentrations to <5 ng/ml (Schukit, 1988).

Since the initial study by Carroll (1968), the DST has generated remarkable controversy (Arana and Mossman, 1988) regarding its diagnostic utility (Carroll, 1982). The rate of cortisol nonsuppression after dexamethasone administration generally has been found to be correlated with the severity of depression; for example, almost all patients with psychotic depression exhibit DST nonsuppression (Evans and Nemeroff, 1983b; Schatzberg et al., 1984; Arana, Baldessarini, and Orsteen, 1985; Krishnan et al., 1985). Hyperactivity of the HPA axis also occurs in patients with bipolar disorder (Kiriike et al., 1988; Stokes and Sikes, 1987), particularly in mixed states (Evans and Nemeroff, 1983a; Krishnan, Maltbie, and Davidson, 1983; Swann et al., 1992), and in rapid-cycling patients (Godwin, Greenberg, and Shulka, 1984; Kennedy et al., 1989). Furthermore, DST nonsuppressors also have higher CSF CRF concentrations than DST suppressors (Roy et al., 1987; Pitts et al., 1995) (Table 6.1).

HPA-axis activity, including the DST, usually normalizes after recovery from

Table 6.1. *Alterations in the activity of the hypothalamic-pituitary-adrenal axis in major depression*

- Increased corticotropin-releasing factor (CRF) concentrations in cerebrospinal fluid
- Blunted adrenocorticotropic hormone (ACTH) and β-endorphin responses after intravenous CRF administration
- Increased density of CRF receptors in frontal cortex of suicide victims
- Pituitary gland enlargement
- Adrenal gland enlargement in major depression and in suicide victims
- Increased cortisol production, hypercortisolemia, and cerebrospinal fluid cortisol concentrations
- Increased plasma glucocorticoid, ACTH, and β-endorphin nonsuppression after dexamethasone administration
- Increased urinary free cortisol concentrations
- Increased 5-hydroxytryptophan-induced cortisol secretion
- Increased ACTH-induced cortisol secretion
- Increased ACTH and cortisol responses to CRF despite dexamethasone pretreatment

depression (Carroll, 1968; Nemeroff, and Evans, 1984), and such normalization may be the harbinger of early relapse or poor prognosis (Arana et al., 1985) as do persistently elevated CSF CRF concentrations (Banki et al., 1992). Increased incidence of DST nonsuppression in depressed patients may, in part, be due to the more rapid metabolism of dexamethasone that occurs in depressed patients (Ritchie et al., 1990). Therefore, the well-documented HPA-axis hyperactivity in depressed patients may be explained by hypersecretion of CRF and secondary pituitary and adrenal gland hypertrophy, although impaired negative feedback of glucocorticoids at various CNS sites and the pituitary also likely contributes. DST nonsuppression, like hypercortisolemia (Sachar et al., 1970), hypersecretion of CRF (Nemeroff et al., 1991; DeBellis et al., 1993), blunting of the ACTH response to CRF (Amsterdam et al., 1988), and adrenal gland hypertrophy (Rubin et al., 1995), all appear, in fact, to be state dependent.

Treatment with glucocorticoid agonists and antagonists

Cushing's syndrome, due to prolonged exposure to excessive cortisol or other related glucocorticoids, is accompanied by psychiatric symptoms of anxiety and/or depression that generally remit with diminution of abnormal glucocorticoid concentrations. Thus, agents that reduce adrenal steroid availability have recently undergone investigation in the treatment of unipolar depression. Metapyrone, an inhibitor of the 11-hydroxylation reaction of steroid synthesis, not only reduces cortisol and corticosterone production but alleviates depression in patients whose symptoms were unresponsive to antidepressant treatment (Murphy et al., 1991). Ketoconazole, an imidazole antifungal drug, also inhibits cortisol synthesis and is a potent glucocorticoid receptor antagonist as well. Hypercortisolemic depressed patients administered ketoconazole experience significant alleviation of their depression in association with lowered serum cortisol concentrations (Wolkowitz et al., 1993). Conversely, depressed patients treated with dexamethasone also experience improvement of their depression (Arana et al., 1994), an effect likely due to a reduction in CRF synthesis and release. Clearly, further studies with glucocorticoid agonists and antagonists are warranted.

Investigations of the hypothalamic-pituitary-gonadal axis in depression

Despite the higher incidence of depression in women than men and the purportedly increased occurrence of depression during and after menopause, the hypothalamic-pituitary-gonadal (HPG) axis has received relatively little scrutiny in patients with mood disorders. As with the HPA axis, the HPG axis is organized in a "hierarchical" fashion. Driven by a "pulse generator" in the arcuate nucleus of the hypothalamus, gonadotropin-releasing hormone (GnRH) secretion occurs in a pulsatile fashion (Knobil, 1990). GnRH causes secretion of luteinizing hormone (LH) and follicle-stimulating hormone (FSH) from gonadotrophs in the anterior pituitary (Midgely and Jaffee, 1971). The ebb and flow of LH concentration in the peripheral circulation is used as an indication of pulses of GnRH secretion (Clarke and Cummins, 1982). In the follicular phase of the menstrual cycle, LH pulses of nearly constant amplitude occur with regular frequency (every 1–2 hours) (Reame et al., 1984). In the luteal phase, LH pulse amplitude (reflecting GnRH secretion) is more variable, with pulse frequency declining to one pulse every 2–6 hours (Jaffe et al., 1990). Through negative feedback, gonadal steroids inhibit the secretion of GnRH from the hypothalamus as well as the secretion of LH and FSH from the pituitary. GnRH secretion is also inhibited by CRF (Jaffe et al., 1990) and β-endorphin (Ferin and Vande-Wiele, 1987).

Sachar and colleagues (1972) measured the plasma concentrations of LH and FSH in depressed postmenopausal women. No significant change in the concentrations of either hormone were observed in 8 postmenopausal women before or after recovery from depression. Moreover, the plasma concentrations of LH or FSH did not differ between these depressed women and a comparison group of nondepressed postmenopausal women (n = 24). However, a group of postmenopausal women suffering recurrent endogeneous depressions (n = 9) exhibited lower LH plasma concentrations than postmenopausal women without depression or postmenopausal women diagnosed before or after a single depressive episode (n = 10).

Rather than measure baseline plasma levels of the pituitary gonadotrophins in depressed patients, other investigators have studied the gonadotropin response to the administered GnRH. Winokur and colleagues (1982) found normal LH and FSH responses to a high dose (250 μg) of GnRH in male and female depressed (pre- and postmenopausal) patients. The sample size was not large enough to analyze baseline LH levels or the response to GnRH stimulation separately for men and pre- and postmenopausal women. Using a lower dose of GnRH (150 μg), Brambilla and colleagues (1990) reported a decreased LH response to GnRH in 15 premenopausal and 32 postmenopausal depressed women. Lower baseline LH concentrations (4 samples obtained over 60 minutes) were observed in the postmenopausal depressed women than in their matched controls. In a depressed cohort including both sexes, Unden et al.

(1988) observed no change in baseline or TRH/GnRH-stimulated (combined 200 μg thyroxin-releasing hormone [TRH] and 100 μg GnRH intravenously) LH or FSH concentrations (analyses of men and pre- and postmenopausal women were not separately performed). Considerable additional research of the HPG axis in depression with greater numbers of subjects of different ages is clearly warranted, including CSF GnRH measures, gonadotropin-induced gonadal steroid secretion, and other measures.

Influence of gonadal steroids upon the HPA axis and age-related changes

Of paramount importance are the increasing data concerning the influence of estrogens (estradiol, estrone, and estradiol) and progesterone upon regulation of the HPA axis. As discussed in Chapters One and Two, estrogen is crucial for the development of female secondary reproductive characteristics, and progestogen is vital in the preparation of the endometrium for maintenance of pregnancy. This section briefly reviews the influence of ovarian gonadal steroids upon the HPA axis, aging of the HPA axis in women, and HPA dysregulation in depressed women.

The biologic activity of any drug or hormone, including cortisol and gonadal steroids, depends upon its circulating concentrations, particularly the fraction that is not bound to carrier proteins and is therefore "free" to interact with its receptor. In addition to their effects upon maintenance of vaginal, uterine, and breast tissue, estrogens have multiple systemic effects, including stimulating the production of proteins by the liver. Indeed, as estrogen concentrations slowly rise during the follicular phase of the menstrual cycle, so do the levels of a hepatic-synthesized carrier protein, corticosteroid-binding globulin (CBG), an α_2 globulin. During the usual 9 months of a human pregnancy, plasma levels of CBG rise, likely stimulated by increased concentrations of circulating estrogens. CBG binds cortisol and thus spuriously raises total cortisol levels in maternal circulation while minimally changing the fraction of unbound cortisol. Estrogens may provide a buffer from stress-induced HPA activity by their stimulation of CBG production, thereby diminishing any acute elevations in unbound cortisol. It is also important to note that the CRF is manufactured in very large quantities by the placenta; a CRF-binding protein prevents very much of an increase in "free" CRF plasma concentrations.

Like estrogens, circulating progesterone is mostly (>90%) bound to the carrier proteins albumin and CBG. In fact, progesterone binds to CBG with an affinity equal to that of glucocorticoids. Progesterone is generally present in much lower concentrations in plasma than is cortisol. However, during the menstrual luteal phase, the concentration of progesterone is greatest (20–25 ng/ml), similar to that of basal diurnal levels of cortisol. At the morning height of cortisol secretion, however, CBG is saturated with cortisol. At such times, progesterone's competition for CBG may subsequently increase concentrations of free cortisol. During pregnancy, characterized by high progesterone levels, it is well known that concentrations of *both* cortisol and CBG are elevated (Carr et al., 1981; Nolten and Rueckert, 1981; Demey-Ponsart et al., 1982). Postpartum progesterone levels fall precipitously, which has been posited to play a role in the development of postpartum depression.

Preclinical studies have determined that, in addition to competing with cortisol for CBG, progesterone binds to and enhances the dissociation of corticosteroids from Type II glucocorticoid receptors (Rousseau, Baxter, and Tomkins, 1972; Suthers, Presley, and Funder, 1976; Svec, 1988), the low-affinity and high-capacity receptors for endogenous glucocorticoids. Furthermore, progesterone demonstrates a significant affinity for the human Type I glucocorticoid (mineralocorticoid-preferring) receptor (Arriza et al., 1987), the high-affinity and low-capacity receptor for endogeneous glucocorticoids. Indeed, progesterone administration has been shown to contribute to the restoration of Type II glucocorticoid receptor reactivity throughout the hippocampus of the female, but not male rat (Ahima et al., 1992). The hippocampus, an integral part of the limbic system, contains a high concentration of both Type I and II corticosteroid receptors, and is well documented to exert an inhibitory influence upon HPA-axis activity (Jacobson and Sapolsky, 1991). Progesterone's competition with corticosterone for glucocorticoid receptors might explain the greater numbers of glucocorticoid receptors within the hippocampus of female rats in comparison to male rats (Turner and Weaver, 1985). Taken together, these observations suggest that estrogen and progesterone exert important actions on certain elements of the HPA axis in women, possibly functioning as a buffer against elevated circulating glucocorticoids, as occur during episodes of major depression.

Evidence for age-related changes in the HPA axis has been reported in animal (Sapolsky, Krey, and McEwen, 1983, 1986; Heroux, Grigoriades, and DeSouza, 1991; Tizabi, Aguilera, and Gilad, 1992) and in human (Halbreich et al., 1984; Pavlov et al., 1986; Heuser et al., 1991) studies. However, most aspects of adrenocortical regulation appear intact in aged humans. Although age is most frequently positively correlated with hyperactivity of the HPA axis in patients with depression or Alzheimer's disease (Jacobson and Sapolsky, 1991), aging in women is not accompanied by increased baseline plasma cortisol concentrations. With menopause, however, comes the loss of the modulatory effects of estrogen and progesterone upon the HPA axis. Depressed postmenopausal women might not experience modulation of depression-induced increases in cortisol secretion as would premenopausal women with higher levels of CBG. The hypothesized beneficial effects of the glucocorticoid antagonist progesterone would also theoretically be diminished in postmenopausal women. In general, depressed women do not exhibit higher rates of β-LPH/β-endorphin or cortisol nonsuppression after dexamethasone administration than do depressed men (Young et al., 1993). However, dexamethasone nonsuppression is indeed more common in postmenopausal women when compared to premenopausal women (Young, 1995).

To determine the antagonistic effects of progesterone upon HPA-axis activity, Young (1995) studied eight premenopausal women and eight age-matched men who were without psychiatric disorders. The effect of an infusion of cortisol (5 μg/kg/minute for 1 hour) or β-LPH/β-endorphin secretion was examined. The β-LPH/β-endorphin responses of the women with increased progesterone concentrations (>5.00 ng/ml) were compared to those of the women with low progesterone concentrations (<1.00 ng/ml). Although estradiol concentrations were similar in both groups of women, the women with low plasma progesterone levels (in the follicular phase) exhibited suppressed β-LPH/β-endorphin plasma concentrations identical to the male controls following cortisol infusion. However, the women with high progesterone plasma levels (in the luteal phase) exhibited a *rebound* increase of β-LPH/β-endorphin concentrations in the second hour after cortisol infusion in comparison to the men. Thus, the increased concentration of progesterone in the luteal phase appears to antagonize the inhibitory effects of cortisol upon the HPA axis in women.

In addition, Young (1995) examined the effects of gender and depression upon morning cortisol plasma concentrations. Morning cortisol concentrations were measured in depressed premenopausal women (n = 8), depressed men (n = 8), and their age- and gender-matched controls (the mean age of patients and controls was identical, 32.5 years). Only the depressed premenopausal women exhibited elevated plasma concentrations of cortisol. The adrenocortical hyperactivity observed in the premenopausal depressed women might be at least partly due to their higher levels of CBG, resulting in lower free cortisol concentrations. Such diminished concentrations of free cortisol probably results in the increased β-endorphin secretion in depressed women following administration of metapyrone, an inhibitor of cortisol synthesis (Young, 1995).

Furthermore, to examine whether the *absence* of ovarian steroids might affect HPA-axis hyperactivity, Young (1995) measured baseline levels of cortisol in premenopausal (n = 38) and postmenopausal (n = 14) depressed women prior to a DST. Adenohypophyseal (e.g., β-LPH/β-endorphin) and adrenocortical (e.g., cortisol) secretion were subsequently measured. Only the premenopausal women who exhibited nonsuppression of β-LPH/β-endorphin exhibited elevated cortisol concentrations at baseline in comparison to those premenopausal women who were cortisol suppressors. Basal cortisol concentrations were similar in the postmenopausal women who were β-LPH/β-endorphin nonsuppressors and suppressors, respectively. Increased basal cortisol concentrations appear necessary for DST nonsuppression in premenopausal depressed women. The premenopausal β-LPH/β-endorphin nonsuppressors did *not* exhibit significantly increased baseline cortisol levels in comparison to the postmenopausal β-LPH/β-endorphin nonsuppressors (10.5 vs. 9.8 ng/ml). However, as CBG is saturated at concentrations of cortisol greater than 10 ng/ml, the cortisol levels in the premenopausal β-LPH/β-endorphin nonsuppressors may be much greater than was assayed. Considering the loss of the protective effects of increased levels of CBG and the antiglucocorticoid effects of progesterone, depressed postmenopausal women most likely exhibit higher rates of dexamethasone nonsuppression due to the resulting lower baseline concentrations of cortisol than premenopausal women who are dexamethasone nonsuppressors.

Pituitary and adrenal imaging studies in affective disorders

Although the data regarding sex differences are still accumulating, structural changes in the various components of the HPA axis (e.g., the pituitary and adrenal gland) have been reported in depressed patients. Other morphologic and functional brain imaging alterations in patients with affective disorders are discussed by Drs. Casper and Marsh in Chapter Four.

Depressed patients exhibit pituitary gland enlargement on magnetic resonance imaging (MRI) (Krishnan et al., 1991). To assess if this and other alterations in HPA axis *morphology* are associated with abnormal *function*, investigators have utilized computerized tomography (CT) and MRI studies of the CNS in conjunction with neuroendocrine stimulation tests, neuropsychological testing, monitoring patients' clinical course, response to treatment, and so on. Indeed, the pituitary gland enlargement exhibited by depressed patients significantly correlates with plasma cortisol concentrations after dexamethasone administration (Axelson et al., 1992). MRI studies determining normative size and shape of the pituitary reveal transient enlargement of the pituitary in periods of intense neuroendocrine activity: pregnancy, the immediate puerperium

(Elster et al., 1991), and adolescence (Elster et al., 1990). Normal maturation of the pituitary gland in adolescence involves a period of physiologic hypertrophy in both sexes, though it is more prominent in females. Other than adolescence and pregnancy, there have been no other documented differences in pituitary size between the sexes (Doraiswamy et al., 1992; Tien et al., 1992). In contrast, reduction of pituitary gland size is associated with increasing age (Lurie et al., 1990; Krishnan et al., 1991) and anorexia nervosa (Doraiswamy et al., 1990). The stability or state dependency of depression-associated pituitary enlargement is unknown.

As mentioned earlier, another HPA-axis structure, the adrenal gland, has been found to exhibit structural alterations in depressed patients. Enlargement of the adrenal gland has been reported postmortem in suicide victims (Zis and Zis, 1987; Szigethy et al., 1994) and in depressed patients using CT and MRI (Amsterdam et al., 1987; Nemeroff et al., 1992; Rubin et al., 1995), a finding probably due to chronic ACTH hypersecretion.

Adrenocortical hypertrophy most likely explains the normal plasma cortisol response to CRF in depressed patients, a sharp contrast to the blunted ACTH and β-endorphin response to the peptide (Gold et al., 1984, 1986; Holsboer et al., 1984; Amsterdam et al., 1987; Kathol et al., 1989; Young et al., 1990; Krishnan et al., 1993). For each pulse of ACTH, depressed patients with an enlarged adrenal cortex would be expected to secrete greater quantities of glucocorticoids than control subjects. Adrenocortical hypertrophy likely underlies the markedly enhanced cortisol response to high doses of ACTH in depression (Kalin et al., 1982; Amsterdam et al., 1983; Linkowski et al., 1985; Jaeckle et al., 1987; Krishnan et al., 1991). Indeed, the significant positive correlation between adrenocortical thickness and increased adrenal gland weight of suicide victims suggests that the increased adrenal mass is due to cortical hyperplasia (Szigethy et al., 1994). Multiple studies have observed that adrenal hypertrophy in depressed patients is significantly associated with body weight and not age or gender (Zis and Zis, 1987; Szigethy et al., 1994). Furthermore, adrenal gland enlargement occurring during an episode of major depression appears to be state dependent in that the adrenal glands revert to the size range of nondepressed control subjects after successful antidepressant treatment (Rubin et al., 1995).

Prospective longitudinal studies should help determine whether patients afflicted with a major mood disorder exhibit structural and functional brain alterations before, during, or as a result of affective episodes, and whether these findings exhibit gender-specific "normalization" with clinical improvement. Further research will also determine the diagnostic specificity of morphologic and functional abnormalities associated with the major affective disorders.

Requiring further scrutiny are those brain structures with corticosteroid receptors or major neuroanatomic connections with the HPA axis (e.g., the amygdala and hippocampus) and relevant cortical areas such as the cingulate and medial prefrontal cortex. Vulnerability to affective dysfunction may derive from disruption of neuronal or hormonal connections between the hippocampus and the HPA axis (Jacobson and Sapolsky, 1991) or from interruption of pathways connecting the limbic system and prefrontal cortex (Alexander, Delong, and Strick, 1986; Krishnan et al., 1991).

Conclusions

In summary, HPA-axis hyperactivity in depressed patients can be explained by hypersecretion of CRF and secondary pituitary and adrenal gland hypertrophy, though impaired negative feedback at various CNS sites and the pituitary also likely contributes. HPA-axis activity, as measured by a variety of parameters, including DST nonsuppression (Carroll, 1968; Nemeroff and Evans, 1984), hypercortisolemia (Sachar et al., 1972), hypersecretion of CRF (Nemeroff et al., 1991; DeBellis et al., 1993), blunting of the ACTH response to CRF (Amsterdam et al., 1988), and adrenal gland hypertrophy (Rubin et al., 1995), all appear to be state dependent, usually normalizing after recovery from depression (Carroll, 1968; Nemeroff and Evans, 1984). Indeed, persistence of DST nonsuppression after treatment may predict early relapse or poor prognosis (Arana et al., 1985), as do persistently elevated CSF CRF concentrations. Thus, it is not surprising that agents which alter steroid availability (metapyrone, ketaconazole, dexamethasone) may alleviate depressive symptoms, though it is difficult to reconcile the effectiveness of both glucocorticoid agonists and antagonists (Murphy et al., 1991; Wolkowitz et al., 1993; Arana et al., 1994). Indeed, premenopausal depressed women have increased quantities of an endogenous glucocorticoid antagonist (progesterone) and CBG, a protein capable of binding free cortisol and whose synthesis is stimulated by estrogen. The decreased amounts of ovarian gonadal steroids in depressed postmenopausal women likely contribute to their increased rates of dexamethasone nonsuppression in comparison to depressed premenopausal women. Undoubtedly, future investigations of affective disorders in women will scrutinize the HPG axis and attend to the interplay of the HPA axis with gonadal steroids. Those brain structures with high concentrations of corticosteroid and/or gonadal steroid receptors should be scrutinized via morphologic and functional imaging in order to further characterize the neuroendocrine pathophysiology of unipolar depression.

Acknowledgments

The authors are supported by NIMH Grants MH-42088, MH-39415, MH-40524, NIH Grant RR-000039, and NIH Grant DK-07298.

CHAPTER SEVEN

THE COST OF STARVATION

EATING DISORDERS

REGINA C. CASPER

Throughout history, famine has been imposed by both natural and human causes – by drought, locusts, war, poverty, or overpopulation – and to this day under-nutrition and malnutrition are the major health problems in India and Africa.

By contrast, in the western hemisphere and increasingly in Asian nations, not undernutrition but overweight is causing health problems. Overconsumption of food has led to an increase in the incidence of obesity, non-insulin-dependent diabetes mellitus, hypertension, cardiovascular diseases, and eating disorders. Easy access to too much palatable food has had the paradoxical effect of self-imposed starvation: Dieting or deliberate food restriction has reached epidemic proportions, especially among female populations, who strive for thinness as their beauty ideal. Dieting in the form of semistarvation is currently the main trigger for the development of the two eating disorders, anorexia nervosa (AN) and bulimia nervosa (BN).

Both disorders are the products of a complex interplay of psychological and physiologic processes. They both belong to a group of heterogeneous psychiatric disorders that can have their onset in childhood, but typically occur during early to middle adolescence (AN) or late adolescence and young adulthood (BN).

AN is a rare but by no means novel disorder, with an incidence rate of 0.7–1.0/10,000/year for females and 0.05/10,000/year for males. Since 1960 an increasing number of new cases, in Denmark as high as 1.9/10,000/year for females and 0.17/10,000/year for males (Nielsen, 1990), have been observed.

Expressed differently, if 85 percent of schoolgirls diet at one time or another during their high school years (Leon, Perry, and Mangelsdorf, 1989), at most 1 percent among them are expected to develop AN. Age at onset currently peaks at about 14 years (Casper, 1996). Whereas the sex ratio in adolescence is about 20:1 (female:male), during prepuberty the proportion of boys who develop AN seems to be higher, with a female:male ratio of 4:1 (Casper, 1995b). Cases in women of middle and old age are uncommon (Beck, Casper, and Anderson, 1996). BN has only recently been classified diagnostically as a syndrome (Russell, 1979; Casper, 1983), although its clinical features were known in antiquity (Ziolko, 1985). The disorder is typically observed in late adolescence and early adulthood with a female:male ratio of 10:1. Population studies have estimated the lifetime prevalence rates for BN to be about 3–4 percent, and up to 8 percent counting bulimia-like syndromes in the female population (Kendler et al., 1991).

The purpose of this chapter is to familiarize professionals with the clinical picture and the medical and endocrine consequences of the two eating disorders. The first section describes the psychological symptoms and physical changes and the second the endocrine disturbances associated with AN and BN. The

Table 7.1. *DSM-IV criteria for anorexia nervosa and bulimia nervosa*

Anorexia nervosa
- Refusal to maintain body weight at or above minimally normal weight for age and height (body weight less than 85 percent of expected) or failure to make expected weight gain during a period of growth
- Intense fear of becoming fat, even though underweight
- Disturbance in the way body weight or shape is experienced; undue influence of body weight or shape on self-evaluation or denial of seriousness of current low body weight
- In postmenarchal females, amenorrhea: i.e., the absence of at least three consecutive menstrual cycles
- Specify type: restricting; binge-eating/purging

Bulimia nervosa
- Recurrent episodes of binge eating:
    Eating, in a discrete period of time, an amount of food definitely larger than most people do
    Lack of control over eating during the episode
- Recurrent compensatory behavior in order to prevent weight gain: self-induced vomiting, misuse of laxatives or other medications, fasting or excessive exercise
- Binge eating and compensatory behaviors occur, on the average, at least twice a week for 3 months
- Self-evaluation is unduly influenced by body shape or weight
- Specify type: purging; nonpurging

last part considers treatment approaches and summarizes the studies on outcome for both disorders.

The criteria for the diagnoses of both eating disorders are listed in the Diagnostic and Statistical Manual – DSM-IV (American Psychiatric Association, 1994) (see Table 7.1). An additional category, termed "eating disorders not otherwise specified," was created for those conditions that do not meet the criteria for either syndrome. The DSM-IV now specifies subtypes of AN, the restricting (nonbulimic) and bulimic types (Casper et al., 1980) and for BN the less well investigated purging and nonpurging types. The International Classification of Diseases – ICD 10 (ICD, 1992) – lists fewer specific criteria, yet includes "dread of fatness" as the central psychopathology of the body image disturbance in AN.

Anorexia nervosa: Psychological symptoms and determinants as risk factors

Historical records have shown that prolonged food abstinence severe enough to induce significant weight loss, such as religious fasting in the Middle Ages or chronic infectious and gastrointestinal diseases, the latter common among women in the late 19th century, can precede the psychological and behavioral symptomatology of AN. Bell (1985) has described an epidemic of AN among Italian women saints who took charge of their own spirituality by living a life of sacrifice, fasting, and self-torment to renounce earthly pleasures. St. Catherine of Siena, who distinguished herself by persuading Pope Gregory XI to return from Avignon to Rome, died of what seems to have been chronic AN at the age of 32. Whatever the reason for the initial weight loss, a strong attachment to the lean body and a deliberate decision to maintain a low body weight are common to all cases. The motivation to pursue a low weight varies with the times and from individual to individual. If the wish to silence bodily desires in order to liberate the soul from the flesh moved medieval young women to excessive fasting, the most common motive among contemporary young women appears to be the culturally sanctioned pursuit of thinness as attractive and fashionable in interaction with a misguided attempt to establish control over one's life through control over one's body size.

The term "anorexia," coined by Gull in the late 19th century, which translates as "no appetite," is a misnomer because patients retain their appetite. About half of all AN patients at hospital admission were found to endorse a good appetite (Casper, 1990a). Famines were feared because hunger is a painful, nagging sensation. With food deprivation thoughts of food crowd the mind and distract from

Table 7.2. *Symptoms in semistarvation compared to symptoms in anorexia nervosa*

	Semistarvation	Anorexia nervosa
Initiative, mood, and hunger	• Lack of initiative • Labile mood, quarrelsomeness • Indecisiveness • Deterioration of personal appearance • Continuous hunger	• Initiative high • Labile mood, alternating with feeling good • "Strong-willed" • Pride in personal appearance, occasional exhibitionistic tendencies • Hunger consciously suppressed
Mental content	• Thinking and dreaming about food • Concentration and interest in food with narrowing of unrelated interests • Daydreaming, reading, and conversing about food	• As in starvation, preoccupation with low weight and anxiety about food continues after weight normalization.
Eating behavior	• Food hoarding • Preference for bulky and hot meals • Picking up crumbs • Bulimia	• As in starvation, but low-calorie foods and fluids are preferred; fat and carbohydrates are avoided.
Activity level	• Fatigue, loss of energy • Avoidance of physical exertion • Restlessness	• Seemingly inexhaustible energy • Physical exercise sought • Restlessness with overactivity
Sexual activity	• Decrease in sexual feelings, interest, and behavior • Amenorrhea, impotence	• Same as in starvation • Amenorrhea, impotence

Reprinted with permission of APA Press from Casper and Davis, 1977.

other thoughts, so that the person can mobilize all resources in search of nourishment to still the hunger. Loss of appetite or "true" anorexia does not give rise to thoughts of food. Thoughts of food impel AN patients to cook or bake, to read and cut out recipes, and to hoard and dream about food (see Table 7.2). AN patients value hunger feelings. They interpret hunger sensations as a signal of their control over food and over their body and hence of self-control. In the restricting or fasting type of AN, hunger can be tamed consistently. In the bulimic type, the urge to eat, especially with exposure to food, becomes irresistible and more often than not leads to episodic uncontrollable eating.

Core symptoms

Lack of concern, denial of illness, and fear of weight gain are the classic symptoms. Clinicians not familiar with AN frequently want to know how AN can be distinguished from mere weight loss due to excessive dieting. One differentiating and still puzzling symptom is lack of concern regarding the gravity of the weight loss combined with emotional inattention to its dangers and physical consequences, typically accompanied by a sprightly mood. Lasègue (1873) gave a telling description of this peculiar state of mind in AN: "What dominates in the mental condition of the patient is above all a state of quietude – I might almost say a condition of contentment truly pathological. Not only does she not sigh for recovery, but she is not ill-pleased with her condition, notwithstanding all the unpleasantness it is attended with, here we have an inexhaustible optimism against which supplications and menaces are of no avail: 'I do not suffer and must then be well'."

This lack of awareness that anything is wrong seems to reinforce the denial of illness, another pathognomonic feature (Casper and Heller, 1991). Denial and unconcern in turn support the body image distortion, the disavowal that the body shape has changed drastically, a third classic feature. Taken together, these misperceptions contribute to and in part explain the refusal to maintain an age-appropriate weight. It must be pointed out that, except for physical illnesses, AN is the only condition that can result in life-threatening weight loss. Occasionally, loss of appetite in severe retarded depressions leads to alarming weight loss, but weight is easily regained once the depression lifts. When AN patients were asked in a survey to date the onset of "feeling more content" retrospectively, patients estimated that it occurred after losing about 10–15 percent of their previous weight (Casper and Davis, 1977). The difference between a dieter who undoubtedly would experience satisfaction and pleasure from losing 20–30 pounds and an AN patient is, on the one hand, that in a dieter this amount of weight loss is rarely achieved and, on the other, that most people would know of and acknowledge the weight loss.

Patients report the appearance of another symptom about the same time: intense anxiety on eating caloric food coupled with dread of becoming overweight if they allow themselves to eat normally. The cognitive counterpart of this anxiety is the "anorectic attitude," a mindset intent on avoiding caloric food and weight gain. Garner et al. (1982) have devised a questionnaire, the Eating Attitudes Test (EAT), that assesses these feelings, thoughts, and behaviors. The total EAT score provides a reliable measure of the severity of the dieting preoccupation. This irrational fear of weight gain has led Crisp (1970) to propose that

AN constitutes a weight phobia. A phobia would account for the irrational fear but does not explain the euphoric state of mind, the body image distortion, and yet another poorly understood symptom set into motion by the starvation – a restless activity, even overactivity, which is contrary to the fatigue observed in other instances of undernutrition (Keys et al., 1950; Casper et al., 1991).

Hyperactivity

This symptom again is not merely culture-bound. Gull (1873 [1964]) described it this way: "The patient complained of no pain, but was restless and active. This was in fact a striking expression of the nervous state, for it seemed hardly possible that a body so wasted could undergo the exercise which seemed agreeable." Lasègue (1873) observed, "Another ascertained fact is that so far from muscular power being diminished, this abstinence tends to increase the aptitude for movement. The patient feels more light and active, rides on horseback, receives and pays visits and is able to pursue a fatiguing life in the world without perceiving the lassitude she would at other times have complained of." Several studies have measured activity levels and confirmed higher than normal activity levels in underweight AN patients. (Blinder, Freeman, and Stunkard, 1970; Casper et al., 1991; Pirke et al., 1991). In rodents an experimentally induced condition called hyperactivity induced anorexia bears some similarity to the phenomenon (Kanarek and Collier, 1983), but the mechanisms that drive the overactive behavior in rodents and in humans in the presence of caloric deficiency remain elusive.

Personality traits

Particular features of the patient's personality seem to contribute to the type of AN and may well play a role in sustaining the disorder. Bruch (1974) thought an early tendency to please others and to conform to rules impaired normal self-development and prevented the anorectic patient from recognizing her own sensations and desires and from acting on self-initiated cues, resulting in the proverbial "good little girl." Research studies have supported this hypothesis, because greater than normal inhibition and rigidity seem to characterize patients who have the restricting form of AN. Restricting AN patients, even after full recovery, reported greater self-discipline, more emotional and social inhibition, and more rigid and perfectionistic attitudes and behavior than their sisters, normal female controls, and BN patients (Casper, 1990b; Casper, Hedeker, and McClough, 1992). Such traits toward reserve and emotional and

Table 7.3. *Predisposing and sustaining factors in restricting anorexia nervosa*

Sociologic	Culture: thinness as beauty ideal	
Physiologic	Caloric restriction gender age race	Loss of appetite due to depression, gastrointestinal disturbances, exercise
	Weight Loss	Genetic factors
Psychologic	Personality tendencies: emotional, cognitive, and behavioral overcontrol; perfectionism	**Anorexia nervosa**
	Poor self-concept: critical self- and body image; negative mood	Comorbid disorders: major depressive disorder obsessive-compulsive disorder anxiety disorder

cognitive restraint – in other words, a greater than normal ability to repudiate needs and sensations and a more exacting conscience – would be expected to facilitate food restriction. Bulimic AN patients did not report such overcontrol, which would be consistent with their difficulty in restraining their appetitive behavior. Gillberg, Rastam, and Gillberg (1994) have observed autisticlike features and an inability to articulate feeling and to empathize significantly more often in AN patients than in a control group. If, as Bruch's (1974) observations suggest, the starved body in AN consolidates a fragile self and conveys a unique sense of strength and confidence, this would explain why patients resist change so much and do not want to take risks in an environment experienced as imposing its own demands and caring little for her wishes. Table 7.3 summarizes the principal risk factors for the development of AN.

Psychiatric comorbidity

Just as AN as a disorder can range in severity, its comorbidity varies. It is important to recognize that many of the psychological symptoms are the sequelae of starvation (see Table 7.2). The restricting type of AN is associated with adjustment disorders, obsessive-compulsive and avoidant personality disorders, symptoms of anxiety and depression, and less commonly with affective or obsessive-compulsive disorders. The bulimic type of AN is more extroverted and shows a closer relationship with affective disorders. The incidence of schizophrenia is not higher than that found in the normal population. Whereas anxiety and depressive symptoms seem to be muted by starvation, obsessive-compulsive symptoms become more apparent with increasing weight loss.

Physical changes in anorexia nervosa

Pathologic weight loss leading to a starved and eventually skeletonlike appearance is the hallmark of AN. Adjustments to the negative energy balance can be found in virtually every system. Inadaequate food intake leads to decreased availability of glucose and amino acids and enhanced lipolysis and gluconeogenesis. Restricting AN patients who are less than 20 percent below normal weight are generally asymptomatic and have few if any laboratory abnormalities. A greater than 30 percent weight loss leads to a host of physical symptoms, usually minimized by the patient (see Table 7.4). Symptom prevalence depends upon the rate of weight loss, the duration of undernutrition or malnutrition, and ultimately the total amount of weight loss.

Bulimia nervosa: Determinants and syndromal and psychological symptoms

BN is an eating disorder characterized by episodic binge eating most often followed by vomiting. BN develops in adolescents or young women who aspire to a lower than normal ideal weight but have difficulty dieting. The strong hunger sensations, induced by fasting, stimulate a powerful urge to eat, so that instead of eating little as intended, patients end up overeating without experiencing sensations of satiety, which under normal conditions terminate eating. The term "bulimia," derived from the Greek *boulimos,* or "ox hunger," is descriptive of behavior induced by a voracious appetite, but the term does not do justice to the syndrome because eventually not only hunger but any distressing emotion, frustration, boredom, annoyance, or insecurity can trigger thoughts of food and a powerful urge to binge. The term "nervosa" points to the psychological component. To prevent weight gain, the majority of patients induce vomiting or abuse laxatives, sometimes diuretics, and least often engage in vigorous exercise. The critical factor for BN seems to be the habituation of these compensatory behaviors, in particular vomiting. The current diagnostic classification of BN (see Table 7.1) includes a frequency criterion of at least two binge eating episodes per week for at least 3 months. Because bulimic patients

Table 7.4. *Physical symptoms and medical complications in restricting anorexia nervosa and bulimia nervosa*

	Anorexia nervosa, restricting subtype	Bulimia nervosa; anorexia nervosa, bulimic subtype
Physical symptoms	Body weight loss (from 15 to 55%) Loss of subcutaneous fat tissue Growth retardation (children)	Body weight fluctuations (2–50 lbs) Parotid enlargement
Metabolic	Hypothermia; hypometabolism Cold intolerance Carbohydrate intolerance Hypercholesterolemia, hyper-carotenemia	Hypothermia; hypometabolism Hypokalemia Hypochloremic alkalosis
Central nervous ssystem	Abnormal EEG; abnormal CAT scan Cerebral pseudoatrophy Peripheral neuritis	Abnormal EEG Seizures
Oral		Dental enamel erosion, pharyn-gitis Swelling of salivary glands
Gastrointestinal	Delayed gastric emptying Superior mesenteric artery syn-drome Constipation	Esophagitis, ↑serum amylase Mallory-Weiss tears Gastric dilation; gastric rupture Diarrhea
Cardiovascular	Hypotension Bradycardia; decreased heart size Acrocyanosis Edema	Hypotension EKG–flat or inverted T waves Arrhythmias; cardiac arrest Edema
Renal	Dehydration Edema Polyuria; nycturia Partial diabetes insipidus	Dehydration Metabolic alkalosis; renal calculi Renal insufficiency or failure Partial diabetes insipidus
Hematologic	Anemia, normochromic, normo-cytic Leukopenia with relative lym-phocytosis Thrombocytopenia, petechiae, ecchymoses Bone marrow hypoplasia	
Pulmonary		Aspiration pneumonia
Skin	Dark, yellowish color, rough texture	Bruises and lacerations over knuckles
Musculoskeletal	Lanugo coat of silky hair Osteoporosis; stress fractures	Ecchymoses on face and neck Cramps; muscle weakness

EEG, electroencephalogram; CAT, computerized axial tomography; EKG, electrocardiogram.

try to fast, they typically do not eat meals, although they might pick at food until the urge to eat and binge eat becomes so compelling that whatever is eaten is experienced as eating out of control or as a binge. Food intake, therefore, alternates between long periods of fasting and binge eating. In chronically bulimic patients, binge eating followed by vomiting is premeditated and becomes part of the daily routine. The day might not proceed as planned because the sight, smell, or simply the presence of tasty food easily overturns any plans. Depending upon the severity of the abnormal eating pattern, body weight can markedly fluctuate, even though most patients tend to remain within a high, rather than a low, weight range. A low weight in a BN patient is cause for alarm because it suggest frequent vomiting, even after trivial amounts of food are consumed. Kendler et al. (1991) identified the following risk factors as associated with BN using the Virginia Twin registry, a population-based register: birth after 1960, low paternal care, a history of dieting, a slim ideal body image, low self-esteem, and high levels of neuroticism. Table 7.5 illustrates factors contributing to BN.

Although we do not fully understand how the bulimic behavior escalates out of control because some but not all women who try this behavior for weight control develop BN, it appears that the ease with which regurgitation and vomiting are achieved, that is, the easier esophageal peristalsis can be reversed, the greater the risk of acquiring the behavior. More important are the level of emotional distress and the presence of psychopathology because both have been found to be related to the severity of the bulimic behavior. Binge eating has been observed as

Table 7.5. *Predisposing and sustaining factors in bulimia nervosa*

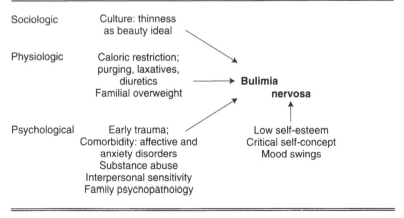

a response to emotional deprivation. Selling and Ferraro (1945) have described excessive eating in refugee children brought from Europe to the United States between 1933 and 1939. As long as the children felt insecure and abandoned, they ate frantically and gorged themselves; once they felt a sense of security in their new homes, they reduced their intake to physiologic levels.

Patients are aware of the abnormal function food plays in their lives. Not infrequently they describe their craving for food and their loss of control over food as an "addiction," even though BN does not really fit the addiction model because tolerance and physical dependence are absent. The amounts of food and calories, up to 5,000 calories, that some patients can consume in one binge are not only astounding, they can be life-threatening and are expensive. On the Minnesota Multiphasic Personality Inventory, BN patients show higher than normal levels of somatic concerns and rebellious deviant behavior, and on the Multidimensional Personality Questionnaire BN patients score in the high normal range for impulsivity (Casper, Hedeker, and McClough, 1992). If patients qualify for a personality disorder, they qualify most often for Cluster B personality disorders (American Psychiatric Association, 1994). Many studies have shown a close relation between BN and affective disorders and an association with behaviors related to impulse control, such as stealing (kleptomania) and substance abuse (Lacey, 1993). Other problems – for example, a history of sexual abuse and disturbed family relationships – seem not to occur more frequently in BN than in other psychiatric populations (Pope and Hudson, 1992). It is important to realize that the psychopathology recorded in any investigation is a function of the sample studied and that many of the published data derive from inpatients (i.e., the most severely impaired group).

Physical changes in bulimia nervosa

The by and large normal body weight in the mostly young BN patients deceives the clinician into expecting no health problems, and many patients tolerate the severe and protracted emesis and the fluid and electrolyte disturbances with minimal clinical or laboratory abnormalities. However, as Table 7.4 indicates, BN can be associated with numerous medical complications. The most serious and potentially life-threatening situation is hypokalemia, which results as much from emesis as from increased renal potassium excretion secondary to the metabolic alkalosis. A combination of vomiting and laxative and diuretic abuse in BN patients presents the greatest danger for significant potassium loss, which is associated with a risk for cardiac arrythmia or cardiac arrest, followed by the combination of alcohol abuse and binge-vomiting behavior with the potential for fatal aspiration pneumonia.

Endocrine changes in anorexia nervosa

Early claims that AN is a primary endocrine disorder, the result of pituitary atrophy (Simmonds, 1914), were not confirmed by research. The thin body in AN is essentially an undernourished and often a malnourished body that has undergone adaptations in virtually every endocrine system as a result of the negative energy balance. Some, but not all, of these adaptations give rise to symptoms. In scope, the hypothalamic-endocrine disturbances vary with the degree of the caloric deficit. Because all hormonal values ultimately return to normal with weight gain and adequate nutrition, no hormonal pathognomonic markers have been identified with certainty. However, the fact that the core symptoms of AN become more pronounced with increasing caloric deprivation and weight loss strongly suggests that one or several of the neurotrtransmitters or hormones might be involved in reinforcing the psychopathology of AN.

In bulimic AN or bulimia nervosa, similar starvation-induced adaptations in hypothalamic areas reverberate throughout the endocrine system, confounded by emesis or laxative abuse. For the most part, physical and hormonal alterations in BN are less pronounced than in AN because cycles of hyperhagia and hypophagia provide, albeit intermittently, more nutrition. Moreover, body weight in BN fluctuates within the normal range.

Adaptations in the hypothalamic-pituitary-gonadal axis

Menstrual dysfunction. Primary or secondary amenorrhea is diagnostic for AN. Some studies have reported the onset of menstrual disturbances early in the illness, before any substantial weight loss (Warren and Vande Wiele, 1973; Mecklenburg, Loriaux, and Thompson, 1974). These findings have been interpreted as evidence for a primary hypothalamic disturbance in AN (Russell, 1977). This conclusion, however, seems premature, not only because most earlier studies dated the onset of amenorrhea retrospectively but because it is now well recognized that substantial stress and gradual food restriction can lead to secondary amenorrhea. Moreover, over 60 percent of cases become amenorrheic concurrent with the onset of anorexia nervosa (Starkey and Lee, 1969).

Similarly, primary amenorrhea in young girls with AN can occur with a weight loss of as little as 10–15 percent, equivalent to a loss of about one third of body fat. Frisch (Frisch and McArthur, 1974; Frisch, 1985) has calculated a critical body fat composition as one of the necessary physiologic preconditions for the initiation of puberty, because adipose tissue is important as an endocrine organ for the aromatization of androstendiol to estradiol. Amenorrhea is generally considered a sign of anovulation, yet sporadic ovulation may occur in sexually active, albeit underweight, patients, and pregnancy has been reported in severely underweight amenorrheic women (Stewart, Raskin, and Garfinkel, 1987). The return of normal regular menstrual cycles or menarche following primary amenorrhea does not always coincide with the restoration of normal weight. One reason for the delay may be that many patients remain diet conscious, becoming selective eaters and occasionally vegetarians (Goldin et al., 1982), shunning fat and carbohydrates, or remain excessively active through exercise (Smith, 1980; Yates, Leehey, and Shisslak, 1983); both situations prevent accumulation of adipose tissue. Some patients with AN who exercise excessively might in fact gain weight through muscle tissue but may not gain sufficient fat tissue for appropriate luteophase activity. Female patients with AN typically, but not always, report decreased sexual interest (Casper and Davis, 1977), and boys experience impotence (Andersen, 1990).

Regulatory changes in the hypothalamic-pituitary-gonadal axis

In anorexia nervosa, as in simple weight loss (Warren and Vande Wiele, 1973; Vigersky et al., 1977; Isaacs et al., 1980; Pirke, Fichter, and Chlond, 1987), the menstrual dysfunction reflects system disturbances at different levels (see Table 7.6). A change in the hypothalamic luteinizing hormone–releasing hormone (LHRH) secretory pattern reduces pituitary luteinizing hormone (LH) secretion and consequently lowers release of estradiol and progesterone from the ovary (Beumont et al., 1974; Boyar, Katz, and Finkelstein, 1974; Sherman and Halmi, 1977). Plasma follicle-stimulating hormone (FSH) levels have also been reported to be depressed in patients, but normal FSH levels have been reported in severely underweight patients (Vigersky, Loriaux, and Andersen, 1976; Vigersky et al., 1977). With increasing weight loss, the adult circadian pattern of LH secretion undergoes regressive changes, which sequentially reactivate the LH pattern typical of mid-, early, and eventually prepuberty (Boyar, Katz, and Finkelstein, 1974). In effect, female patients whose weight loss exceeds 45 percent invariably display the low-sleep-dependent LH secretion reminiscent of prepuberty. Following weight gain, patients can be primed with endogenous LHRH to restore normal responsiveness of the pituitary and to induce ovulation (Beumont et al., 1974; Bringer, Hedon, and Jaffiol, 1985), suggesting that

Table 7.6 *Hypothalamic-pituitary-adrenal, -thyroid, -gonadal, and human growth hormone regulation in anorexia nervosa*

	Corticotropin-releasing hormone	Thyrotropin-releasing hormone	Luteinizing-follicle stimulating-releasing hormone	Growth hormone—inhibiting factor
Hypothalamus	↑ CRH	→ TRH	↓ LH-FSH-RH	↓ GIF
Pituitary gland	Adrenocorticotropin → ACTH ↑ beta-endorphin	Thyrotropin TSH delay ↑ GH secretion → Prolactin	Prepubertal LH and FSH secretion pattern	Human growth hormone ↑ HGH secretion
End organ and plasma	↑ Cortisol ↑ Urinary free cortisol	→ T_4[a], ↓ T_3[b] ↑ rT_3 : 3, 3', 5-triiodothyronine	↓ Estradiol ↓ Progesterone → Testosterone ↑ (2-OH) Estrone ∼ Androstendione/etiocholanolone ∼ Dehydroepiandrosterone	

[a]Thyroxine.

[b]Triiodothyronine.

the primary defect is at the hypothalamic level. Furthermore, a higher proportion of plasma estradiol is metabolized to 2-hydroxyestrone at the expense of estradiol, whereas testosterone levels remain about the same (Boyar, Hellman, and Roffwarg, 1977; Katz et al., 1978; Casper, Chatterton, and Davis, 1979). This obervation is important physiologically because 2-hydroxyestrone has a normal binding affinity for estrogen receptors, but less than 0.1 percent of the biologic activity of estradiol and therefore functions as an antiestrogen. Catecholestrogens also inhibit the release of LH/FSH as well as of enzymes that are crucial for the synthesis and disposition of catecholamines and thus might have an effect on brain dopamine levels. When weight is restored to normal levels and corresponds to the premorbid constitutional weight of the individual patient, in virtually all patients the prepubertal LH pattern converts to the adult LH secretory profile (Katz et al., 1978). Thus, as AN patients gain weight, they undergo in an orderly sequence all maturational changes in LH and, to a lesser extent, FSH secretion, initiating, in those who have secondary amenorrhea, puberty for a second time. At 70 percent of ideal body weight, an exaggerated FSH response has been reported (Beumont et al., 1974). At about 90 percent of ideal body weight, normal pituitary gonadotroph responsiveness is restored in most patients.

Not enough studies have examined the reproductive function of recovered patients with AN to draw any conclusions about the effects of the illness on fertility (Starkey and Lee, 1969; Stewart, Raskin, and Garfinkel, 1987). If full (i.e., physiologic and psychological) recovery occurs, reproductive function can be expected to be within the individual's normal range.

Low estradiol levels have been associated with osteoporosis (Ettinger, Genant, and Cann, 1985). However, the high level of physical activity seems to protect AN patients from bone loss, and bone fractures are uncommon. Nevertheless, absorption studies have shown evidence of decreased bone density (Rigotti et al., 1984; Szmukler, Brown, and Parsons, 1985). In young, physically active patients with a good chance for full recovery, prophylactic estradiol administration would be contraindicated, especially because no systematic studies have demonstrated the value of hormone replacement to increase bone density under conditions of protein caloric malnutrition during adolescence.

Adaptions in the hypothalamic-pituitary-adrenal axis

Boyar and Bradlow (1977) have shown that an activation of the hypothalamic-pituitary-adrenal axis in AN leads to increased cortisol production relative to body mass and body surface area. Urinary free cortisol and plasma cortisol levels are typically increased in emaciated patients and remain elevated throughout the 24-hour cycle (Boyar and Bradlow, 1977; Walsh et al., 1978; Casper, Chatterton, and Davis, 1979; Ferrari et al., 1989). When urine volume is controlled, urinary free cortisol content has been calculated to be double or triple in AN patients (Boyar, Hellman, and Roffwarg, 1977). Doerr, Fichter, and Pirke (1980) have described increases in the number of secretory episodes and in the time spent in cortisol seretory activity during the 24-hour cycle. Other factors that contribute to increased plasma levels of cortisol are prolongation in the half-life of cortisol due to a reduced metabolic clearance rate and alterations in steroid metabolism (Zumoff et al., 1983). As a result of the hypercortisolemia, patients with AN fail to suppress morning or afternoon cortisol levels after dexamethasone administration (Gerner and Gwirtsman, 1981). Unfortunately, little is known about the absorption, metabolism, or disposition of dexamethasone in AN, although the 1-mg dose usually administered at night would be expected to suffice for suppression, given the patient's emaciated condition.

Studies by Gold, Gwirtsman, and Avgerinos (1986) suggest that the hyperactivity of the adrenal cortex might be caused by increased release of corticotrophin-releasing hormone (CRH). With stimulation tests a significantly reduced net corticotrophin (ACTH) response to CRH administration, but normal mean basal ACTH levels even among patients with the highest cortisol levels, were found. Following short-term weight recovery, the ACTH response to CRH continued to be markedly attenuated. Patients with a long-term recovery had normal cortisol plasma levels, a normal ACTH response, and a normal ACTH:cortisol ratio on stimulation with CRH. The data suggest that the hypercortisolism in AN is related to a regulatory defect at or above the hypothalamic level and normalizes with weight restoration (Walsh et al., 1978; Kennedy, Brown, and McVey, 1991). A reduced caloric intake has been shown to increase diurnal plasma cortisol levels in fasting normal volunteers (Fichter and Pirke, 1984) and in depression (Casper, Chatterton, and Davis, 1979). Cortisol stimulates gluconeogenesis and thus plays an important role in maintaining adequate blood glucose concentrations necessary for central nervous system function.

Adaptations in the hypothalamic-pituitary-thyroid axis

Emaciated AN patients display clinical symptoms consistent with hypothyroidism, such as a low basal metabolic rate; dry, rough skin; hypothermia; cold intolerance; bradycardia; and elevated cholesterol and carotene plasma levels. The TSH peak release can be delayed or attenuated (Miyai et al., 1975; Moshang, Parks, and Balsor, 1975; Moshang and Utiger, 1977; Macaron,

Wilber, and Green, 1978; Casper and Frohman, 1982; Kiriike, Nishiwaki, and Izumiya, 1987). In AN alternate pathways of peripheral T_4 metabolism are activated. Thyroxine (T_4) production in AN has been reported as normal or occasionally decreased, whereas triiodothyronine (T_3) serum concentrations in emaciated patients are reduced (Miyai et al., 1975; Moshang and Utiger, 1977; Macaron, Wilber, and Green, 1978; Casper and Frohman, 1982; Kiriike, Nishiwaki, and Izumiya, 1987). Because 80 percent of T_3 is produced by extrathyroidal deiodination of T_4, the decrease in serum T_3 in AN is thought to be a result of reduced activity of the Type I 5-deiodinase present in liver and kidney. Such reduction has been documented in other starvation states (Vagenakis et al., 1975). At the same time an alternate pathway served by Type II deiodinase is activated and leads to the formation of reverse T_3 ($3,3',5'$-triiodothyronine), which has less biologic activity. Basal TSH levels have been generally described as normal and sometimes as increased (Miyai et al., 1975; Casper and Frohman, 1982). Increased TSH levels would suggest hypothyroidism, whereas normal TSH serum levels in the presence of low serum T_3 suggest a readjustment of the homeostatic control of TSH secretion, probably through T_4 feedback. This syndrome is known as the sick euthyroid syndrome and resembles changes observed in serious nonthyroidal illnesses (Bermudez, Surks, and Oppenheimer, 1975) and in other starvation states (Vagenakis et al., 1975). Low T_3 values have been related to the markedly reduced metabolic rate in AN (Casper et al., 1991). During weight gain temporary rises of T_3 into the hyperthyroid range (Leslie et al., 1978) and exaggerated TSH responses have been reported. Hypercholesterolemia and hypercarotenemia are common in severe AN and may be related to the hypometabolic adaptation (Casper et al., 1991). The increased cholesterol levels are accounted for by an increase in low-density lipoprotein cholesterol and are reversible with weight gain (Crisp, Blendis, and Pawan, 1968).

Human growth hormone

Raised plasma growth hormone levels are common in starving AN patients, and elevated levels can persist throughout the 24-hour day (Mecklenburg, Loriaux, and Thompson, 1974; Casper, Davis, and Pandey, 1977; Macaron, Wilber, and Green, 1978; Fullerton, Swift, and Getto, 1986; Kiriike, Nishiwaki, and Izumiya, 1987). Growth hormone release is stimulated by other forms of malnutrition or undernutrition and even by short-term fasting. Growth hormone levels normalize promptly with refeeding, especially with carbohydrates (Cahill et al., 1966; Pimstone, Barbezat, and Hansen, 1968; Alvarez et al., 1972). Following a glucose load, elevated growth hormone levels can generally be suppressed in patients with AN (Casper, Davis, and Pandey, 1977). Pathologic growth hormone release in response to administration of TRH has been reported by Macaron, Wilber, and Green (1978). Marked growth hormone elevations can also be observed in response to emotional stress, although the levels might not be as high as those recorded in AN. Under normal conditions, growth hormone secretion is augmented during slow-wave sleep onset. This association can be disturbed in patients with AN in whom nocturnal growth hormone surges can be prolonged or decreased in amplitude (Kalucy et al., 1976). Elevated growth hormone levels in states of starvation are believed to conserve protein precursors necessary for linear growth and thus play an important adaptive role. Growth hormone also stimulates the mobilization of fat from fat tissue and plays a synergistic role with sex steroids in the adolescent growth spurt (Brasel, 1976) in conjunction with insulin-like growth factor-1 (IGF-1) (Phillips and Vassilopoulou-Sellin, 1980).

Insulin-like growth factor-1

Children who develop AN during prepuberty or early puberty frequently suffer impaired linear growth (Ettinger, Genant, and Cann, 1985). Because somatomedin, or IGF-1, produced in the liver, mediates the effects of growth hormone in the periphery (Phillips and Vassilopoulou-Sellin, 1980; Berelowitz et al., 1981), the reduced plasma somatomedin activity as reported by Rappaport, Prevot, and Czernichov (1980) in 8 of 12 underweight adolescent patients with AN very likely contributes to the growth arrest.

Prolactin and vasopressin

Prolactin secretion is not much altered during the course of AN or in malnutrition (Wakeling et al., 1979; Isaacs et al., 1980; Casper and Frohman, 1982; Kiriike, Nishiwaki, and Izumiya, 1987). Normal prolactin levels would speak against the dopamine deficiency theory of AN if pituitary dopamine concentrations reflect central nervous system dopamine levels. Plasma prolactin release in response to TRH administration has been reported as normal (Beumont et al., 1974; Wakeling et al., 1979), although some investigators (Vigersky, Loriaux, and Andersen, 1976) found a temporal delay in the peak prolactin response. Kalucy et al. (1976) described the nocturnal surge in prolactin as significantly diminished in AN compared with controls. Regarding vasopressin secretion during the emaciated state, Gold et al. (1983) found low basal and unstable arginine vasopressin responses to sodium stimulation in AN. With weight improvement, the instability of the arginine vasopressin response persisted in three patients, but seven other patients showed normal vasopressin responses to sodium loading.

Melatonin

The data on the circadian rhythm of plasma melatonin in AN are conflicting. Ferrari and co-investigators (Ferrari et al., 1989; Ferrari, Fraschini, and Brambilla, 1990) reported higher mean 24-hour melatonin plasma levels compared with normal controls and obese patients. In anorectic patients, the timing, amplitude, and duration of the melatonin varied widely, and abnormal daytime secretory peaks were observed. By contrast, Kennedy, Brown, and McVey (1991) found similar melatonin secretion rates in underweight and weight-improved AN patients and in normal controls, although patients who had the lowest weight tended to display the highest nocturnal melatonin levels.

Neuroendocrine alterations in bulimia nervosa

Normal-weight patients with BN, whose caloric intake is well balanced, show few if any endocrine abnormalities (Casper et al., 1988; Weltzin et al., 1991). As in AN, endocrine changes are generally due to a low caloric intake or malnutrition. Pirke, Pahl, and Schweiger (1985) described elevated blood levels of beta-hydroxybutyric acid and free fatty acid in bulimic patients compared with normal controls as metabolic indexes of starvation. In the same study, lower than normal plasma T_3 levels were observed as well as decreased norepinephrine responses to orthostatic testing. TSH responses to TRH can be blunted in some patients with BN (Mitchell and Bantle, 1983), with a trend toward lower weights in patients with blunted TSH responses. Altemus et al. (1996) have shown a positive relation between caloric intake and TSH levels in BN patients, suggesting that food binging stimulates thyroid acitivity. Elevated plasma cortisol levels have been described with a failure of dexamethasone suppression in about 20–40 percent of patients (Hudson, Pope, and Jonas, 1983; Musisi and Garfinkel, 1985; Kiriike, Nishiwaki, and Izumiya, 1987) and in 100 percent of patients in one study (Levy, Dixon, and Malarkey, 1988). Others have described normal hypothalamic-pituitary-adrenal–axis activity (Walsh, Roose, and Katz, 1987). Fullerton, Swift, and Getto (1986) attributed the greater than normal beta-endorphin release in response to glucose ingestion in BN patients to stress.

Menstrual disturbances are not infrequent in patients with BN, and oligomenorrhea is common. Pirke and co-workers (Pirke, Pahl, and Schweiger,

1985; Pirke, Fichter, and Chlond, 1987) found progesterone concentrations above 3 ng/ml during the luteal phase in only three out of eight patients with BN. FSH levels were also diminished. Kiriike, Nishikawa, and Izumiya (1987) found normal prolactin levels, whereas Levy, Dixon, and Malarkey (1988) reported reduced basal prolactin concentrations in patients with BN. The observations suggest that weight fluctuations associated with intermittent dieting or irregular food intake and loss of food due to vomiting contribute to highly variable endocrine changes and to disturbances of the menstrual cycle in BN, not unlike those seen in AN and other starvation states.

Treatment of anorexia nervosa

The treatment of AN (see Table 7.7) includes in order of priority:

1. Renutrition
2. Individual psychotherapy and family therapy
3. Medication for comorbid disorders.

Table 7.7. *Anorexia nervosa: Indications for hospitalization and hospital treatment*

Indications for hospitalization
- Body weight below 75th percentile for age and height
- Abnormal laboratory values and physical symptoms of malnutrition
- Signs of an organic brain syndrome
- Inability to function in school or job; physical debility
- Refusal to drink fluids (more likely among children)

Hospital treatment
- The ultimate target weight should be a return to an individually determined healthy body weight at which normal reproductive function resumes and calcium loss ceases. Determine body weight as Body Mass Index (BMI), kg/m2 (normal range 18–25).
- Supervised refeeding program to ensure weight gain to low normal weight for age and height with liquid nutrient, 1,800–3,300 cal/day depending on metabolic rate, level of activity
- Experienced and caring nursing staff
- Indications for hyperalimentation: chronicity, life at risk
- Individual psychotherapy: monitor therapeutic alliance, explore motivation for weight loss; raise self-esteem, reduce self-critical attitude and perfectionism.
- Family therapy: explore dysfunctioning family interaction, and help parents care for and support patient.
- Peer group participation to improve interpersonal skills
- Behavioral strategies: privileges and passes linked to food intake/weight gain
- Pharmacotherapy for comorbid disorder

It is not feasible within the scope of this chapter to describe the complex treatment process and the adjustments necessary to treat young adolescents or children or to do justice to all approaches discussed in the literature, so we refer the reader to a selection of articles and books for an overview of strategies and programs on nutritional management, psychotherapy, and family therapy (Bruch, 1974; Selvini-Palazzoli, 1978; Garfinkel and Garner, 1982; Beumont, Burrows, and Casper, 1987; Werne and Yalom, 1996). Among experts, the consensus about the treatment approach is so close that the practice guidelines for eating disorders (Guidelines, A.P.A.P., 1993) were the first in the series developed by the American Psychiatric Association.

We describe here certain points important to consider in the evaluation and the treatment recommendation. With its effort to build an alliance with the patient against the disorder, the evaluation actually serves as an introduction to treatment. The patient's strong identification with her starved body, her failure to perceive her body as wasted, and her dread of fatness, not surprisingly, make her resist treatment. For this reason, virtually all AN patients are brought in by the family or by friends. Aside from establishing the diagnosis, the evaluation seeks foremost to engage the usually antagonistic patient. A conversation about the patient's opposition to treatment and how the patient was persuaded to come as an opening gives the patient a chance to speak her mind and backs up her hopes that she will be heard. This is followed by a review of the past and developmental history; her interests, personality, friendships, and talents; and only then is her physical condition – which includes her weight, her symptoms, and the severity of her weight loss – discussed, along with her future plans, hopes, and ambitions. At this point the patient cannot evade the realization that continued weight loss is not a viable solution and that maintaining the status quo perpetuates her emotional isolation and prevents her from having a normal life. The patient is then asked to reflect on her motivation and reasons for losing weight, which usually reveal a lifelong unhappiness, a sense of inadequacy, and a fragile self-esteem. Although these negative emotions have been relegated to the background by the patient's discovery of a new sense of mastery and achievement through successful weight control, the patient is still aware of them.

An explanation of AN is offered before a treatment plan is proposed. Treatment needs to teach the patient more effective ways of dealing with her self- and body dissatisfaction and life's problems and thus must offer an alternative to AN as a lifestyle. Because the family has not been able to provide their child with sufficient emotional nurturing for her to grow and mature without adopting weight loss to bolster her self-esteem, it is of utmost importance to assess the family's strengths, limitations, and weaknesses in the patient's presence. A more detailed explanation of this step-by-step approach has been published (Casper, 1982, 1986). Based on the outcome of the patient and family interview, a final treatment recommendation is worked out with the patient and her family. Usually it involves first an outpatient trial, if the patient is medically stable, and a proposal to hospitalize, if outpatient treatment fails (i.e., the patient cannot gain weight). A verbal contract for a minimum weight is negotiated with the patient. The patient and the family vastly underestimate the enormous obstacles to treating AN because they assume that eating food and gaining weight is merely a matter of will power. If the weight loss exceeds 25 percent of normal body weight, outpatient treatment is effective only if the patient is fairly healthy (i.e., there is no serious psychiatric comorbidity) and if the parents are caring, flexible, and willing to change and to collaborate in treatment.

Either way, renutrition and weight gain are the foundations for treatment. Food is the most effective "medication" for AN. Nutrition is initially offered in the form of liquid dietary supplements. Eliminating food has several advantages: It provides the patient with control over the caloric information without fretting over the caloric content of every bite of food, is easily supervised, supplies sufficient fluids, and offers ample vitamins and minerals for rebuilding tissues. With this supervised regime no medical complications have been encountered. Treatment needs to be flexible and continuously renegotiated with a terrified, often oppositional patient. The patient requires daily, sometimes hourly, support and gentle persuasion to deal with her anxiety over losing her most precious possession, her starved body, and to deal with her terror that she will end up "fat" and deformed.

Numerous drug trials have been conducted, but no drug has been shown to be effective, and no FDA-approved drug exists for AN (Casper, 1986). Because in a severely emaciated patient the psychological symptoms can mimic depression, the patient is best reevaluated after about 10 percent weight gain for the presence of any comorbid condition that might be drug responsive. The newer antidepressants can be useful for treating a major depressive disorder or an obsessive-compulsive disorder, but they do not significantly improve the patient's obsession with food and weight and her dread of overweight. Unless weight can ultimately be restored to the low normal range, chances for relapse remain high. Treatment needs to be continued as long as the patient feels uncomfortable with her body and cannot easily maintain a normal weight.

Outcome from anorexia nervosa

To understand the information on the outcome of AN, one needs to know that virtually all sizable follow-up studies are derived from consecutively admitted patients hospitalized in specialty programs in teaching hospitals. Depending on the referral pattern, such patients generally constitute a severely ill group. AN patients who never needed hospital admission and could be treated safely and effectively in pediatric or psychiatric clinics would be expected to show the best prognosis; unfortunately, their long-term outcome has not been studied.

Methodologically well-designed follow-up evaluations that apply explicitly stated diagnostic criteria (e.g., have more than 25 subjects in the sample and less than a 20 percent attrition rate, with subjects assessed after a minimum of 4 years using direct interviews and standardized rating scales) have shown considerable variation in course and long-term outcome. As the summary information from outcome studies that fulfilled these requirements (Table 7.8) shows, about 40–60 percent of patients evaluated after 5–10 years have reached a normal weight and regained cyclical menstrual function. From 20 to 30 percent are significantly better, while between 10 and 30 percent live with chronic AN (Theander, 1970; Steinhausen, Rauss-Mason, and Seidel, 1991; Eckert et al., 1995; Casper and Jabine, 1996). AN has a remarkably high mortality rate – from 5 to 8 percent, rising up to 15–17 percent after 20 years. The two long-term studies, which conducted follow-up assessments at 20 and 24 years, respectively, show markedly different outcomes. The discrepant findings may in part be attributable to differences in the patient population. The 20-year outcome, given in Table 7.8, describes 41 AN patients hospitalized on a specialized treatment unit at the Maudsley Hospital in London (Ratnasuriya et al., 1991), whereas the second, with over 75 percent of patients showing a good outcome, is a population-based study by Theander (1985) of 94 AN patients from regions in southern Sweden, limited to hospitalized cases. Interestingly, another in part population-based prospective study of adolescent AN patients at a 6-year follow-up, conducted by Gillberg, Rastam, and Gillberg (1994) in Goteburg, Sweden, showed recovery rates not much different from those in other intermediate (5- to 10-year) follow-up studies based on hospitalized samples. The outcome from AN with an onset before age 13 was examined in two prospective studies (Walford and McCune, 1991; Bryant-Waugh et al., 1996). Even though the overall recovery rate appears similar to that found in intermediate-term adolescent outcome studies (Deter and Herzog, 1994; Herpertz-Dahlmann et al., 1996), more young patients would be expected to have improved if the follow-up had been longer (Theander, 1985).

Table 7.8. *Physical outcome from anorexia nervosa (in percentages)*

Physical outcome	Follow-up after		
	3 years[a]	5–10 years	20/24 years
Good	50	40–60	29/76
Regular menses			
Ideal body weight > 85%			
Intermediate	27	20–30	32/1
Menstrual disturbance or			
Body weight not sustained at 85%			
Poor	22	10–30	37/7.4
Amenorrhea, oligomenorrhea			
Ideal body weight < 85%			
Died	0–7	5–8	17.5/16

[a]Age at onset < 13 years.

Indeed, Bryant-Waugh et al. (1988) observed a higher recovery rate in a retrospective 14-year outcome study of children with AN.

Physical recovery does not always coincide with psychological recovery. In point of fact, from 35 to 60 percent of the physically well display some abnormal eating, and from 10 to 30 percent can still have signs of an eating disorder at follow-up. Physically recovered patients tend to qualify more often than normal controls for an anxiety disorder, a social phobia, and/or an obsessive-compulsive disorder, and if they had bulimic AN for an affective disorder (Halmi et al., 1991; Rastam, Gillberg, and Gillberg, 1996) and for substance abuse disorder (Strober et al., 1996). The studies suggest that on average 20–40 percent have fully recovered from AN (Eckert et al., 1995; Casper and Jabine, 1996).

Most outcome studies have searched for prognostic indicators. A short duration of illness, a good relationship with parents, and absence of psychopathology predict a good outcome (Tolstrup et al., 1985; Steinhausen, Rauss-Mason, and Seidel, 1991). Conversely, chronicity, a lower minimum weight, premorbid maladjustment, a greater number of hospitalizations, and bulimic symptoms are associated with a poorer outcome (Eckert et al., 1995; Strober et al., 1996). Although an early age at onset in most psychiatric disorders augurs a poor prognosis, this does not seem to apply to AN; in fact, some studies have claimed a better outcome for younger patients (Swift, 1982), although Bryant-Waugh et al. (1988) described a less favorable prognosis for young AN patients. This controversy may be resolved only if a consensus about the operational definition of "early onset" (childhood vs. early puberty) can be reached and if long-term prospective studies drawn from the general population can be conducted.

Treatment of bulimia nervosa

The primary goals of treatment are:

1. The elimination of dieting and the establishment of healthy eating habits
2. Reduction in the patient's emotional distress and improvement in interpersonal functioning
3. Drug treatment for comorbid disorders.

Like AN patients, BN patients constitute a psychopathologically heterogenous group, and in severity BN can range from mild to severe. The main challenge is to assist the patient to reestablish control over a chaotic eating pattern, improve a poor self-concept, explore and address dysfunctional interpersonal relationships, and treat the comorbidity – most often dysthymia, major depressive disorder, panic disorder, and/or substance abuse. Table 7.9 lists indications for hospitalization and some guidelines for in-hospital treatment. The BN patient is more disposed than the AN patient to want help, but many BN patients do not want to give up binging and vomiting entirely. A careful evaluation and a psychiatic diagnostic assessment, including an evaluation of the severity of the bulimic behavior, are the cornerstones for designing a treatment plan with which the patient can agree. Psychological treatment solicits the patient's active participation and works well in the highly motivated, moderately disturbed patient. Psychotherapy alone with monitoring binging/vomiting frequency can lead to remission (Johnson and Connors, 1987). Two approaches, a behavioral self-monitoring approach combined with supportive psychotherapy (Lacey, 1983) and a cognitive behavioral approach designed by Fairburn (Fairburn and Wilson, 1993), which is currently undergoing another efficacy trial (Fairburn, Marcus, and Wilson, 1993), have both proven effective in reducing bulimic symptoms on systematic follow-up at 2 years. A meta-analysis of 25 treatment studies comparing a total of 447 BN patients found evidence that psychotherapy, especially combined with dietary management, was superior to drug treatment for controlling bulimic symptoms. In older and more chronically ill patients the advantages of psychotherapy were less pronounced (Laessle, Zoettle, and Pirke, 1987). Because only two of the drug studies monitored drug plasma levels, impaired drug absorption might have been a problem. For

Table 7.9. *Bulimia nervosa: Indications for hospitalization and hospital treatment*

Indications for hospitalization
- Inability to function independently, suicide attempt
- Intractable overeating and vomiting several times daily, loss of control
- Excessive or dangerous emetic, laxative, or diuretic abuse

Hospital treatment
- Regulated, supervised food intake during meal times to gain control over weight and eating; limited access to bathroom to prevent vomiting
- Psychotherapy to improve personality maladjustment and self-esteem
- Family therapy to explore dysfunctional relationships, focus on father
- Peer and support groups to foster age-appropriate functioning
- Pharmacotherapy for bulimic symptoms and comorbid disorder

Pharmacotherapy
- Monoamine oxidase inhibitors: phenelzine sulfate, tranylcypromine
- Other antidepressant drugs: tricyclics, fluoxetine

more seriously disturbed patients, who cannot or will not agree to weight maintenance, regular meals, or monitoring truthfully their eating behavior (provided that they still want treatment), psychological treatment needs to be combined with medication to address the psychiatric disorder, as well as with group treatment and, if feasible, family therapy.

Drug treatment

Drug absorption in BN patients is unpredictable due to habitual vomiting and diuretic or laxative abuse. This might explain why monoamine oxidase inhibitors (MAOIs), which bind irreversibly to the enzyme, have been found to reduce binging/vomiting frequency if taken regularly in recommended doses (Walsh et al., 1984). Similarly, the long half-life of fluoxetine and its metabolite norfluoxetine, the only drug currently approved by the FDA for the treatment of BN, might explain its effectiveness for reducing bulimic symptoms in conventional and in higher doses. With both drugs the antibulimic effects are not solely a function af the drugs' antidepressant effects. Other antidepressants, such as the tricyclic drugs, have been shown to reduce bulimia in short-term drug trials. Most experts agree that psychological treatments, including group and family therapy, need to be combined with drug treatment (Mitchell et al., 1990) to achieve significant and long-lasting improvement or remission of severe bulimic behavior and to help the patient experience greater emotional stability through mutually caring personal relationships.

Outcome from bulimia nervosa

Although BN is at least four times more prevalent than AN, its outcome is just beginning to be investigated. In a 10-year follow-up of 50 BN patients who were originally involved in a study with the antidepressant Mianserin, 52 percent had recovered fully, 39 percent had some symptoms, and 9 percent continued with the full syndrome (Collings and King, 1994). In a prospective 5.8-year reassessment of 89 BN outpatients by Fairburn et al. (1995), 46 percent still met criteria for an eating disorder but few had signs of other psychiatric disorders. The outcome for those who had received cognitive therapy or focused interpersonal therapy was markedly better than for those who had received behavior therapy. Premorbid and paternal obesity predicted a poor outcome. Another 5-year follow-up of 32 out of 50 BN clinic patients found being in a satisfactory stable relationship, having a fulfilling social life, and being in a higher occupational class independently related to a good outcome, defined as no bulimic behavior or at a frequency of less than monthly (Reiss and Johnson-Sabine, 1995).

Conclusions

Dieting in the form of deliberate semistarvation or intermittent food abstinence, which has reached epidemic proportions in the United States, appears to account for the rise in disordered eating and eating disorders in the Western world. AN, well documented as a nosologic entity for centuries, remains uncommon. Without intervention AN perverts life processes and takes on a progressively fatal course. Prolonged self-starvation and weight loss are the sine qua non for triggering AN. So far our knowledge about other factors that contribute to the acquired and/or innate susceptibility to AN is limited. In a culture that values thinness in women, being female, undergoing puberty and adolescence, having a low self-esteem, and having personality features of overcontrol, rigidity, and perfectionism increase chances that dieting will be used for self-improvement. It is conceivable, although there is no firm evidence, that some of the starvation-induced endocrine adaptations abet the core psychopathologic processes in AN. Paradoxically, in the presence of widespread physiologic, metabolic, and endocrine signs consistent with the emaciation,

AN patients retain a remarkable physical and mental energy that supports their anxious desire for bodily sameness and their dread of fatness.

From an endocrine perspective, virtually every hormonal system undergoes energy-sparing adaptations in AN. The underweight and undernourished body regresses to prepuberty with low or absent circulating gonadal hormones. The body's excessive exposure to glucocorticoids, which are overproduced and too slowly degraded, bears some similarity to changes seen under severe stress and in depression. Thyroid economy is altered to the sick euthyroid syndrome in terms of TSH secretion, but signs of hypothyroidism, dry skin, a low basal metabolic rate, bradycardia, and hypercholesterolemia suggest that the metabolic impact of thyroid hormones in peripheral tissues is decreased. Many more hormonal alterations, among them in human growth hormone, melatonin, and vasopressin, have been recorded. AN patients bear a heavy cost for the exposure to starvation. Follow-up studies have shown that by fixing their whole being on a single interest, even those 30–40 percent who recover fully, physically and psychologically, pay dearly with a disruption of their lives for many years. In chronic cases an unremitting lifelong obsession with thinness ensues and emotional and psychological development comes to a standstill, even though study and work performance might remain high. In a few the arrest in physical maturation leads to stunted growth. Outcome studies after 20 years show a significant mortality rate.

Dieting for body weight and shape control also precedes the development of BN, a disorder four to five times more prevalent than AN. Its symptoms, recorded under various names such as kynorexia, can be traced to antiquity. Failure to maintain dietary restraint eventually leads to an overwhelming desire for food and binge eating, terminated usually by vomiting. Once established, this cycle of over- and underconsumption seems to trigger psychological and physiologic processes that interfere with satiety and facilitate binge eating. Not only do intermittent abstention and the loss of food through vomiting disrupt satiation, the sense of deprivation leads to food being regarded, cognitively and emotionally, as a quick, albeit fleeting, remedy for distressing feeling states. Many studies have established a link between psychopathology and the frequency and severity of bulimic behavior. The negative energy balance as a result of the irregular food intake and loss of food through vomiting produces usually less extensive and less pronounced endocrine changes similar to those observed in AN.

CHAPTER EIGHT

CORONARY ARTERY DISEASE AND WOMEN

ESTROGENS AND PSYCHOSOCIAL AND LIFESTYLE RISK FACTORS

JOAN M. FAIR, KATHLEEN A. BERRA,
AND REGINA C. CASPER

Cardiovascular disease is the leading cause of death in women as it is in men. The lower incidence of coronary artery disease (CAD) in young and middle-aged women compared to men has unfortunately led to the exclusion of women from nearly all randomized controlled studies on risk factors, treatment, and outcome from coronary heart disease (CHD). To make matters worse, when the protective effects of endogenous estrogen in women were recognized, high doses of estrogen were given to male survivors of myocardial infarction in the Coronary Drug Project, resulting in a high incidence of coronary and thromboembolic complications in the estrogen-treated men (Coronary Drug Project Research Group, 1973). The recent identification of different forms of estrogen that bind to different types of receptors in the heart, bone, and reproductive organs is beginning to finally offer an explanation for this calamity (Mack and Ross, 1989; Washburn et al., 1993; Auchus and Fuqua, 1994).

Incidence and prevalence in women and men

Before the age of 60, CHD affects women about half as often as men. Among women aged 55–65, mortality rates from CHD triple compared to those aged 45–55 (U.S. Department of Health and Human Services), and after the seventh decade, the rate of CHD for women equals that of men (Orencia et al., 1993). Of the more than half a million persons who die each year from heart disease, almost half are women (Packard and Eaker, 1987), and they incur 58 percent of the health care costs related to CHD (Eaker et al., 1994). Hospitalization rates for CHD account for 10 percent of the primary hospital discharge diagnoses for women aged 45–64 years and for 20 percent after age 65 (Pagley and Goldberg, 1995). Because women outlive men in the United States by an average of 7 years, they tend to incur a disproportionate burden of CHD disability and health care costs (Kinsella, 1992). In spite of these alarming statistics, most women erroneously perceive their risk of heart disease to be low (Pilote and Hlatky, 1995). The proportion of women in the United States 45 years of age and older is expected to rise to 38 percent of the population by the year 2000 and to 45 percent by the year 2015. These numbers provide a compelling reason to collect more information about those risk factors that contribute to coronary disease and treatment outcome in women. Table 8.1 highlights some of the known facts and gender differences related to CHD.

Recognition, diagnosis, and management

Not only health professionals but women themselves tend to perceive angina pectoris as a benign problem, even though women are more likely to experience angina and atypical chest pain syndromes and to report more symptoms of fatigue, dyspnea, and disability than men (Murabito et al., 1990; Nickel and Chirikos, 1990; Pinsky et al., 1990; Wiklund et al., 1993). Angina with angiographically normal coronary arteries (Prinzmetal), which carries a favorable prognosis, is more common among women than among men (Scholl et al., 1988). Nonetheless, women have a higher rate of early death and subsequent heart attacks after myocardial infarction than do men (Kannel and Abbot, 1987). There is increasing evidence that women undergo diagnostic procedures and receive treatment substantially less often than men. Women are less likely to be admitted to intensive care monitoring units (Green and Ruffin, 1993), to receive coronary angiograms or bypass surgery (Steingart, Packer, and Hamm,

Table 8.1. *Gender and heart disease facts*

1. Within 6 years after a heart attack
   - 23 percent of men and 31 percent of women will have another heart attack.
   - 9 percent of men and 18 percent of women will have a stroke.
   - 20 percent of men and women will be disabled with heart failure.
2. In 1992
   - 48.1 percent of cardiovascular deaths occurred in men and 51.9 percent in women.
   - All cardiovascular diseases combined accounted for 479,000 female deaths. Cancer accounted for 246,000 deaths.
   - Death from stroke was 77.3 percent higher in black females compared to white females.
3. Coronary heart disease
   - Is more frequent in the least educated.
   - Death rates are 32.6 percent higher in black females compared to white females.
   - 27 percent of men and 44 percent of women will die within 1 year after having a heart attack.
   - At older ages women who have a heart attack are twice as likely as men to die within a few weeks.

Source: American Heart Association, 1996.

1991), and to participate in cardiac rehabilitation programs (Boogaard, 1984), and they are at least two to ten times less likely to undergo cardiac catheterization (Ayanian and Epstein, 1991). A lower rate of diagnostic evaluation would be expected to lead to delayed referral for coronary artery bypass surgery and potentially more severe disease at the time of myocardial infarction or cardiac arrest, and may account for the higher in-hospital mortality rates observed in women who undergo coronary angioplasty and bypass surgery (Bickell et al., 1992). Certainly, other factors – the smaller diameter of the coronary arteries in women, their older age, and coexisting hypertension or diabetes mellitus – contribute to the excess mortality.

Women are also less frequently advised to take daily aspirin, but are more frequently prescribed diuretic medications (Wenger, Speroff, and Packard, 1993). These prescription differences may be explained in part by the fact that the use of aspirin as a secondary preventive measure for CHD has shown proven effectiveness in double blind studies in middle-aged men, whereas the data on outcome in women are still outstanding (Hennekens, Buring, and Sandercock, 1989). Because women do not generally present with symptoms of CHD until their mid-60s, few, if any, have been included in clinical trials. Several studies in women have now been initiated by the federal government and the National Institutes of Health (NIH) in response to public and scientific appeals for more information and research on women's health issues. (Mastroianni, Faden, and Federman, 1994).

What do we know about coronary risk factors and women?

Since women have been included in trials, coronary risk factors similar to those for men have emerged, even though the onset of clinical coronary heart disease is delayed by 10–20 years in women compared to men (Wenger, 1985). This delay is thought to be due in part to the protective effects of premenopausal endogenous female hormones. Increasing age combined with postmenopausal status are hallmarks of rising CHD risk in women.

Of the coronary risk factors shared by men and women, cigarette smoking remains the major treatable cause of increased risk. Smoking has been found to be a serious risk factor for myocardial infarction and sudden cardiac death in young women (Myers et al., 1987). There is an alarming synergism for young women between cigarette smoking and oral contraceptive use, increasing CHD risk fivefold (American Heart Association, 1996) Cardiovascular risk is greatly reduced if women, especially young women, stop smoking, although cultural trends go in the opposite direction, showing a 31 percent increase in the number of young female smokers in the United States since 1965 (Eaker, Packard, and Thom, 1989).

Other risk factors, such as low-density lipoprotein (LDL) and high-density lipoprotein (HDL) cholesterol, differ in women compared to men, not solely because estrogens affect the lipid profile (Bush, Fried, and Barrett-Connor, 1988). At least two subspecies of HDL have been identified based on apolipro-tein composition. HDL_2 has higher levels of apoprotein AI (ApoAI), whereas HDL_3 has higher levels of apoliprotein AII (ApoAII). ApoAI acts to increase lipoprotein catabolism and enhances the removal of atherogenic LDL particles from the circulation. Subspecies of the HDL containing both ApoAI and ApoAII (AI:AII) convey higher CAD risk than the subspecies containing AI without AII. Women have higher concentrations of apolipoprotein AI but not of AI:II (Fruchart, Ailhaud, and Bard, 1993). An increased level of HDL cho-lesterol is a particularly strong predictor of a reduced risk of CHD in women (Jacobs et al., 1990). Cholesterol-lowering studies have concluded that LDL cholesterol is a strong risk factor for the development of CHD in men (Lipid Research Clinics Program, 1984; Gordon, Knoke, and Probstfield, 1986), but a relatively weaker risk factor for women, based on the Lipid Research Clinics

Prevalence Data and the Framingham Observational Trial (Lipid Research Clinics Program, 1984; Gordon, Knoke, and Probstfield, 1986; Kannel, 1987), perhaps because LDL cholesterol levels are low in premenopausal women. In contrast, both studies identified low HDL cholesterol as an important risk factor for women. The National Cholesterol Education Adult Treatment Panel II (NCEP II, 1993) recognizes low HDL cholesterol (<35 mg/dl) as a risk factor for both women and men.

Prior to NCEP II, "being male" was considered a risk factor. In NCEP II, age replaced gender as a coronary risk factor. Men are now designated at risk after their 45th year and women after their 55th year. This change recognizes the risk of CHD death and disability in older postmenopausal women. Similar considerations apply to calculating the risk from family history data. For instance, having a first-degree male relative who develops CHD before the age of 55 or a first-degree female relative who develops CHD before the age of 65 increases the risk of developing CHD.

Women with diabetes mellitus are at high risk for the development of CHD (Kannel, 1987; Abbott et al., 1988). Premenopausal women with diabetes lose their apparent protection from endogenous estrogens and, as men do, develop clinical CHD at a significantly earlier age (Gordon, Castelli, and Hjortland, 1977). High triglycerides, commonly found in the presence of diabetes, have been shown independently to predict CHD in women (Lipid Research Clinics Program, 1984; Walsh et al., 1991). Elevated triglycerides are associated with small, dense, atherogenic LDL cholesterol molecules and with a downregulation of HDL cholesterol, thereby further adding to CHD risk (Austin, 1989; Barrett-Connor, 1994).

Obesity and physical inactivity convey an equal risk for CHD in women and men. Women who are obese, especially if they carry fat on the upper body (truncal type or male pattern obesity), are more likely to have high blood pressure, high triglycerides, low HDL cholesterol, and diabetes, and to die from CHD compared to women of equal weight whose adiposity is carried on their hips and thighs (Kissebah et al., 1982). Two measures of obesity, Body Mass Index (BMI)[1] and Waist to Hip ratio (W:H),[2] are useful in evaluating CHD risk. In women with a BMI above 27 kg/m^2 and a W:H ratio above 0.80, the risk for CHD rises steeply (Lapidus et al., 1984).

Hypertension is a major risk factor for both CHD and stroke for women. In women and men, systolic blood pressure is strongly associated with increased risk

[1] BMI = weight in kg/height in meters squared.
[2] W:H = waist measured in cm:hip measured in cm at the widest point.

of acute myocardial infarction as well as cardiovascular mortality (Brezinka and Padmos, 1994). Hypertension is a potent risk factor for young black females, especially in the presence of diabetes (Maynard et al., 1993). Women who drink more than two glasses of alcohol per day and women smokers who have higher blood pressures than their nondrinking and nonsmoking counterparts increase their risk (Leer, Seidell, and Kromhout, 1994). These findings apply equally to men.

Interesting work has recently been reported on the influence of race and gender on blood pressure. Psychological and social states appear to be strong predictors of hypertension among women of all races and ethnicity; moreover, high blood pressure is more prevalent in persons with lower educational and income levels (American Heart Association, 1996). Ewert and Kolonder (1994) demonstrated in black and white adolescent students that trait effects of depression and anger predicted blood pressure levels. This prediction persisted after accounting for obesity, smoking, and alcohol use. Kreiger (1990) reported a positive correlation between internalized anger, measured as responses to unfair treatment plus failure to mention race and gender discrimination, as a risk factor for hypertension in black women. The American Heart Association (AHA, 1996) reports that black, Puerto Rican, Cuban, and Hispanic women are more likely to be overweight and develop high blood pressure than white women. In 1992, 58 percent of all deaths from high blood pressure in women occurred in black women.

A sedentary lifestyle is considered a risk factor for women and for men. Observational studies suggest that not only cardiovascular but all cause mortality is inversely related to levels of physical fitness (Blair et al., 1989; Blair, Kohl, and Barlow, 1993). Even modest exercise can improve physiologic parameters. Owens and co-workers (1992) examined the effects of exercise on aging in middle-aged women as part of the Healthy Women's Study. Women without clinical CHD who were more physically active at baseline gained the least amount of weight over the 3 years of the study. Women who increased their activity level, even a modest amount, showed the smallest decrease in HDL cholesterol, and women who increased their activity the most during the 3 years had the smallest increase in depression and stress scores over time. Women with clinical CHD who participated in cardiac rehabilitation programs showed improvements in exercise capacity and quality of life measures similar to those of male participants (Lavie and Milani, 1995), even though they had lower baseline scores than men for exercise capacity, function, energy, and total quality of life. The authors added that women may have the most to gain from participation in cardiac rehabilitation programs (Lavie and Milani, 1995).

Food high in saturated fat, high in cholesterol, and low in fiber is associated with a greater risk for CHD in both men and women (NCEP II, 1993).

Reductions in saturated fat and cholesterol have been shown to retard the angiographic progression of CHD, and total elimination of fat from the diet can in some cases result in regression of atherosclerotic lesions (Ornish et al., 1990; Schuler et al., 1992; Watts et al., 1992; Haskell et al., 1994).

Does hormone replacement therapy prevent coronary heart disease in women?

The lower CHD risk in premenopausal women has been attributed to the beneficial effects of estrogen on lipoprotein profiles. Furthermore, levels of reproductive hormones affect the magnitude of stress responses. During pregnancy blood pressure responses to psychological and physical challenges are diminished (Matthews et al., 1989), and premenopausal women have lower stress-induced increases in systolic and diastolic blood pressure than men or postmenopausal women. (Owens et al., 1992).

In postmenopausal women, estrogen replacement therapy (ERT) reduces LDL cholesterol and raises HDL cholesterol by approximately 15 percent (Cauley et al., 1983), and lipid profiles more closely resemble premenopausal values (Writing Group for the PEPI Trial, 1995). This study, one of the first randomized placebo-controlled double blind trials, evaluated the influence of a variety of hormone replacement therapy (HRT) regimes on several physiologic parameters and showed that estrogen alone provides greater benefit to lipid profiles than a combination of estrogen and progestin. Unfortunately, estrogen given alone increases the chances of developing endometrial hyperplasia, which is associated with a 33 percent increased risk of endometrial cancer. For this reason, women with an intact uterus require the estrogen/progestin combination in order to mimic physiologic hormone exposure and to induce periodic withdrawal bleeding. The short duration of the study and the relatively young age of its participants did not provide data to assess the incidence of CHD and all cause mortality. Atherogenic apolipoproteins such as Lp(a) would be reduced with ERT (Soma et al., 1993), and in animal studies, ERT decreases lipid accumulation in arterial walls (Wagner et al., 1991).

Long-term studies in women on ERT have found a lower mortality rate from CHD compared to women not taking estrogens. A recent meta-analysis reported a relative risk of myocardial infarction of 0.56 (95 percent CI, 0.050 to 0.061) for ERT users compared to nonusers (Grady et al., 1992). Another piece of evidence is data from the Nurses' Health Study, which have shown that estrogen reduces the risk of severe CHD (Stampfer et al., 1985).

Alterations of vasomotor responses following ERT may be related to cardio-vascular perfusion. In both human and animal studies, coronary and peripheral vascular reactivity responses to vasodilators such as acetylcholine and nitric oxide differ based on estrogen status (Williams, Adams, and Klopfenstein, 1990; Mugge et al., 1993; Collins et al., 1994; Gilligan et al., 1994, 1995). Forearm blood flow and peripheral vascular resistance have been evaluated in women fol-lowing an acute infusion of 17-beta estradiol and following 3 weeks of transder-mal 17-beta estradiol therapy (Gilligan et al., 1994, 1995). Compared to base-line measures, acute estrogen infusion resulted in increased blood flow and decreased peripheral vascular resistance. Animal studies have shown little differ-ence in coronary diameters following acetylcholine infusion in ovarectomized monkeys treated with 26 months of 17-beta estradiol (Williams, Adams, and Klopfenstein, 1990). By contrast, when ovarectomized monkeys did not receive estrogen replacement, acetylcholine infusion produced significant vasoconstric-tion. The data suggest that estrogen use modulates vasoconstrictor responses, perhaps by enhancing endothelial-dependent dilating mechanisms.

Only a few studies have examined the effect of HRT on measures of myocar-dial ischemia. A study of women with CAD, who were given sublingual 17-beta estradiol immediately prior to exercise testing, found that 17-beta estra-diol improved measures of exercise ischemia (Rosano et al., 1993). Time to 1-mm ST segment depression (indicative of myocardial ischemia) and time to peak exercise (indicative of functional capacity) were increased in the estrogen-treated group as compared to the placebo group, suggesting that acute estrogen use favorably influences exercise test responses.

Social support, social networks, coronary heart disease, and women

Social factors such as living alone and social isolation have been linked to increased CHD morbidity and mortality (Case et al., 1992; Williams et al., 1992). For both women and men, no or few social ties increase the mortality risk twofold (Berkman, Vaccarino, and Seeman, 1993). Widowed men experi-ence increased morbidity and mortality, whereas widowed women do not (Hels-ing, Szklo, and Comstock, 1981; Stroebe and Stroebe, 1983; Berkman, Vac-carino, and Seeman, 1993). It has been speculated that women cope more easily with the loss of a spouse because women are more likely to be close to other family members and more likely to have relationships with other widowed women (Baum and Grunberg, 1991). Because women live approximately 7 to

10 years longer than men and tend to marry men older than themselves, women with CHD are likely to live alone longer. A prospective study of elderly myocardial infarction patients found that a lack of emotional support was a stronger predictor of mortality in both men and women than was living alone or being unmarried (Berkman, Leo-Summers, and Horwitz, 1992).

Socioeconomic status, heart disease, and women

Low socioeconomic status (SES) has negative health outcomes for both women and men. A recent study of Finnish men used carotid ultrasound to examine the association of carotid intimal thickening and SES (Lynch et al., 1995). A significant graded inverse association of SES and amount of intimal atherosclerosis was observed. This held true whether SES was measured as occupation, income, or education and persisted after controlling for traditional coronary risk factors. In the U.S. population, the least educated women have up to 80 percent higher CHD mortality rates than do women with some college education (LaCroix, 1994). In a study of middle-aged women residing in Allegheny County, Matthews et al. (1989) found that the less education the women reported, the higher their blood pressure, LDL cholesterol, triglycerides, apolipoprotein B, glucose and insulin levels, body mass index, and cigarette consumption, and the lower their HDL cholesterol and exercise level.

Type A behavior, psychosocial status, coronary heart disease, and women

The Type A behavior pattern, a constellation of behaviors and personality characteristics of impatience, time urgency, competitive job overinvolvement, anger, and hostility related to an increased incidence of CHD, was originally identified in men (Friedman and Rosenman, 1959). Within this construct, hostility and anger expression have emerged as key dimensions (Booth-Kewley and Friedman, 1987; Helmer, Ragland, and Syme, 1991; Smith, 1992). A meta-analysis of 16 early research studies identified specific Type A behaviors associated with CHD outcomes (Booth-Kewley and Friedman, 1987). The correlations ranged from −0.02 for job involvement to 0.19 for behaviors categorized as hard-driving or aggressive. Hostility measures had the largest effect size across all studies, with correlations ranging from 0.14 to 0.21. When the four studies including women were combined, the observed effect size of 0.27 for

Type A and CHD suggested that this relationship is at least as strong in women as it is in men.

The Framingham study represents the only longitudinal study to include gender comparisons of Type A behaviors and CHD morbidity and mortality (Haynes et al., 1978; Haynes and Feinleib, 1980; Eaker, Pinsky, and Castelli, 1992). The initial cross-sectional analysis was performed separately for women and men and compared cases (those with CHD) to noncases (those without CHD). The CHD cases scored higher than controls on the Type A behavior scale. For women in the age group of 45–64 years the difference between cases and controls was significant ($P < 0.01$), whereas in women older than 65, no significant differences were found. An 8-year follow-up analyzed differences between working women and housewives (Haynes and Feinleib, 1980). In this analysis, CHD incidence did not differ in working women as compared to housewives. However, women with clerical jobs (i.e., in subordinate positions) were almost twice as likely to have CHD (10.6 vs. 5.4 percent, $P < 0.06$). The most significant predictors of CHD in clerical workers included suppressed hostility ($P < 0.05$), a nonsupportive boss ($P < 0.01$), and decreased job mobility, measured as job changes over the past 10 years ($P < 0.01$). Using multivariate techniques to control for traditional risk factors, a 20-year follow-up showed that symptoms of anxiety and tension were associated with increased CHD risk (RR = 2.9, CI = 1.3–6.8) (Eaker, Pinsky, and Castelli, 1992). Among homemakers, only loneliness and lack of vacations predicted risk of CHD events (RR = 4.0, CI = 1.8–9.2; RR = 16.2, CI = 1.9–135 respectively). The authors suggest that these predictors indicate a coronary-prone situation, where homemakers report loneliness and tension due to lack of perceived options to change the situation. Judging from the Framingham data, anger suppression seems to be an important risk dimension for women. Observations that Type A housewives reported less self-esteem, more marital disharmony, and greater tension and physical health problems (Houston and Kelly, 1986) suggest that Type A behavior in part represents a coping style in response to psychosocial pressures. This interpretation is supported by a review by Booth-Kewley and Friedman (1987), who suggested that the person likely to develop CHD is characterized by one or more negative emotions.

Reactivity testing in association with hostility surveys has been studied in an attempt to link physiologic, behavioral, and emotional responses. Reviews of this literature point to different cardiovascular responses for women as opposed to men (Thoresen and Graff-Low, 1990; Dimsdale, 1993). Men appear to have greater blood pressure responses to reactivity testing than women (Burns and Katkin, 1993; Lawler et al., 1993), whereas women may have a greater heart rate response (Girdler et al., 1990; Allen et al., 1993). In a study of 48 men and 48 women, reactivity was measured by blood pressure and heart rate response to a timed forced choice test conducted under a harassment condition or a social evaluation condition. The harassment condition is hypothesized to result in expressive anger on hostility surveys and to raise heart rate and blood pressure responses. No interaction between assessments of expressed anger (Cook-Medley Hostility Inventory) and cardiovascular reactivity was found for women, and in men reactivity was associated with the harassment condition only.

In a study that directly compared reactivity in a group of men and women who had CHD, hostility surveys were performed prior to thallium exercise testing and ambulatory monitoring to determine if hostility and gender were associated with ischemic responses (Helmers et al., 1993). In female patients only, hostility scores were significantly associated with the frequency of ischemia and the total number of minutes of ischemia determined by ambulatory monitoring (r^2 = 0.51 and 0.90 respectively, P < 0.05). In contrast, the thallium measures of ischemia did not relate significantly to the hostility scores. These data suggest a relationship between hostility and CHD ischemia in women with established CHD, but they do not permit a prediction of risk for CHD development because insufficient evidence was provided to determine whether disease severity was similar for women and men. It is conceivable that increased severity of CHD and symptom experience may be the triggering factors eliciting the hostility responses in women. It has also been suggested that Type A behavior is a masculine construct and does not capture the emotional repertoire of women (Friedman and Booth-Kewley, 1987; Thoresen and Graff-Low, 1990). In an investigation that included an equal number of men and women from the Family Heart Study, in a 5-year dietary intervention program, the relationship between Type A behavioral measures and total and HDL cholesterol was significant for men but marginal for women. However, when hostility was examined separately, strong significant relationships were found in both men and women (Weidner et al., 1987). Education and depression may be other critical variables because in less educated women a higher atherogenic risk profile was associated with greater depression and less social support, yet fewer Type A behaviors (Matthews et al., 1989).

An important observation was reported in the meta-analysis of Type A behavior and CHD by Booth-Kewley and Friedman (1987). By combining the results from three studies that included depression measures, an effect size of 0.20 was found for depression and CHD. This effect size was as high as those found for Type A behavior and for hostility. Such observations suggest that the effect of psychosocial responses on CHD cannot be evaluated without considering other measures of emotional distress, among them depression.

Negative emotional states, depression, coronary heart disease, and women

A growing body of literature suggests that expression of emotion and experience of emotional distress are associated with disease outcomes (Fielding, 1991; Adler and Matthews, 1994; Scheier and Bridges, 1995). Of course, in some women, chest pain and tachycardia may be the somatic manifestations of depressive and anxiety disorders. Within the cardiovascular literature, negative emotional states such as depression and anxiety have been linked to adverse CHD outcomes following a myocardial infarction or bypass surgery (Carney et al., 1988; Schleifer et al., 1989; Lesperance, Frasure-Smith, and Talajic, 1995). After controlling for indicators of disease severity, patients with major depression were three to four times more likely to die within the first year following a myocardial infarction (MI) compared to those with mild or no depression (Frasure-Smith, Lesperance, and Talajic, 1993). As with most cardiovascular studies, the number of women included in this study was not sufficient to conduct gender comparisons. In the general population, in age groups comparable to the CHD population, the prevalence of depression is estimated at 6 percent, with the rates in women more than double those for men (Weissman and Klerman, 1977; Greenberg et al., 1993). Depression is significantly more prevalent in the CHD population, where the rate of clinical depression can be as high as 24.6 percent among women and 13.3 percent in men (Frasure-Smith, Lesperance, and Talajic, 1993).

If women with CHD experience more psychosocial distress than men, their social disadvantage may offer one reason. A study by Powell et al. (1993) provides evidence linking social position to adverse CHD outcomes in post-MI women. In this study, being divorced and being employed without a college degree were univariate predictors of premature CHD mortality (RR = 6.9, P = 0.003). In multivariate analysis, divorce and in a negative association the personality trait "time urgency" remained significant predictors for mortality. The authors suggest that the unexpected finding of an inverse relationship between time urgency and mortality may be explained if low time urgency is a marker for malaise or fatigue associated with symptoms of CHD. Chesney (1993), in an editorial accompanying the study by Powell and colleagues, proposes that the inverse relationship with time urgency suggests a lack of emotional arousal or withdrawal, which would be consistent with a state of depression. Interestingly, social support has been shown to reduce blood pressures and heart rates in normotensive women exposed to a high-stress condition (Gerin et al., 1995). Conversely, cynomologus monkeys separated from their social groups and housed in single cages had significantly more coronary artery atherosclerosis that those housed in social groups (Shively et al., 1989). The fact that such monkeys often react with agitation and behavioral depression to social isolation points to depression as one of the mediating variables.

More research is needed to determine whether depressive disorder per se is a risk factor for CHD. Appels and Mulder (1988) described a rise in cardiovascular death in the year following a diagnosis of "vital exhaustion" in men, which could conceivably have been an undiagnosed depressive disorder. Talbott et al. (1977) noted a sixfold increase in sudden cardiac death during the first half-year following the death of a spouse.

In an extension of this study, the population of MI women (n = 83) was compared to a group of randomly selected healthy women (n = 73) in order to evaluate the contribution of depression, anxiety, and Type A behavior to subsequent CHD events (Graff-Low et al., 1994). CHD women had significantly higher anxiety, depression, and hostility scores than healthy control women. Among the post-MI women with complete follow-up data (n = 65), total anxiety score and time urgency correlated with subsequent events (r = 0.28, P < 0.01 and r = −0.22, P < 0.05 respectively). A study of 173 post-MI men and 49 post-MI women similarly observed that both anxiety and depression were independent predictors of CHD events (Frasure-Smith, Lesperance, and Talajic, 1995). Negative emotional states such as anxiety and depression may therefore be predictive of adverse outcomes in both women and men. Further studies are needed to determine the mechanisms through which negative emotional states influence CHD outcomes.

The effectiveness of coronary risk reduction strategies in women

Several angiographic clinical trials have examined the effect of lifestyle and risk reduction interventions on the progression and regression of CAD (see Table 8.2). Studies that included women have found that women and men equally benefit from interventions (Kane et al., 1990; Haskell et al.; 1994, Waters et al., 1995). Two studies used a lipid-lowering medication intervention, and one used a multifactor lifestyle and medication intervention. The rate of CAD progression observed in untreated women who served as controls was approximately twice that of the treatment groups and was similar to the rates observed in men. Table 8.3 shows angiographic changes in two studies that used similar angiographic end-point measurements but had differing lengths of follow-up. In both studies, lipid therapy medication and multifac-

Table 8.2. *Changes in lifestyle that have been documented to reduce the risk of coronary heart disease*

Intervention	Estimated mean reduction in risk
Smoking cessation	70% within 3 to 5 years
Avoidance of obesity	50%
Increased aerobic exercise	80%
Reduction in caffeine	Unknown
Moderate alchohol use	Unknown
Postmenopausal estrogens	44%
Aspirin, 100 mg alternate days	Under study
Stress reduction, relaxation	50%
Treatment of depression	Unknown
Social and group support	Unknown

torial risk reduction reduced the rate of CAD progression by 35 to 50 percent, regardless of gender.

Lipid-lowering medications, therefore, seem to be as effective in women as in men (Bradford et al., 1993). Feasibility studies have found that women adopt and maintain low-fat and low-cholesterol diets. For example, among 144 women randomized to a diet of less than 20 percent of calories from fat, 70 percent reached this goal within 3 months and maintained this diet for 3 years (Bowen et al., 1994). Men appear to have more success than women in entering and maintaining exercise programs, although among women who stay in cardiac rehabilitation programs, the improvements in physiologic measures of exercise

Table 8.3. *Angiographic change in minimal coronary diameters[a] in women*

Angiographic measure	Women		Men	
	Treatment	Control	Treatment	Control
CCAIT[b] average minimum diameter change over 24-month follow-up	–0.05	–0.09	–0.05	–0.10
SCRIP[c] average annual minimum diameter change	–0.016	–0.046	–0.026	–0.045

[a] Change in minimum diameter = follow-up minus baseline diameters in mm (a larger negative number indicates more progression).

[b] CCAIT, Canadian Coronary Atherosclerosis Trial (Waters et al., 1995).

[c] SCRIP, Stanford Risk Intervention Project (Haskell et al., 1994).

capacity and cardiac function are of similar magnitude to those observed in men (Ades et al., 1992; Cannistra et al., 1992; Lavie and Milani, 1995). Women do have higher dropout rates from exercise programs and lower attendance rates than men (O'Callaghan et al., 1984; Schuster and Waldron, 1991; Ades et al., 1992), and they report more guilt feelings about the time spent on recovery versus performing their normal roles when compared to men (Boogaard, 1984). Differences in expectations, beliefs, and attitudes about exercise may explain some of the differences in exercise adoption between men and women. For example, some women do not like physical exercise and the accompanying sensations of sweating and shortness of breath. Other predictors for women include years of education, family support, support from friends, and a lower BMI. Predictors for men include age, neighborhood environment, and cigarette smoking (Sallis, Hovell, and Hofstetter, 1992). Research on health concepts found that women emphasized the importance of diet, appearance, and caring for or love of friends and family, whereas men emphasized physical performance, work performance, and control over their body (Saltonstall, 1993). It follows that measures aimed at prevention, which would include changes in lifestyle, need to consider gender differences in health concepts and values.

Conclusions

Disease prevention starts with the recognition of health risks by health care professionals and by women themselves. In the case of CAD, widely held misconceptions about women's resilience to CHD need to be modified. Chest pain in women always warrants a thorough diagnostic evaluation. Although CAD is less common and occurs at a later age in women, women have the same and some unique risk factors for the development of CHD. Cigarette smoking carries increased hazards, especially in young women who take oral contraceptives, a combination that promotes thrombogenesis. Overweight occurs more often in women and tends to be associated with hypertension and non-insulin-dependent diabetes mellitus, each risk factors for CHD. There is increasing evidence that the coronary-prone Type A pattern of behaving and coping, especially hostility and time urgency, are as predictive of CHD development for women as they are for men. Additional features identified in women are repressed hostility and depression. It appears that the overall lower social status of women, their social isolation following divorce and separation, and ultimately their longevity increase the risk for CHD. On the positive side, social support, in particular under conditions of high stress, has been shown to reduce blood pressure and heart rate responses in women. Estrogen replacement therapy favorably influences important coronary risk factors, such as LDL cholesterol and HDL cholesterol and appears to modulate cardiovascular responses to exercise and stress. Finally, more research will be needed to understand the basic mechanisms underlying the development of CAD and how reproductive homones or psychosocial factors reduce the risk of CAD.

Education about cardiovascular disease will hopefully motivate the young generation of women to initiate health-related behavioral changes early and encourage all women to seek timely health care in response to symptoms suggestive of CAD.

CHAPTER NINE

THE PSYCHOPHYSIOLOGY OF BREAST CANCER

DISEASE, HORMONES, IMMUNITY, AND STRESS

SARA L. STEIN, KAYE HERMANSON,
AND DAVID SPIEGEL

Introduction

Breast cancer is a major public health problem in the United States, with an estimated 182,000 new cases occurring in women in 1994. It is the leading cause of cancer death among women 54 years of age or younger and overall accounts for 18 percent of female cancer deaths (Boring et al., 1994). At the time of diagnosis, in 47 percent of women with breast cancer the disease has spread to the lymph nodes or beyond, compared with 72 percent of those with ovarian cancer. Early detection of both diseases may allow for cure in up to 95 percent of breast cancers (Tabar et al., 1992) and 90 percent of ovarian cancers (Young et al., 1990a).

For most women, a diagnosis of breast cancer marks the beginning of a life-long struggle. The disease and treatments become physical-psychological stressors whose effects linger long after the individual is tumor-free. The effects are often widespread. Breast cancer is associated with anxiety and depression, not only in those who are affected but in their families and loved ones as well (Holland, 1989). Newer studies in animals indicate that marked stress can shift the neuroendocrine axis. For example, increases in cortisol levels are associated in animals with more rapid tumor growth (Sapolsky and Donnelly, 1985; Ben-Eliyahu et al., 1991). Effects of stress on components of the immune system that are associated with cancer progression, such as natural killer cells (Levy et al., 1987), have also been documented (Kennedy, Kiecolt-Glaser, and Glaser, 1988). In some studies, serious life stress such as bereavement or job loss has been found to be associated with higher risk of relapse of breast cancer (Ramirez, 1989). The implications of this mind–body connection in breast cancer include the possibility that if stress can activate a hormonal response that leads to immunosuppression and possibly tumor progression, can relief of stress modify or even reverse the process?

These issues are explored systematically in this chapter. In discussing "breast cancer" we refer to the overall process of this illness rather than the tumor alone, a process that includes risk, treatment, disease, and psychosocial implications. The majority of studies cited in this chapter are taken from the vast literature on breast cancer; their results are not necessarily applicable to other gynecologic or primarily female cancers. This chapter is designed to familiarize the clinician with the experience of breast cancer, the physiologic implications of stress on tumor growth, and the possibility that stress-reducing interventions can ultimately affect survival time in cancer patients. The first section discusses the breast cancer experience, including treatment, risk, and psychological sequelae. The second section explores the effects of stress on the hormonal environment and the secondary effect on tumor kinetics. This background sets the stage for the third section, an examination of the components of psychosocial stress, interventions designed to minimize that distress (social support, emotional expression, and relaxation), and the possibility that interventions may help prolong survival time from cancer.

Psychophysiologic effects of breast cancer and treatment

In this country, 1 in 9 women will develop breast cancer in her lifetime (11 percent). An estimated 80–85 percent of breast cancer cases are "sporadic," with patients having no prior family history of the disease. Women with familial histories of breast cancer compose 20 percent of new cases, with 15 percent having one or more affected first-degree relatives (mother, sister, daughter). In women with two affected first-degree relatives, lifetime risk is elevated to 25–28 percent (Cramer et al., 1983; Love, 1989; Grover, Quinn, and Weideman, 1993).

The prognosis for breast cancer is based on a number of variables including

(1) size of tumor and spread to lymph nodes or distant metastases, (2) tumor histology and cellular differentiation, (3) hormone receptor status, and (4) age and risk status of the individual. Standard treatment for breast cancer includes varying combinations of surgical, cytotoxic, immunologic, and radiotherapies with endocrine adjuvant therapy (Castiglione-Gertsch et al., 1994). In a world-wide collaborative review of 75,000 women in 133 randomized clinical trials of adjuvant hormonal, cytotoxic, or immunotherapy treated prior to 1985, 32 percent had died of their disease and another 10 percent had recurrences (Early Breast Cancer Trialists' Collaborative Group, 1992). Newer treatments include immunotherapy and autologous bone marrow transplantation.

Exogenous hormone therapy and cancer risk

Considerable controversy exists regarding the relationship between exogenous hormone therapy and breast and endometrial cancer risk in both pre- and post-menopausal women (Colditz et al., 1995; Stanford et al., 1995). Only one third of breast cancers are accounted for by known risk factors, including hormone therapy (Krieger, 1989). In premenopausal women, the use of combination oral contraceptives may confer some protection against development of both endometrial and ovarian cancers, with mixed results regarding breast cancer (Schneider and Birkhauser, 1995; Schuurman, van den Brandt, and Goldbohm, 1995). Progestogen usage in premenopausal women with benign breast disease may be protective against breast cancer; however, different derivative forms of the hormone (such as 19-nortestosterone vs. other derivatives) may have differing cancer risk profiles according to their potencies (Plu-Bureau et al., 1994).

A review of the literature by Hulka (1994) confirms a common finding that estrogens cause cell proliferation in vitro and enhance tumor progression in animals. In postmenopausal women on hormone replacement therapy (HRT), the addition of progestin reduces the risk for endometrial cancer, which is estrogen related, but not the additional risk of breast cancer (Hulka, 1994; Schairer et al., 1994). Nonetheless, both endometrial and breast tumors formed while on HRT may be lower grade. Bonnier and colleagues (1995) noted that women on HRT developed fewer locally advanced cancers and better-differentiated tumors and had a lower incidence of receptor negative tumors.

Hormonal expression of breast tumors

Both adrenal and sex steroids have been implicated in breast cancer risk (Recchione et al., 1995; Berrino et al., 1996). In a review of women with breast cancer, Zumoff (1994) noted four patterns of endogenous hormonal production: (1) decreased adrenal androgen production in women with premenopausal breast cancer; (2) ovarian dysfunction at all ages (luteal inadequacy plus increased testosterone production); (3) increased 16 alpha-hydroxylation of estradiol; and (4) evidence that prolactin is a permissive risk factor for breast cancer. The presence of prolactin and prolactin receptors in breast epithelium suggests that an autocrine/paracrine stimulatory loop exists within malignant breast tissues (Clevenger et al., 1995). One study suggests that there may a steroid gradient across malignant breast tissue, with sex and adrenal steroids stored in the cancerous breast (Massobrio et al., 1994). Previous pelvic radiotherapy is related to a lowered breast cancer risk in both pre- and postmenopausal women, suggesting that decreases in both estrogen and ovarian androgen production may be protective (Inskip, 1994).

Estrogen antagonists

The precedent for hormonal therapy in breast cancer began a century ago with the observation that bilateral oophorectomy caused tumor regression in premenopausal breast cancer patients (Schneider, Jackisch, and Brandt, 1994). The most widely used antiestrogen agent to prevent or delay the growth of breast tumors is tamoxifen, an estradiol receptor antagonist. Currently, over 10,000 women have been enrolled in the National Surgical Adjuvant Breast and Bowel Project Breast Cancer Prevention Trial, a multicenter chemoprevention trial testing the efficacy of tamoxifen in prevention of breast cancer recurrence or development of contralateral breast cancer (Ganz et al., 1995). In vitro, tamoxifen inhibits the uptake and metabolism of estrone sulfate to estradiol (Lonning et al., 1995). In addition to the direct antiestrogenic effect, use of tamoxifen in combination with chemotherapy may delay the development of resistance to selected agents (McClay et al., 1994).

Side effects of tamoxifen

Tamoxifen and cancer risk. The role for tamoxifen as adjuvant therapy is far from standardized. Subject selection may be crucial to survival because certain breast or ovarian tumors may be stimulated rather than inhibited by the presence of tamoxifen (Boccardo et al., 1984; Osborne et al., 1994; Cohen et al., 1996). This weak estrogenic effect may provide a mechanism for relapse or tumor resistance among women receiving standard antiestrogen adjuvant therapy. Cytologic sampling of breast cancer patients who have taken tamoxifen for a minimum of 3 years revealed a mild estrogenic effect, with endocervical hyperplasia and a trend toward increased endometrial thickness (Rayter et al., 1994). In addition, tamoxifen may impair quality of life without conferring a compensatory survival advantage in some patients. Gelber and colleagues (1996) undertook a meta-analysis of nearly 4,000 women over 50 with node-positive breast cancer, using a technique of combined quality of life and survival analysis. Their findings indicate that quality-adjusted survival did not differ between those who underwent adjuvant chemoendocrine therapy and those who took tamoxifen alone.

Tamoxifen and mood. Two studies indicate that depression may be a side effect of tamoxifen treatment. Cathcart and colleagues (1993) assessed 257 patients with node-negative breast cancer who were on tamoxifen therapy and found that 15 percent of those on tamoxifen had major depression versus only 3 percent of the control group. Symptoms in the tamoxifen group appeared to be related to initiation of therapy. Shariff and colleagues (1995) noted an increase in depression over an 8-month period in women with early stage (I or II) breast cancer receiving adjuvant tamoxifen, despite no significant increase in state anxiety or anger levels. The source of this depression is unclear because other neuroendocrine alterations have been reported following tamoxifen therapy. Mamby, Love, and Lee (1995) noted that tamoxifen therapy in postmenopausal women results in altered thyroid function, specifically an increase in thyroid-binding globulin with secondary increases in T_3 orthiodothyronine uptake and free T_4. However, a number of studies have suggested a relationship between thyroid disorders and breast cancer independent of treatment regimen (Giani et al., 1996).

There is recent evidence that endocrine therapy for breast cancer with tamoxifen or antiestrogenic agents may be modulated by the addition of other hormones. Current endocrine research includes the efficacy of progesterone antagonists (including RU-486), which have been shown to interrupt mitotic division of cancer cells in vitro (Michna et al., 1992; Klijn et al., 1994; Shi et al., 1994). Concomitant administration of melatonin with tamoxifen in hormone-resistant metastatic breast cancer may induce tumor regression through synergistic decrease of tumor growth factors (Lissoni et al., 1995).

Hereditary breast and ovarian cancers

At least three different genes have been identified and linked with early onset hereditary breast and ovarian cancers: (1) the *BrCA1* gene, located on chromosome 17q (Hall et al., 1990; Easton et al., 1993); (2) *BrCA2*, localized to chromosome 13q12-q13 (Wooster et al., 1995); (3) the *p53* gene, linked to the multi-cancer Li-Fraumeni syndrome (Li and Fraumeni, 1982; Li, Correa, and Fraumeni, 1991). Genetic forms account for only 5–10 percent of breast and ovarian cancer cases, but lifetime risk is strikingly elevated. Estimates of lifetime risk in female *BrCA*1 carriers have been estimated at up to 59 percent by age 50 and fully 87 percent by age 70 for breast cancer and 44 percent for ovarian cancer by age 70 (Easton et al., 1993; Claus, Risch, and Thompson, 1994; Ford et al., 1994).

Surveillance of women with elevated breast and breast-ovarian cancer risk often encompasses difficult and personal decisions, which may not be clearly defined due to the lack of sensitive predictive biomarkers (Zurawski et al., 1988; Bast, 1993). This inability to readily predict precancerous conditions has led to the use of two management approaches: (1) surveillance with early detection and (2) chemical or surgical prophylaxis as prevention (Love, 1989; Sclafani, 1991; Cruickshank et al., 1992). Early induction of menopause through prophylactic oophorectomy or tamoxifen may lead to additional health risk in other areas, including cardiovascular and cerebrovascular disease and osteoporosis (King, Rowell, and Love, 1993; Levin, 1993). Watchful waiting involves frequent physical and radiographic examination. However, diagnostics are limited by an absence of early signs and symptoms in both cancers (Gallion and Bast, 1993; Lynch et al., 1993), as well as the technical limitations of surveillance by mammography and breast examination.

Psychological distress in patients with cancer

Approximately 20–50 percent of cancer patients have coexisting psychiatric diagnoses, most often depression and anxiety (Derogatis et al., 1983; Bukberg, Penman, and Holland, 1984; Massie and Holland, 1990). The presence of symptoms of depression and anxiety in cancer patients falls well within the range of normal human response to catastrophic life events, making it difficult to distinguish between a "normal" reaction to a diagnosis of cancer and one that manifests psychiatric illness. In addition, many of the symptoms of cancer or cancer therapy mimic depression, such as hopelessness, low energy, or anorexia (Kathol, Mutgi, Williams et al., 1990; Kathol, Noyes, Williams et al., 1990).

Difficulties in diagnosing psychological distress

In addition to the diagnostic dilemma of cancer with its inherent psychic distress, there are descriptive dilemmas in the psycho-oncology literature. Followers of cancer-related psychosocial research find that it is often difficult to distinguish between "psychosocial adjustment" and "quality of life," two interrelated constructs that are often used synonymously by researchers. Generally, quality of life instruments contain considerably more physical symptoms and activities of daily living rather than measures of psychological distress. In a small but illustrative study, Roberts and colleagues (1992) demonstrated that psychosocial adjustment and quality of life are not like terms. In a study of 32 women following radical gynecologic surgery, quality of life was rated high by most patients, who also reported significant levels of psychological distress on the Symptom Checklist-90-Revised (SCL-90-R).

The findings regarding depression and anxiety in similarly staged breast cancer patients are not consistent. Nevertheless, the stage of disease and treatment burden seem to be the primary variables associated with mood disorder among cancer patients (Bukberg, Penman, and Holland, 1984). In addition, both preexisting psychological morbidity and prior stressful life events may influence an individual's adjustment to cancer. In an analysis of newly diagnosed breast cancer patients assessed for levels of psychological distress, a high correlation was found with prior history of depression (Maunsell, Brisson, and Deschenes, 1992). The level of distress also correlated with the number of stressful life events in the 5 years preceding diagnosis. Early stage breast cancer patients who exhibited psychological distress a year after diagnosis were found to have healing problems, difficulty communicating with partners, a negative body image, and sexual dysfunction (Schag et al., 1993).

The psychological impact of mastectomy versus breast conservation

Treatment regimens and stage of life may also affect psychological response to cancer. In a Swedish study examining the difference between women who had received mastectomy or lumpectomy, the onset of therapy in both groups was associated with anxiety rather than depression, as measured by the Hospital Anxiety and Depression scale (Maraste et al., 1992). Although sample numbers were small, a subset of mastectomized women ages 50–59 demonstrated morbid anxiety, raising the question of an unexplored menopausal relationship.

Surprisingly, breast conservation does not always lessen the psychosocial impact of treatment when compared with modified radical mastectomy (Spiegel, 1992; Rijken et al., 1995). Using the Profile of Mood States (POMS) and the Karnofsky scale of physical functioning, Levy and colleagues (1992) followed 129 early stage breast cancer patients following either mastectomy or lumpectomy and found that while breast conservation patients were rated as more functional by others, they suffered more psychological distress in the first 3 months and perceived that they had less social support than women who underwent more radical surgery. This finding, consistent with an earlier report from Fallowfield and colleagues (1991), suggests that a surprising cost of breast salvage is higher levels of denial and reduced support from spouses (Spiegel, 1992). Greater anxiety about recurrence may also accompany the more conservative procedure (Fallowfield et al., 1991). Not surprisingly, mastectomy patients had greater difficulty with body image issues and sexuality. Interestingly, in an exploration of 83 women who underwent delayed breast reconstruction at Memorial Sloan-Kettering Hospital in New York City, a majority felt that reconstruction had helped them forget about having cancer, and half felt "less worried" about their health than they did prior to surgery (Rowland et al., 1993).

The role of choice

Even the decision-making process may have an impact on a patient's level of distress. Degner and Sloan (1992) compared 436 newly diagnosed cancer patients with 482 nonpatients (general public) in terms of the degree of control they wanted over treatment selection. A majority (64 percent) of the public imagined that they would want to select their own treatment if diagnosed with a serious illness, but a majority (59 percent) of cancer patients wanted physicians to make their treatment decisions. There is suggestive evidence that women who were free to choose their own treatment plan for breast cancer had higher life satisfaction at 3 months than those who were directed, but that difference was not evident at any later time (Pozo et al., 1992). However, a study at Johns Hopkins Oncology Center revealed that women with breast cancer often wrongly estimate their prognoses with standard available treatment and choose not to participate in randomized clinical trials as a result of misinterpretations (Sheldon, Fetting, and Siminoff, 1993). Some of the difficulty with information processing may be a result of anxiety. In a study of 67 breast cancer patients receiving surgical consultation, those who had tape recordings of the meetings demonstrated clearer knowledge of their treatment after 2 weeks and had fewer doctor visits and less postoperative anxiety (Hogbin, Jenkins, and Parkin, 1992).

Treatment-related distress

The physiologic side effects of undergoing chemotherapy, radiation, surgery, hormonal manipulation, or bone marrow transplantation as a treatment for breast cancer are universal. Although there may be a behavioral, psychological, or even environmental component to the degree of discomfort experienced by an individual, certain patterns are well established and should be considered by health professionals working with cancer patients. Despite the discomfort of both the disease and its treatment, the benefit of prolonged survival can modulate added distress (Fraser et al., 1993).

Nausea. Perhaps the best-known and most widely feared side effects of cancer treatments are nausea and vomiting. Chemotherapy-induced nausea and vomiting influence both treatment selection and patient quality of life (Lindley et al., 1992) and, in turn, may ultimately affect compliance and survival. Fortunately, chemotherapy-induced emesis is less than universal. Many chemo- or radiotherapy patients will develop transient, nonspecific food aversions without treatment significance (Mattes et al., 1992). Unfortunately, treatment-related nausea may become anticipatory. Anticipatory nausea and vomiting (ANV) has been associated with chemotherapy in 25–30 percent of all patients and has been significantly associated with both state and trait anxiety (Redd, 1989). Morrow, Lindke, and Black (1991) analyzed 530 chemotherapy outpatients and found two different types of correlations with anticipatory side effects: (1) learned associations based on prior experience and severity of nausea and vomiting and (2) age and prior susceptibility to motion sickness, suggesting a physiologic predisposition.

There is abundant evidence for both behavioral and physiologic mechanisms of anticipatory nausea. The level of side effects and the clinic setting are related to the severity of symptoms, suggesting classical environmental conditioning (Sabbioni et al., 1992; DiLorenzo et al., 1995). In a longitudinal study of 70 chemotherapy patients, those with ANV had higher measures of intellectual absorption and autonomic perception, perhaps suggesting a difference in perceptual sensitivity (Challis and Stam, 1992). This may aid in explaining the biofeedback and relaxation training intervention study by Burish and Jenkins (1992), in which chemotherapy patients who were randomly assigned to relaxation therapy experienced diminished nausea and postchemotherapy physiologic arousal, whereas electromyographic biofeedback and skin temperature biofeedback groups showed no effect. Other studies have suggested an increased autonomic response in some ANV patients (Kvale et al., 1991), with equivocal response to attempted treatment by noradrenergic blockade with clonidine (Fetting et al., 1992).

Pain. A common problem in many cancer patients, particularly those with bone metastases, is severe, unrelenting pain. Pain affects approximately one third of primary cancer patients and two thirds of those with metastatic disease (Bonica, 1990). Pain interferes with an individual's ability to perform regular activities of daily living as well as with the ability to sleep. The psychological side effects that result from chronic or severe pain also impede quality of life. Peter Strang studied 93 inpatients with cancer pain and found that half expressed anxiety as a result of pain and 71 percent reported feeling depressed due to their pain intensity. Strang (1992) also noted a serious tendency toward isolation and withdrawal from social contacts. Pain and depression co-occur and reinforce one another (Spiegel, 1996). In one study of metastatic breast cancer patients, the intensity of pain was significantly related to mood disturbance on the POMS and patients' interpretation of the pain as a signal of advancing disease, but not to site of metastasis (Spiegel and Bloom, 1983).

The degree of breast pain experienced by an individual may be perceptual rather than physiologic. Kroner and colleagues (1992), in an attempt to determine the incidence of "phantom breast syndrome" following mastectomy, prospectively studied patients over a 6-year period. They found a significant relationship between preoperative pain and postoperative phantom breast syndrome. Nearly one third of patients had pain in the scar at 6 years postoperatively, and 12–18 percent of patients had phantom sensation or pain in the mastectomized area.

Psychopharmacologic therapy has been shown to be an effective adjuvant therapy for cancer pain. Antidepressant analgesia is successful both in treating depression and pain directly and in potentiating opioid effects (Breitbart, 1992). In a critical review, Breitbart distinguished between physical and psychological components of pain such as anxiety or neuropathy and suggested creative augmentation using psychostimulants or neuroleptics as well as antidepressants or antiemetics.

The sedating and often disorganizing effects of large amounts of narcotics in cancer patients are generally tolerated in exchange for analgesia. Bruera, Miller, Macmillan, and Kuehn (1992) studied the effects of methylphenidate on patients receiving continuous subcutaneous narcotic infusion in a double blind crossover trial and noted improved cognitive functioning in those patients receiving psychostimulant augmentation. This Canadian group also studied 61 bedridden patients receiving parenteral narcotics and noted that 76 percent of them received most of their extra doses between 10 A.M. and 10 P.M., suggesting the possibility of a circadian rhythm to pain, although the authors admit that the findings are likely multifactorial (Bruera, Macmillan, Kuehn, Miller et al., 1992). Once affected, human beings appear to have a natural tendency to augment pharmacologic therapy with behavioral interventions, with over 40 behaviors noted in one study of cancer pain patients (Wilkie et al., 1992). Nonpharmacologic techniques such as hypnosis are also effective in reducing cancer pain and related anxiety. In one randomized study, training in self-hypnosis coupled with group therapy resulted in a 50 percent reduction in pain intensity over the course of 1 year on comparable and low amounts of analgesic and psychotropic medication (Spiegel and Bloom, 1983).

Fatigue. Fatigue, usually attributed to the effects of chemotherapy and radiation, is common in cancer patients. However, it is also a symptom of depression. In a small but important study of early stage breast cancer patients undergoing localized radiotherapy, Greenberg and colleagues (1992) outlined a fatigue pattern that did not correlate with either depression or radiation dose. Fatigue seemed to plateau midway through therapy and diminish within 3 weeks after therapy, consistent with a pattern of adaptation to a continuous physiologic stress.

Sexual dysfunction. The presence of sexual disturbance in cancer patients has been well documented and is multifactorial. Primary discomfort may result from surgically or chemically induced menopause, disfiguration, or chemo- and radiotherapies, as well as the extent of the disease. Secondary psychosexual dysfunction may result from mood disturbance or anxiety as well as interpersonal and environmental upheaval brought on by the cancer diagnosis.

The anatomic range and treatment burdens of genitourinary cancers prevent generalization of psychosexual predictions. One model of estimating sexual morbidity in women with gynecologic cancer divided patients into low, moderate, and high risk for psychological distress based on the severity of disease and treatment (ranging from cervical dysplasia to pelvic exenteration) (Andersen, 1993). Corney and colleagues (1993) assessed 105 survivors of radical pelvic surgery, of whom 90 percent had been sexually active prior to surgery. Three quarters of the subjects reported postoperative sexual difficulties, with lack of desire named at the most common problem. However, it may be the presence or absence of malignancy rather than the actual surgery that has the greater impact on postsurgical sexual adjustment. In a study of female patients who had undergone ileal conduit urinary diversion, women with malignant disease experienced more sexual dysfunction than those who had nonmalignant disease, many of whom increased sexual functioning after surgery (Nordstrom and Nyman, 1992).

The psychosexual impact of surgery in breast cancer patients is less clearly defined. Eligible patients with operable breast cancer are frequently offered the choice between the more disfiguring modified radical mastectomy and breast conservation (lumpectomy) with adjuvant radiotherapy. Breast cancer patients in general demonstrated significant levels of psychosocial distress, impaired sexual functioning, and disturbed body image when compared with patients with benign disease (Goldberg et al., 1992), as did a subset of breast conservation patients (Sneeuw et al., 1992). Three separate studies examined psychosexual functioning in women following either mastectomy or breast conservation with varied findings. It is not surprising that distress over breast loss, scarring, and appearance in clothing were greater in the mastectomy group (Levy et al., 1992). A greater number of mastectomy patients were more likely to have ceased sexual intercourse completely at 1 year; however, these findings have been contradicted in a second study (Omne-Ponten et al., 1992). Pozo and colleagues (1992) noted significant sexual disturbance in mastectomy patients at 6 and 12 months post-surgically, but no difference in overall well-being between the two groups during the same time periods. They wisely pointed out that this discrepancy may reflect the weightier impact of 1-year survival on patient outlook.

Bone marrow transplantation and gonadal dysfunction. One of the current treatments of poor-prognosis or metastatic breast cancers includes autologous bone marrow or stem cell transplantation. Treatment includes high-dose ablative chemoradiotherapy prior to infusion of the "transplanted" marrow or cells. In one study of adult male and female survivors of bone marrow transplantation for heterogeneous cancers, 65 percent indicated some degree of sexual satisfaction on a questionnaire; however, most patients had some gonadal dysfunction, including altered levels of estradiol and follicle-stimulating hormone (FSH) in women (Wingard et al., 1992). Mumma and colleagues (1992) compared the psychosexual functioning of leukemia survivors treated with either high-dose chemotherapy or heterologous bone marrow transplantation. No difference was found between the two treatment groups; however, when compared with healthy adults, both groups demonstrated impaired sexual functioning. Women tended to have decreased sexual frequency and satisfaction, and both genders reported poorer body image.

Cancer cachexia. In many cancers, progression of tumor leads to cancer cachexia, a hypermetabolic, hypercatabolic state of starvation. Cachexia is typified by simultaneous, coexisting, contradictory states of weight loss and tumor growth. In a "normal" host, the "work" of starvation is characterized by a compensatory resting state manifested by (1) lowered energy requirements in the form of decreased basal metabolism and (2) a shift in substrate utilization from glucose to fat in an attempt to preserve muscle mass. In a cachectic cancer host, however, the requirement for energy and protein is increased, and protein (in the form of muscle mass) rather than ketones becomes the preferred substrate for glucose production (Dills Jr., 1993).

Endocrinologic alterations in this state of deranged metabolism include a markedly activated hypothalamic-pituitary-adrenal axis, with increased secretion of "stress hormones" such as cortisol, ACTH, epinephrine, and glucagon. These changes progress and expand with increased physical stress, implying that there is a "window of opportunity" in which lowering the burden of psychosocial stress may translate into delayed tumor progression. In a study of neuroimmunoen-docrine parameters in 50 patients with advanced malignancy, Lechin and colleagues (1990) noted that patients with continuous physical symptoms (such as pain and nausea) demonstrated increased baseline levels of plasma noradrenaline, adrenaline, and cortisol as well as decreased platelet serotonin levels when compared to similar subjects who were symptom-free. During periods of symptom exacerbation, additional increases occurred in plasma dopamine and free serotonin, along with reduction in cytotoxic natural killer cell activity and lymphocyte number. Those patients in terminal stages showed an overall lack of responsiveness of these mechanisms, with maximal decreases in all neurotransmitters and immunologic parameters, an ultimately irreversible downward spiral.

Neuroimmunoendocrine effects of stress on cancer progression

The first section reviewed the literature which demonstrated that there are a multitude of stressors including the disease, the treatments, and the related psychosocial effects of the illness, for an individual diagnosed with cancer. Such physiologic and psychological stressors have been shown to profoundly influence neuroimmunoendocrine functioning. In turn, these alterations may lead to potentiation of existing tumor growth and subsequently reduced survival time. This section first reviews the literature indicating the effects of stress and support on immune function and then addresses the crucial issue of the clinical significance of these findings for cancer.

Stress-induced immunosuppression

The delicate balance between physical and psychological stress and the immune system has led to the emergence of psychoneuroimmunology as a field of study. Physical stressors such as aging, chronic infection and inflammation, cancer, surgery, and malnutrition, as well as overtraining in athletes, have all been shown to alter immune function (Goodwin, Searles, and Tunk, 1982; Fong et al., 1990; Irwin and Strasbaugh, 1992; Naito et al., 1992; Sharp and Koutedakis, 1992; Sternberg et al., 1992). Environmental stressors such as noise, smoke, pollution, and alcohol in humans suppress immune function, as do acute foot shocks, noise, and rotation in rats (Sklar and Anisman, 1979; Dantzer and Kelley, 1989; Sieber et al., 1992). Psychological stressors such as traumatic life events (e.g., loss of a spouse, unemployment, marital discord, disruption of social support, anticipation of a cancer diagnosis, caring for a loved one with Alzheimer's disease) have all been demonstrated in multiple studies to adversely affect immunologic cell activity and function (Arnetz et al., 1987; Irwin et al., 1987; Kiecolt-Glaser, Fisher, Ogrocki et al., 1987; Kiecolt-Glaser, Glaser, Dyer et al., 1987; Eysenck, 1988; Kennedy et al., 1988; Weisse et al., 1990).

The measurement of the interaction between psychosocial factors such as stress and support and immune functioning is complex, requiring laboratory measurement of cellular activity, number, and function (Temoshok et al., 1985; Spiegel et al., 1989). Uncomplicated bereavement has been associated with elevated mortality, change in immune cell numbers (altered T helper and T suppressor cell counts, decreased total lymphocyte count), and altered function – impaired natural killer cell cytoxicity and decreased lymphocyte mitogen activity despite steady-state numbers of T and B cells (Bartrop et al., 1977; Pagel, Bicher, and Cappel, 1985; Irwin et al., 1987). Even an external event as seemingly trivial as an academic examination altered both cellular function (decreased lymphocyte mitogen and reduced natural killer cell activity, increased plasma titers of viral antigens, decreased cytokine production) and number (alterations in T-cell subpopulations) in medical students (Dorian et al., 1982; Glaser et al., 1986; Kiecolt-Glaser et al., 1986). This effect was modulated by good social support, demonstrating the complexity of the immune response.

Effects of internally perceived stressors

Although stress-induced immunosuppression is more commonly described, internally perceived stressors such as job strain or poor social support may also result in overactivation of the immune system, with an increase in immunoglobulin production rather than a decrease (Theorell, Orth-Gomer, and Eneroth, 1990). Dobbin and colleagues (1991) found that although examination stress led to both decreased levels of gamma-interferon and decreased lymphocyte mitogen response, it also led to increased production of the cytokine interleukin 1-beta and monocyte blast transformation under the same conditions. Certain rheumatoid and collagen-vascular diseases have long been felt to reflect activation of an immunologic/inflammatory system, with treatment often centered around exogenous suppression of activity with glucocorticoids (Laue, Loriaux, and Chrousos, 1988).

Subtle psychological factors have also been shown to influence immune functioning. These include how one copes with adversity, including negative mood, self-blame, and perceived loss of situational control (Lazarus and Folkman, 1984; Pagel, Bicher, and Cappel, 1985; Stone et al., 1987; Temoshok and Dreher, 1992). Sieber and group (1992) noted that not only did the perception of lack of control over a stimulus cause a decline in natural killer cell activity, the simple desire to be in control had a similar effect. Poor adjustment and negative affect resulting from maladaptive coping styles such as blaming, fantasy, or avoidance also had an immunosuppressive effect (Felton, Revenson, and Hintrichsen, 1984). Passive stoicism, apathy, and lack of social support correlated with decreased natural killer cell activity (Levy et al., 1987). Surprisingly, positive personality variables such as optimism and an optimistic explanatory style seem to suppress immune function, leading to decreased cutaneous responses to delayed hypersensitivity testing and diminished lymphoproliferative response to mitogenic challenge (Temoshok, 1985; Kamen et al., 1991; Sieber et al., 1992).

Mechanism and timing of stress-induced immunosuppression

Significant evidence indicates that there exists a complex feedback loop between the immune system and the central nervous system via the hypothalamic-pituitary-adrenal (HPA) axis, mediated principally by cytokines and modulated by neuroendocrine hormones, catecholamines, endogenous opioids, and corticosteroids (Keller et al., 1983; Dantzer and Kelley, 1989; Meyerhoff et al., 1990; Sternberg et al., 1992). Early studies revealed that administration of antigen to rats produced increased corticosterone levels at 72 hours, which then lasted up to 10 days (Besedovsky et al., 1986; Eskay, Grino, and Chen, 1990). Chronic changes in glucocorticoid levels were not associated with changes in cell number such as total lymphocyte counts or T-cell subpopulations. Chronic exposure to stressors even led to immunologic adaptation or enhancement of immune function (Sklar and Anisman, 1979; Monjan, 1984).

Immune variability. There may be an innate variability in the immune system's recovery from stress-induced changes. Bovjberg and Valdimarsdottir (1993) studied women with family histories of cancer and noted that those with such a history had lower cytotoxic activity. This suppressed activity was also seen in women with greater emotional distress, independent of family history. Impaired cellular response to stress, whether genetic or reactive, may lead to accelerated progression of the disease. In a series of studies, Levy and colleagues (1985,

1987, 1990, 1991) related sustained psychosocial stress and decreased natural killer (NK) cell activity with increased breast cancer progression and axillary lymph node and estrogen receptor status. Ben-Eliyahu and colleagues (1991) administered laboratory stress to disease-free rats, significantly reducing their NK cytotoxicity levels. The animals were injected with mammary (MADB-106) tumor cells, and lung metastases were assessed 12 days later. The stressed, immunosuppressed rats demonstrated rapid metastatic spread of mammary tumor to lung in addition to increased plasma levels of cortisol and ACTH.

Systemic immune function may not reflect cellular activity, however. In a study of preneoplastic mammary tissue from nonstressed tumor-bearing mice, NK cell activity was elevated, not diminished, and waned as spontaneous tumors developed (Wei and Heppner, 1987). Suppression of NK activity led to longer tumor latency and slower progression, suggesting that a differential signal exists between normal and malignant tissue (Wei et al., 1989).

Can stress-related immunosuppression lead to cancer?

The relationship between stress and immunosuppression raises a twofold question: Can the occurrence of major life stressors (1) lead to the development of cancer in healthy persons or (2) accelerate disease progression in patients with preexisting cancer? There is considerable controversy in the literature about the long-term physiologic sequelae of painful life events in cancer patients. Some of the variability in results stems from the lack of methodologic uniformity and the relatively limited duration of follow-up in studies looking at this connection. A number of retrospective case-controlled or matched studies have attempted to correlate greater severity of life events with the occurrence of malignancy (breast cancer and melanoma) 5 or 6 years later (Forsen, 1991; Geyer, 1992; Havlik et al., 1992; Chorot and Sandin, 1994). However, circumstances of life stressors differ among the studies, making comparison difficult.

The following two opposing studies further illustrate the confusion surrounding the findings related to major life stressors and breast cancer progression. In the first study, Ramirez (1989) studied a matched sample of relapsed versus non-relapsed breast cancer patients and observed a higher prevalence of major life stressors in the recurrent group. These serious stressors included divorce, job loss, and forced relocation. The severity of stressor was crucial, with only major stressors contributing to an elevated risk of relapse. In contrast, in the second study, Barraclough and colleagues (1992) prospectively studied a group of breast cancer patients in which 51 percent experienced such major life events during the 42 months of the study and 23 percent had disease progression and found no correlation between stressors and disease progression. One possible explanation for the equivocal results between the studies may be the failure to correlate the level of stress during the stressor with the level of stress years later, when varying degrees of individual adaptation may have occurred.

Chronic exposure to stressors may also lead to immunologic adaptation (Sklar and Anisman, 1979). One study of over 2,000 women presenting at a breast-screening clinic for routine check-up indicated that while experiencing a single, acute major life stressor may be associated with malignancy, regular exposure to stress (implying adaptation) may actually reduce the risk of malignancy (Cooper and Faragher, 1993).

Having cancer can be considered a chronic stressor. Reminders of the illness are a daily occurrence, with arduous treatments providing additional sources of stress. For some, cancer is also a traumatic stressor. The existence of traumatic symptomatology such as intrusive thinking, dissociation, and avoidant behavior has been associated with the diagnosis of cancer (Alter et al., 1996), surviving cancer (Levy et al., 1991), and diagnosis of recurrence (Cella, Mahon, and Donovan, 1990). Gruber and colleagues (1993) found that women with node-negative stage I breast cancer who underwent relaxation, guided imagery, and biofeedback training for stress relief demonstrated improved immune function over an 18-month period.

Depression, immune function, and cancer

Researchers have been unable to clearly establish a causal or progressive link between depression and cancer. Although it is well known that rates of depression are high among cancer patients (Derogatis et al., 1983; Spiegel, Sands, and Koopman, 1994), the idea that depression may be associated with cancer incidence or progression has not been clearly established. Shekelle and colleagues (1981) initially showed that depression predicted higher cancer incidence. However, several later studies failed to confirm this finding (Fox, 1989; Zonderman, Costa, and McCrae, 1989; Friedman, 1994).

Depression has been clearly linked to diminished neurotransmitter (norepinephrine and serotonin) levels, decreased immunologic function, and endocrine aberrations. For example, a number of studies have demonstrated that baseline serum cortisol levels are elevated in acute endogenous depression (Sachar et al., 1973; Linkowski et al., 1987; Rubin et al., 1987, 1989). This activation of endocrine activity is associated with a corresponding decrease in natural killer cell activity found in other studies (Sapolsky and Donnelly, 1985). Sachs and colleagues (1995) found that lymphokine-activated killer cell (LAK) activity was reduced in breast cancer patients with depression and anxiety prior to surgery, but not at 1-year follow-up, where the only predictive factors of LAK activity were tamoxifen use and chemotherapy.

Immunosuppression and aging

Some of the difficulty in clarifying the immunoendocrine response to depression and cancer is confounded by simple aging. Sapolsky and Donnelly (1985) noted that endocrine flexibility decreases in normal aging, leading to prolonged elevation of cortisol under stress. They demonstrated that aged rats show increased tumor proliferation as well as slower recovery of corticosterone secretion after exposure to a stressor. Normal aging is also associated with a blunted immune response, leading to age-related immunosuppression (Goodwin et al., 1982). In a study of depressed adults, cortisol elevation and related immunosuppression were strongest in the elderly and were not noted in younger adults (Schleifer et al., 1983). This suggests that immunosuppression in the elderly may be secondary to aging rather than depression.

Endocrine effects on tumor proliferation

The association between psychosocial stress, endocrine shifts, and tumor proliferation was first established in a set of classic animal experiments. Riley (1981) and colleagues demonstrated that animals reared in crowded environments had much more rapid tumor progression than those raised in less stressful environments. The endocrine response to stress involves a cascade of hypothalamic-pituitary-adrenal activity, in which cortisol, the classic stress hormone, is elevated. This stress response appears constant despite the nature of the stressor, with the same endocrine pattern being elicited from either physical or emotional stress. However, the degree of endocrine shift varies relative to the severity of the stressor. For example, both acute medical illness and spousal bereavement (Irwin et al., 1987, 1988) are associated with increased secretion of ACTH (Drucker and McLaughlin, 1986), dehydroepiandrosterone (DHEA), and cortisol (Parker, Levin, and Lifrak, 1985), and lowered DHEA/cortisol ratios (Ozasa et al., 1990). Milder psychological distress does not elicit the same degree of stress response, as is shown by the elevated cortisol levels that accompany spousal bereavement (Irwin et al., 1987), but not examination stress (Glaser et al., 1994).

Several theories predominate that explain the mechanisms by which stress-induced hypercortisolemia stimulates tumor progression – including immunosuppression, angiogenesis, differential gluconeogenesis, and the effects of other adrenal hormones:

1. Glucocorticoids exert an immunomodulatory effect. Chronic stress and elevation of glucocorticoids may result in immunosuppression and therefore tumor proliferation (Sapolsky, Krey, and McEwen, 1983; Sapolsky and Donnelly, 1985; Sternberg et al., 1990).

2. Elevated cortisol stimulates angiogenesis, leading to subsequent tumor vascularization and growth (Folkman et al., 1983).

3. To maintain high circulating levels of glucose under stress, glucocorticoids stimulate gluconeogenesis and inhibit intracellular transport of glucose into healthy cells. However, because tumor cells have greatly increased intracellular energy needs in order to sustain rapid growth, they are believed to become resistant to glucocorticoid inhibition of intracellular transport, which leads to much of the glucose being shunted to the tumor (Romero et al., 1992). The tumor cells exhibit a shift in glucose metabolism from aerobic to anaerobic glycolysis during which glucose is converted to lactate, which is then returned to host cells as a nonusable waste product (Dills Jr., 1993). The end result of these cycles is to greatly facilitate the noninhibited tumor cells in obtaining necessary cellular nutrition, to the detriment of healthy cells.

4. Other steroid hormones, especially the adrenal hormone dihydroepiandrosterone (DHEA), may directly oppose the action of cortisol and exert an inhibitory effect on dysplastic transformation and malignant proliferation. Rats who were adrenalectomized following inoculation with mammary tumor had greater tumor progression than those with normal adrenal glands (Carter and Carter, 1988). The addition of DHEA in the diet of rats with mammary tumor led to a significant decrease in both tumor promotion and progression (Ratko et al., 1991). However, in ovariectomized rats, the addition of DHEA enhanced rather than slowed tumor growth, suggesting that the interaction with ovarian androgens may also play a role in tumor growth (Boccuzzi et al., 1992).

Psychosocial influences on disease progression

The first two sections of this chapter examined the inherent psychosocial stressors that accompany a cancer diagnosis and the psychophysiologic effects that may occur as a result of these stressors. Some recent evidence indicates that psychosocial interventions designed to alleviate the cancer patient's distress may affect disease progression and survival time, as well as improve quality of life. Three domains that may play a role in moderating health outcome are personality and coping characteristics, level of emotional expression, and social support.

Personality and coping styles

Although some have argued that certain forms of coping, such as stoic acceptance, are unhealthy coping responses to cancer (Greer, 1991), most breast cancer patients are psychologically healthy individuals and choose psychologically healthy coping strategies in response to a devastating illness (Greer et al., 1992; Ellman and Thomas, 1995). Jarrett and colleagues (1992) reported that following a diagnosis of cancer, many patients increase their use of positive reappraisal as well as cognitive avoidance strategies. They also conclude that the coping strategies employed may reflect the context of the stressful situation rather than trait coping styles. In another study by Rodrigue and colleagues (1993), bone marrow transplant candidates were assessed for negative coping styles, mood, and personality variables prior to hospitalization. Passive coping styles were related to higher levels of anxiety and depression. The literature has suggested that individuals with "fighting spirit" show longer survival than those characterized by "stoic acceptance" or "anxious preoccupation and helplessness" (Greer et al., 1992). This picture is complicated by the fact that patients who exhibited the less putatively adaptive defense of "denial" also lived longer. A prospective study of breast cancer progression in 52 women and 32 controls suggested that cancer progression over a 2-year period was associated with repression, reduced expression of negative affect, helplessness/hopelessness, chronic stress, and comforting daydreaming (Jensen, 1987). Studies have suggested associations of some of these traits with immunosuppression (Temoshok and Dreher, 1992). Levy and colleagues (1985) found that not only was lower NK activity predictive of breast cancer spread to axillary lymph nodes, lower NK activity also correlated with an observer to patient rating of "well adjusted to their cancer." Women with higher NK activity were considered distressed or "maladjusted" by observers. It seems that when the patient appears to be pleasantly quiet, the immune system reacts. Expression of intrapsychic distress is a major component in relief of stress and may contribute significantly to delay in tumor progression as described later in this chapter (Derogatis, Abeloff, and Melisaratos, 1979).

Emotional expression

Emotional expression in a supportive, empathic environment is a key component in the reduction of psychological distress in cancer patients (Spiegel et al., 1989; Fawzy et al., 1990a, 1990b; Spiegel, 1993). Pistrang and Barker (1992) studied the patterns of self-disclosure and perceived empathy for 77 women with breast cancer. Most women confided preferentially in women friends or relatives and in partners rather than seeking out mental health care settings. Recent studies have begun to explore the relationship between nonexpression of strong emotion and cancer progression. Women with more advanced breast tumors at the time of diagnosis demonstrated a tendency to suppress emotion, to trivialize, and to display self-pity (Neuhaus et al., 1994). In a study of 2,000 women seen in a breast cancer screening clinic, the correlation between malignancy and a recent single acute life stressor was strongest in those women who were unable to express their emotions (Cooper and Faragher, 1993).

Although the association between expression of affect and neuroendocrine immune function has been only preliminarily explored and is yet unclear, the probability exists that normal expression of emotion is accompanied by endocrine and, perhaps, immune alterations. In breast cancer patients undergoing an educational and coping intervention, improvement in psychological distress was related to both immediate and longer-term decreases in cortisol levels and increases in lymphocyte numbers (Schedlowski et al., 1994). In a study of laboratory mood-induction in healthy female subjects, serum cortisol levels increased significantly during conditions of both sadness and elation, independent of arousal, but showed no change under neutral conditions (Brown et al., 1993). In another study of normal subjects, those who suppressed emotion (high on conformity and low in experienced distress) had lower early morning cortisol levels (Brown et al., 1996).

The act of disclosure as a component of expression also appears to be "good for one's health." Subjects who disclosed personal trauma in journal form as part of a study design had both fewer doctor visits and improved immunologic function (Pennebaker, Kiecolt-Glaser, and Glaser, 1988). These data suggest that repression of strong emotion may compound the effect of a stressor, thereby affecting immune and endocrine function, either transiently or chronically.

Social support

Human beings are naturally social animals, and lack of community has been associated with elevated mortality of all causes (House, Landis, and Umberson, 1988). Studies in both animals and humans have shown that the presence of social support buffers the effects of stress, although not universally. To achieve a beneficial effect, the social support must be both adequate in quantity and non-confrontational in quality. In examining the differential response to added social support, three different models can be identified: loneliness, commonality, and stability. Loneliness itself may be a sufficient stressor to impair immune response. For example, in one study of cynomolgus monkeys, those assigned to unstable social conditions with constant rearrangements of social groupings showed weaker mitogen proliferation responses. This immunosuppressive effect was strongest among those monkeys that, from the beginning, demonstrated very little affiliative behavior (Cunnick et al., 1991). In studies of heterogeneous cancer patients, increased mood disturbance, decreased life expectancy, and decreased natural killer cell activity all correlated with a lack of social support (Jensen, 1991; Ell et al., 1992; Levy et al., 1992; Waxler-Morrison et al., 1992). Reynolds and Kaplan (1990), in a reanalysis of the Alameda County data, showed that poor social support in the form of few social contacts was related to higher cancer incidence in women and more rapid disease progression in men.

Buffering effect of social support

Shared social support may buffer the effects of stressful events. Support groups have been shown to (1) reduce feelings of isolation by providing a sense of universality among the members (Spiegel, Bloom, and Yalom, 1981; Yalom, 1985); (2) decrease traumatic and psychological distress symptoms in both trauma victims and cancer patients (Spiegel, Bloom, and Yalom, 1981; Marmar, 1991); and (3) buffer the effects of the stressful conditions (Kiecolt-Glaser and Greenberg, 1984). In a study of squirrel monkeys subjected to an aversive conditioned stimulus, the resultant stress-related elevation of plasma cortisol was reduced when the animal had the company of a friend during administration of the stressor (Coe, Rosenberg, and Levine, 1988). The cortisol increase disappeared entirely when the monkey was surrounded by five such friends. These conditions may be replicated in support groups for cancer patients. The stability of a secure social environment may reduce the physiologic impact of a full neuroendocrine immune stress response. Medical students who scored as well supported on the UCLA Loneliness Scale did not have stress-induced immunosuppression at examination time, whereas those who reported themselves to be lonely did (Kennedy, Kiecolt-Glaser, and Glaser, 1988). Even the lowest vertebrates demonstrate this effect. In a study of aggressive fish, social confrontation in the nonaggressors produced leukocyte immunosuppression (nonspecific cytotoxicity and mitogen-stimulated response). Some of this immunosuppression was reversed by administration of naltrexone, an opioid antagonist, implicating at least partial mediation by endogenous opioids (Faisal et al., 1989).

Family environment

The demands and side effects of cancer and its treatment tend to decrease the accessibility of social support. Both the quality of relationships and the ability of the patient to interact with others may be affected. Strang (1992) found that cancer-related pain led to decreased physical and social activity. Although patients reported feeling supported by friends and family, 85 percent of patients in the sample reported less self-initiated contact with friends, and 65 percent reported that they isolated themselves due to the intensity of their pain. Lewis and Hammond (1992) found that breast cancer patients' psychosocial adjustment remained stable over time. Depressed patients, however, suffered impaired marital and family relationships when the depression became chronic.

Coyne and colleagues (1987) have provided considerable documentation of the difficulty that friends and family have in maintaining good relationships with depressed individuals. However, difficulties that family members have in coping with a loved one's illness could also have an impact on patient mood. A, 1992 study by Ward and colleagues demonstrated a peculiar thing: For some cancer patients, increased communication about the cancer with "supportive" others was related to lower self-esteem. However, sensitizing the supportive others to the emotional and physical needs of the cancer patient eliminated the relationship between communication and low self-esteem. Unfortunately, a good relationship with another individual did not compensate for a difficult or inadequate relationship with one's partner (Pistrang and Barker, 1995). This raises three points. First, not all social relationships are supportive, nor are all supportive relationships consistent in the level of support provided at all times. Second, relationships may change after one member is diagnosed with cancer. Many patients report feeling isolated within previously close relationships due to the existential issues facing them. Third, brief interventions within the family system can often produce large positive effects on the quality of support received. It appears likely that patient coping patterns may show a variable course as patients adjust to varying amounts of new and often distressing information.

Timing of psychosocial intervention

The interactions among social support, emotional expression, coping, and physiologic variables such as T-cell function and cortisol levels suggest that psychosocial intervention that addresses these domains might plausibly have some effect on disease progression. Early psychosocial intervention can reduce postoperative psychiatric morbidity in newly diagnosed cancer patients undergoing surgery (McArdle et al., 1996). However, Edgar, Rosberger, and Nowlis (1992) found that an earlier intervention was less effective. Patients receiving an intervention 28 weeks postdiagnosis reported considerably less anxiety and worry and had regained more feelings of control at the first follow-up assessment than patients who received a psychosocial intervention within 10 weeks of diagnosis.

Psychosocial interventions: Impact on cancer progression and survival

Three of six published studies have demonstrated that both the psychosocial and physical sequelae of malignant disease can be modulated by psychosocial interventions. The three studies that demonstrated improvement in both disease progression and overall survival all had strikingly similar interventions. In these studies, patients were provided with social support, an arena for emotional expression, and direction in facing and coping with life-threatening illness.

Spiegel and colleagues (1989) randomly assigned 86 women with metastatic breast cancer, all receiving standard medical care, to conditions of either treatment (weekly group therapy) or control (nonintervention). The intervention technique used, supportive–expressive group psychotherapy, consisted of a weekly support group designed to encourage expression of strong emotion; deal with fears of death and dying; intensify mutual support; improve relationships and doctor–patient communication; and manage pain through self-hypnosis. Women assigned to the intervention group showed reduced mood disturbance and pain over the initial intervention year and lived an average of 18 months longer than those in the control group. By 48 months after the study had begun, all of the control patients had died, whereas one third of the intervention subjects were still alive.

Richardson and colleagues (Richardson, Marks, and Levine, 1988; Richardson et al., 1990) randomly assigned lymphoma and leukemia patients to one of two conditions: (1) an active intervention consisting of home visiting by a professional trained to deliver both education and empathic support or (2) a control group that received routine care. Not surprisingly, the intervention group demonstrated significant improvement in adherence to medical treatment. However, independent of that effect, the intervention group had significantly longer survival time. This suggests that the educational benefits were extended by an enriching patient–caregiver relationship that included support, coping, and empathy. Neither the duration of intervention nor the method of delivery (individual vs. group) appears to negatively influence the beneficial effect on both psychological outcome and prolonged survival.

Fawzy and colleagues (1990a) randomly assigned 80 malignant melanoma patients either to routine care or to 6 weeks of an intensive group psychotherapy that included educational, expressive, and supportive components. They found that at the 6-month follow-up, the intervention patients had significantly better alpha-interferon-augmented natural killer cell activity (Fawzy et al., 1990b). This effect was not evident at the 1-year follow-up. However, at the 6-year follow-up, the intervention group had fewer recurrences and significantly fewer deaths (Fawzy et al., 1993). In this study, intervention status correlated with medical outcome, whereas baseline natural killer cell activity predicted rates of recurrence. This raises the question of whether the timing of intervention (i.e., the time from diagnosis or treatment) may influence outcome years later.

Three published studies of psychosocial intervention in cancer patients demonstrated no survival benefit in the intervention groups (Linn, Linn, and Harris, 1982; Gellert, Maxwell, and Siegel, 1993; Ilnyckyj et al., 1994). In an early study by Linn, Linn, and Harris (1982), terminally ill patients were randomized to counseling that focused on quality of life issues. Despite an improvement in quality of life, there was no difference in either functional status or survival between the two groups: Most of the patients died within a year. One possible explanation is that psychosocial intervention cannot alter cancer progression in the setting of overwhelming tumor burden.

In the two other studies, however, the psychological intervention was problematic. Gellert, Maxwell, and Siegel (1993) followed up on the Exceptional Cancer Patient Program developed by Dr. Bernie Siegel (1986) by matching participants with breast cancer in the Exceptional Cancer Patient Program to others receiving routine care at 10-year follow-up. There was no difference observed in subsequent survival time. In the three previously cited studies with survival advantage (Spiegel, Richardson, and Fawzy), the expressive components of the interventions consisted of open patient expression of "negative thoughts" (such as fear of dying, anger, hopelessness). In the Gellert study, the intervention, which centers around the use of "positive" thoughts, places much of the "work" of fighting cancer in the patient's own internal psyche. This may potentially increase rather than relieve the individual's stress response by making the patient feel responsible for the occurrence or progression of her cancer.

The third study was a randomized trial in which breast cancer patients received a poorly defined assortment of group therapies led by a mixture of trained and untrained therapists. The patients received no psychological benefit; thus, it is not surprising that there was also no survival advantage (Ilnyckyj et al., 1994). These results suggest that the skill and training of the therapists in conducting the psychotherapy also play a role in outcome.

Conclusion

Tumor biology alone is insufficient to fully understand the course of malignancy. The disease affects a variety of physiologic systems, which in turn moderate the somatic response to invasion by tumor cells. Cancer is a series of stressors, not only the illness itself, but its implications for possible premature mortality, social isolation, and stimulation of strong affect. A given individual's resources and abilities to handle these stressors may in turn moderate the effects of the disease on psychological and somatic function. The available literature suggests that active and direct confrontation with the problems associated with cancer, expression rather than suppression of emotion related to these problems, and mobilization of social support facilitate coping and may have a positive effect on the rate of disease progression. Interventions designed to facilitate active coping and to enhance social support clearly benefit cancer patients emotionally and may improve medical outcome as well.

CHAPTER TEN

THE PSYCHOPHARMACOLOGY OF WOMEN

REGINA C. CASPER

Women are the principal recipients and have been shown to be the major "consumers" of drugs (Cafferata, Kasper, and Bernstein, 1983; Dworkin and Adams, 1984). By contrast, drug toxicity studies have almost exclusively used male rats as experimental animals (Kato and Yamazoe, 1992), and drug efficacy and safety trials typically have been conducted in men. Not until 1993 did the Food and Drug Administration (FDA) drop its mandate that women be excluded from drug trials. Of course, utmost precautions must be taken to avoid exposing pregnant women to investigational drugs. The decision by the FDA came at a time when other changes in drug development, for instance, in chirotechnology, impacted drug efficacy and safety studies. Because nearly half the organic compounds on the market as drugs consist of isomers (i.e., they contain the dextro- or levorotating forms of the same molecule – for example, the L form of limonene gives lemons their taste, whereas the D form flavors oranges) and because the two forms almost always differ in their action or pharmacologic activity, the FDA began in 1992 to require information about both isomers of a drug. Studies into gender or age effects of racemic compounds are in the initial phases (Hooper and Qing, 1990). Some evidence for subtle sex differences in enantiomer protein binding has emerged (Gilmore et al., 1992).

To produce its pharmacologic effects, a drug must be present in sufficient concentration at its site(s) of action. Ideally, one wants to reach the sites that mediate therapeutic efficacy without immersing peripheral and central neuronal receptors in a sea of drug molecules. It is now well recognized that given the same dose, individuals respond to drugs differently and experience different side effects. Among the many factors contributing to this variation are genetic make-up, sex, age, body weight, and tobacco or alcohol use. Precise control of these factors would allow individualization of drug doses so that medications could be effective with a minimum of toxicity. Psychotropic drugs typically act within a broad therapeutic "window," that is, a wide range of therapeutically effective drug concentrations. Fine-tuning the optimal pharmacodynamic dose for each individual would be particularly important for women given the higher incidence and prevalence of anxiety and depressive disorders in women, which result in more frequent use of anxiolytic and antidepressant drugs.

This chapter is divided into three sections: First, it considers the evidence for sex-related influences on drug disposition, absorption, distribution, and metabolism from studies in humans. It then provides an overview of drug safety during pregnancy and breast-feeding. Finally, it discusses the information from studies that have examined gender differences in treatment response to antidepressant and antipsychotic drugs. A brief summary of some of the studies describing age effects on pharmakokinetics concludes the chapter.

Sex-related differences in uptake, distribution, and metabolism of psychotropic drugs

Absorption

Most psychotropic drugs are administered orally and hence are absorbed from the gastrointestinal tract. Virtually all psychotropic drugs, a notable exception being lithium, are lipophilic nonpolar compounds and are esterified by the liver. Gastric acid secretion is lower in women than in men (Grossman, Kirsner, and Gillespie, 1963), and gastric emptying time is delayed during pregnancy (Davison, Davison, and Hay, 1970). Men taking salicylates reach peak plasma concentrations faster than women, although the plasma concentration area under the curve (AUC), half-life, and protein binding were found to be similar. The extent of drug absorption (Datz, Christian, and Moore, 1987) is a function of gastrointestinal transit time. Drugs that are dissolved slowly and absorbed slowly can be affected more by alterations in gastrointestinal transit time than drugs that are rapidly and completely absorbed. Conversely, an increase in gut motility will lead to decreased absorption of drugs, whereas a decrease in motility may actually increase the extent of absorption. Gastrointestinal transit time has been shown to be prolonged in pregnancy and in the luteal phase, when

Table 10.1. *Drug disposition – definition of terms*

Pharmacokinetics	Time course of a drug as it passes through the body ("what the body does to the drug")
Pharmacodynamics	Relationship between blood and tissue concentrations and pharmacologic effects ("what the drug does to the body")
Effect kinetics	Time course of a drug's action on the body
Oral bioavailability	Fraction of a drug that enters the circulation when taken orally
Volume of distribution (V_d)	The extra- or intracellular space into which drugs distribute; V_d can be a multiple of body weight.
Clearance (Cl)	Rate at which body clears a volume of body fluid, usually plasma from a drug
Half-life ($t^{1/2}$)	Time it takes for one half of the amount of the drug to be eliminated from the body
Steady-state concentration	Concentration at which the rate of drug administration equals the rate of drug elimination, usually after more than four half-lives have passed

progesterone levels are increased compared with the follicular phase (Wald et al., 1981). Once absorbed by the gut, drugs enter the portal circulation and the liver, where a portion of the drug is eliminated before reaching the systemic circulation. This hepatic removal, called first-pass elimination, accounts for the need to give larger oral than parental doses of most drugs to achieve equivalent pharmacologic effects. As a matter of convenience, this phenomenon is called oral bioavailability. The drug fraction that reaches the systemic circulation after oral administration ranges from 40 percent to 60 percent for most drugs. Table 10.1 lists and defines terms that describe drug action and distribution.

Distribution

Once absorbed into the systemic circulation, the drug must distribute throughout the body. Nearly all drugs are highly bound (95–98 percent) to plasma proteins. Among the psychoactive drugs, venlafaxine, from 20 to 30 percent protein bound, is an exception. Usually free drug levels in the plasma and drug bound to proteins are in equilibrium. Special caution is required if a person is taking multiple drugs because drugs compete for the same protein-binding sites and displace one another, leading to variations in free drug concentration, even though total drug concentrations remain the same. Small but statistically significant sex-related differences in protein binding have been reported for imipramine and for some of the benzodiazepines (BZDs), with the extent of protein binding being lower in women than in men of comparable age. Studies that have observed no significant sex-related differences in protein binding might have failed to control for age and smoking habits.

The decrease in plasma protein binding of many drugs during pregnancy, with the greatest decline being noted during the third trimester (Adams and Wacher, 1968; Dean, Stock, and Patterson, 1980), is probably due to decreased levels of albumin (Yoshikawa et al., 1984).

Among the mechanisms responsible for differences in drug protein binding are differences in albumin, which binds acidic drugs, in alpha-1-acid glycoprotein (AAG), a protein that binds weakly basic drugs, in nonesterified fatty acids (NEFAs), and in sex hormone–binding globulins. Whether AAG is a significant determinant in the binding of psychotropic agents is uncertain. Plasma levels of AAG vary with the menstrual cycle (Parish and Spivey, 1991), and oral contraceptive users seem to have lower AAG concentrations (Walle et al., 1993). Sex hormone–binding globulin is generally elevated in women compared to men. Another type, the lipoproteins, especially apoliprotein B and complement C_3, has been shown to be important in the binding of tricyclics, such as imipramine (Kristensen, 1983) and chlorpromazine (Bickel, 1975). The degree of protein binding can have a major effect, as it is the free or unbound fraction of the drug that becomes available to tissues. By measuring drug concentrations in plasma at various times after a drug is administered, a curve can be described from which distribution and elimination can be quantified. Plasma drug levels are a composite of an early distribution phase during which the drug rapidly disappears from the circulation and a later elimination phase during which the drug in the blood is in equilibrium with drugs in the tissue and is more gradually eliminated from the body. The pharmacodynamic effects of most drugs are related to the plasma concentration during the elimination phase. The apparent volume of distribution (V_d) is the relationship between the amount of drug in the body and the concentration of drug in the plasma. For many drugs, the V_d exceeds blood volume (about 5 L in adults), reflecting drug distribution outside the systemic circulation.

Volume of distribution, plasma half-life, and plasma clearance

Few studies have identified sex-related differences in V_d, half-life, and clearance when calculations were controlled for body weight, smoking, drinking habits, and age (Giudicelli and Tillement, 1977). Women have a lower V_d for alcohol and a higher V_d for diazepam (Harris, Benet, and Schwartz, 1995). Gender effects on hepatic drug metabolism and drug elimination are best documented for the BZDs. Total and unbound clearance of diazepam, desmethyldiazepam, and alprazolam were found to be higher in women than in men when smoking and body weight were controlled (Greenblatt et al., 1980; Ochs, Greenblatt, and Otten, 1981; Kristjansson and Thorsteinsson, 1991). The observation that oxazepam (Greenblatt et al., 1980), temazepam (Divoll et al., 1981), and chlordiazepoxide (Greenblatt et al., 1989) clearances were higher in men than in women suggests that for some drugs glucuronyltransferase activities are higher in men than in women because these drugs depend on conjugation with glucuronic acid. Diazepam and alprazolam are first hydroxylated by cytochrome P_{450} (CYP) enzymes, which seem to be more active in women, as was shown originally by O'Malley et al. (1971), using phenazone as a substrate. For five BZDs – chlordiazepoxide, diazepam, desmethyldiazepam, oxazepam, and temazepam – the plasma half-life was found to be consistently longer in women than in men. However, the findings are highly variable. For instance, Greenblatt et al. (1980) observed sex to be an important determinant for the clearance of diazepam and desmethyldiazepam, yet an age-related decline in clearance was found to be larger in men than in women (Greenblatt et al., 1982). It seems, therefore, that BZDs, which are metabolized by oxidative pathways, are sensitive to both age and sex effects. In a phase II study of the new 5-HT_3 antagonist Odansetron, slower clearance was observed in female compared to male subjects and in elderly versus young subjects (Pritchard, 1992).

Drug metabolism

Once in the circulation, drugs are eliminated from the body by two major processes: hepatic metabolism leading to biliary excretion and renal filtration leading to secretion in the urine. For the most part, the rates of hepatic and renal elimination are directly proportional to the concentration of the drug in plasma. The liver is quantitatively the major organ involved in the in vivo metabolic disposition of most compounds. Psychotropic drugs are metabolized by about 20 different enzymes. The primary, phase 1, structural modification of a drug, which involves the addition of a functional group, is mainly carried out by the CYP isoenzymes. The conjugation of the compound and its metabolite with endogenous substrate, such as sulfate, glucuronic acid, or glutathione, is termed phase 2 metabolism. Extrahepatic tissues, such as the brain, the kidneys, and the lungs, also dispose metabolically of drugs. Metabolism depends not only on access to the metabolizing cell but also on the affinity of the substrate to the active site of the enzyme, the availability of essential cofactors, and the hormonal status. Smoking, age, and sex influence drug-metabolizing enzymes. The least conflicting data exist for nicotine. The polycyclic aromatic hydrocarbons contained in cigarette smoke induce hepatic CYP oxidative enzymes and lead to a decreased half-life and increased clearance of drugs (Mac-Donald, 1981). Administration of nicotine has been shown to induce selectively brain CYP enzymes (Anandatheerthavarada, Williams, and Wecker, 1993).

Fewer data exist for sex and age; moreover, effects can vary from drug to drug (Barr and Skett, 1984). In mouse and rat brain, sex-related differences have been observed in total CYP, with the female rat brain showing significantly lower enzyme levels than the male rat brain. These differences were abolished by the administration of testosterone to female rats (Ravindranath and Boyd, 1995). Alcohol dehydrogenase activity (ADH) has been shown to be decreased in women (Frezza et al., 1990). Reduced ADH activity and the lower V_d for alcohol in women might explain why women reach higher peak blood alcohol levels faster, which in turn might explain why women are more susceptible to alcoholic liver disease with a shorter duration of heavy drinking.

The CYP system is a large group of genetically controlled isoenzymes that are known to be involved in the oxidative metabolism of most psychoactive drugs. The CYP isoenzymes most relevant for the metabolism of psychiatric drugs and their substrates are listed in Table 10.2. CYP isoenzymes found on microsomal membranes in the liver and gut mediate the metabolism of exogenous drugs and hormones; those localized on the inner mitochondrial membrane occur in brain and are involved in steroid synthesis. More than 30 CYP isoenzymes have been identified (Butler, Lang, and Young, 1992). In the nomenclature the CYP root is followed by a Roman numeral to denote the family (CYPII), followed by a capital letter for the subfamily (CYPIID) and an Arabic numeral to designate the gene (CYPIID6). Competitive binding to enzymes can lead to significant drug–drug interactions. Compounds such as nicotine can increase the particular activity of an enzyme and lead to enzyme induction, and others such as the selective serotonin reuptake inhibitors (SSRIs) can reduce the metabolic activity of an enzyme and lead to enzyme inhibition. These interactions have become important because the SSRI antidepressants, which have a relatively superior safety profile in vitro, inhibit many of the CYP isoforms and hence can turn normal into poor metabolizers and increase the risk for clinically significant drug interactions. The theoretical potential for drug interactions needs to be kept in mind, even though in clinical practice many drug combinations seem to be well tolerated and safe.

Table 10.2. *Drugs and substrates competing for cytochrome P$_{450}$ enzymes*

Microsomal cytochrome P$_{450}$ isoforms	Substrates	Inhibitors	Inducers	Poly-morphism	Gender	Interactions can lead to:
1A2	Demethylation tertiary TCAs, caffeine, haloperidol, theophylline	Fluvoxamine	Nicotine		M > F	↑ Haloperidol levels (dystonia)
2C	Demethylation TCAs, warfarin, phenytoin, diazepam	Ketoconazole, fluvoxamine, fluoxetine, sertraline, norethindrone	Rifampin	2% Caucasians 20% Japanese	2C19: M > F	
2E	Ethanol, acetaminophen	Disulfiram	Ethanol			

	Substrates	Inhibitors	Inducers	Genetic/Sex variation	Clinical consequences
2D6	Haloperidol, risperidone, thioridazine, perphenazine, clozapine, hydroxylation TCAs, fluoxetine, venlafaxine, paroxetine, codeine, beta blockers	Erythromycin, fluoxetine, paroxetine, sertraline, nefazodone		7% Caucasians; F > M	↑ Antiarrhythmic levels (torsade de pointes)
3A3	Sertraline, estrogens	Progesterone		F > M	False-positive dexamethasone suppression ↓ Contraceptive levels (ineffective contraception)
3A4	Diazepam, alprazolam, triazolam, nifedipine, verapamil, erythromycin, carbamazepine, quinidine, testosterone, dexamethasone, terfenadine	Nefazodone, fluvoxamine, fluoxetine, sertraline, paroxetine, venlafaxine, cimetidine	Carbamazepine phenytoin, phenobarbital, rifampin, dexamethasone		

Several excellent reviews describe in more detail the CYP enzyme system and the pharmacokinetics of drug–drug interactions (Ciraulo et al., 1995; Ketter et al., 1995; DeVane, 1994).

Elimination

The clearance of drugs by the liver and kidney can be influenced by the blood flow to the organ, the binding of the drug to plasma proteins, and the activity of the processes responsible for drug metabolism, such as hepatic enzyme activity, glomerular filtration rates, and renal secretory processes. A useful term to describe elimination is the drug's elimination half-life, which is the time required to reduce the plasma concentration of the drug and the body load of

Table 10.3. *Half-life, volume of distribution, and clearance of antidepressants and their active metabolites*

Antidepressant drugs	Half-life (hours)	V_d (L/kg)	Clearance (L/hour)	Age
Tricyclic antidepressants				
Imipramine	6–28	9–23	32–102	↑ half-life
Desipramine	12–28	12–40	35–110	
Nortriptyline	18–48	15–23	17–79	
10-Hydroxynortriptyline	18–48			
Serotonin reuptake inhibitors				
Fluoxetine	4–6 days	12–42	6–42	↑ half-life
norfluoxetine	7–16 days			
Sertraline	24	20	96	
Desmethylsertraline	2–4 days			
Paroxetine	24	3–28	15–92	↑ half-life
Fluvoxamine	15	5–12	60	
Other				
Venlafaxine	3–6	5–19	50–144	
0-desmethylvenlafaxine	8–12			
Buproprion	10–21	27–63	126–140	
Hydroxyproprion	22			
Erythrobuproprion	27			
Threohydrobuproprion	22			
Trazodone	6–13	1–2	2–4	↑ half life
m-Chlorophenylpiperazine	4–8			

V_d, volume of distribution.

the drug to half the initial concentration. Both V_d and drug clearance influence half-life. For practical purposes, most drugs can be considered to be eliminated completely when less than 10 percent of the effective concentration remains in the body, requiring three to four half-lives. The maintenance dose reflects a steady state, which is achieved when the rate at which the drug is administered equals the rate of drug elimination. Table 10.3 lists the half-life, V_d, and clearance of currently used antidepressant drugs and their metabolites.

Body composition and obesity

Estimates of all pharmacokinetic parameters are derived from an "average," usually male, patient. By nature men and women have different body compositions. Men are typically taller and weigh more, but they carry lower percentages of body fat than women. Remarkably, studies have shown that body composition variations within the normal range have little effect on drug availability. Differences in body composition in adults can be accounted for by normalizing the drug dose or by adjusting kinetic parameters to body weight, to body mass index (BMI: kg/m^2; normal range 18–25 and 19–27 for females and males, respectively), and to ideal body weight for age and height or body surface area. Controlling for body size is important at low extremes of body weight, such as cachexia or anorexia nervosa, where in addition hepatic or renal function may be impaired and cardiac output may be low.

High or excess body weights, in other words obesity (BMI > 30), have been found to have small effects on drug pharmakokinetics. Obese subjects have a greater blood volume and a higher cardiac output, but because the blood flow to adipose tissue is lower than in muscle, fat tissue acts as a storage site for lipophilic drugs. Most of the pharmacokinetic information about obesity deals with drug distribution. Caffeine and antipyrine have been reported to occupy a similar total V_d in obese and lean individuals, but when values were corrected for body weight, obese subjects had a smaller V_d and a reduced AUC (Caraco et al., 1995). However, for more lipophilic drugs (BZDs, carbamazepine (CBZ), trazodone) the V_d and elimination half-life are moderately increased (Cheymol, 1993). Similarly, Dunn et al. (1991) reported a 40 percent reduced clearance in obese subjects for methylprednisolone. They suggest that for drugs with distribution to lean tissue, the loading dose should be based on ideal body weight and the dosing interval should be lengthened because of the decreased clearance. In general then, for drugs metabolized by oxidation, reduction, and conjugation and for those with flow-dependent hepatic clearance, total clearance is not markedly diminished in obesity.

Menstrual cycle and pregnancy

Alcohol is the "drug" best studied during the menstrual cycle. Women obtained significantly higher peak blood alcohol concentrations than men at the time of ovulation and immediately before menstruation, once blood alcohol levels were corrected for body weight (Jones and Jones, 1976). Covarying for weight, Kirkwood et al. (1991) observed no differences in single-dose alprazolam (1 mg po) pharmacokinetics during menstrual cycle phases; however, for nitrazepam, Jochemsen et al. (1982) reported increased clearance. Menstrual cycle effects on lithium are well documented (Chamberlain et al., 1990). Conrad and Hamilton (1986) reported a premenstrual decline of serum lithium levels leading to an exacerbation of a bipolar psychosis.

Influence of oral contraceptives on drug kinetics

Clinically most important are observations that a number of drugs interfere with the efficacy of oral contraceptives (OCs) (Back et al., 1988). Drugs that induce CYP enzymes (see Table 10.2) increase hepatic metabolism and the rate of elimination and consequently lower OC plasma concentrations. Of concern is a report by Haukkamaa (1986), who described conception in epileptic women with subdermal Norplant capsules. Drugs that reduce the intestinal bacterial flora and hence the bacteria-induced hydrolysis of OCs, such as antibiotics, can inhibit the enterohepatic recirculation and intestinal reuptake of OCs. By and large, studies of estrogen–drug interactions have involved younger women on and off OCs. Long-term administration, even of the new, low-dose oral contraceptives, has been shown to inhibit drug-metabolizing enzymes competitively and to prolong the plasma half-life of aminopyrine, nitrazepam, and chlordiazepoxide (Wilson, 1984). Considerable interindividual variation in drug half-life in response to oral contraceptive administration has been observed, suggesting that enzyme inhibition varies depending on the nature of the contraceptive and dosage. OCs have been shown to decrease the clearance and inhibit absorption of BZDs. These observations are consistent with reports that pregnant women show delayed clearance of chlordiazepide as opposed to not pregnant women (Rey et al., 1979). OCs decrease plasma albumin levels and increase alpha-acid glycoprotein levels (Wilson, 1984). Oral contraceptive–induced endocrine and metabolic changes are less well characterized. OCs have been shown to suppress insulin-like growth factor (Jernstrom and Olsson, 1994), to induce insulin resistance, leading to glucose intolerance, and to raise serum lipid and lipoprotein concentrations (Shen et al., 1994). Thyroid function may be activated. In a study of 200 healthy women who received low-dose contraceptives containing 30–50 µg ethinylestradiol, T$_4$ and thyroid-binding globulin increased, and 16 percent had triiodothyronine levels in the hyperthyroid range (Sorger, Schenck, and Schneider, 1992).

Psychotropic drug use during pregnancy

Drug use in pregnancy has shown a downward trend in the United States and in Western Europe (Collaborative Group on Drug Use in Pregnancy, 1990), reflecting an attitude of caution among prescribers and users (Bonati et al., 1990). In a European survey 15 percent among 9,714 pregnant women took no drug at any time of the pregnancy; on average 2.6 drugs were used (Collaborative Group on Drug Use in Pregnancy, 1991, 1992). In England and Western Europe fewer than 5 percent of women take any drug during the first trimester. This compares to an earlier prospective study in the United States by Doering and Stewart (1978), who reported that 35 percent of pregnant women had received at least one psychotropic compound. In a large-scale survey covering 22 countries and 148 maternity wards, Marchetti et al. (1993) found that 3.5 percent of women used psychotropic drugs during pregnancy. BZD use was most common (444/520, or 85 percent, with 7 percent reporting chronic use).

Drug effects on the fetus

The nature of the drugs' effects on the fetus is the overriding concern for drug use in pregnancy. Overall the incidence of major birth defects is about 2–3 percent, and in two thirds of malformations the cause is unknown (Kalter and Warkany, 1983). Pharmaceutical companies warn against drug use, because all drugs are released for human use without establishment of a safety profile in pregnancy. A drug's teratogenic potential is tested in animals, but as the thalidomide experience showed, the test results cannot always be extrapolated to humans. Case reports or retrospective case control studies have been the major source for detection of teratogenic effects. As a rule, psychoactive drugs ought to be used in pregnancy only if the mother's condition is drug responsive and does not improve with psychosocial therapies. Medication ought to be administered at the lowest therapeutically effective dose for the shortest time possible. The physician, who will be expected to provide information about potential risks to the fetus, needs to consider several points:

1. Altered pharmacokinetics during pregnancy.
2. The timing of drug use – in the first, second, or third trimester.
3. The nature of the drug, its relative risk, and which drugs should be avoided at all cost.

Drug absorption changes little during pregnancy except for slower gastric emptying and longer transit time, both of which are more pronounced during the third trimester (Davison, Davison, and Hay, 1970). Reduced plasma albumin concentrations during pregnancy set more drug free, which is then available for passage into tissues including the placenta. On the other hand, the expansion in plasma volume increases the V_d by up to 50 percent in late pregnancy for polar drugs, and additional adipose tissue provides extra storage for lipophilic drugs. This is somewhat compensated for by the higher cardiac output with a corresponding increase in tissue perfusion including the kidney, which is relevant for drugs with high renal clearance rates.

Little is known about the combined and conceivably opposite effects of the high estradiol and progesterone blood levels during pregnancy on metabolizing enzyme systems. Higher doses of antiepileptic drugs seem to be required to maintain therapeutic plasma levels, suggesting increased elimination (Bologa et al., 1991); in contrast, caffeine clearance has been shown to be decreased (Aldridge, Bailey, and Neims, 1981). However, drawing conclusions from total drug levels may be misleading, due to differences in the disposition between protein-bound and free drug. For instance, CBZ clearance was found to be unchanged except for a slight decrease in CBZ concentrations during the third trimester, whereas total phenytoin levels steadily decreased by 39 percent with only an 18 percent decrease in free phenytoin levels (Rey et al., 1979).

The placental transfer of drugs from maternal to fetal circulation occurs by diffusion. Like the liver, the placenta can metabolize drugs, but how this capacity for drug metabolism might affect drugs that pass on to the fetus is not known. For most chronically administered drugs, 50–100 percent of steady-state maternal drug levels will be found in the fetus. For some drugs, such as diazepam, fetal plasma levels can be double or triple the maternal plasma levels. Taken together this means that in pregnant women a dose increase might be necessary to maintain a clinical response, and hence the fetus might be exposed to higher drug levels.

Prescription drugs and drug overdose

Drug exposure during conception and pregnancy has been associated with miscarriage (spontaneous abortion), abruptio placentae, fetal growth retardation, premature labor, and abnormal organ or limb development. Table 10.4 lists the most commonly reported malformations attributed to psychotropic drugs taken during the first trimester. Because cells are undifferentiated in the first 2 weeks following conception, drug effects are likely to interfere with the integrity of the embryo and lead to embryonic loss rather than malformation. Correy et al. (1994) conducted a large-scale survey of 56,000 births in Australia. Among the women 30 percent had used prescription drugs and 40 percent had used alcohol. The overall rate of 1.85 percent malformations was not different from rates observed in subgroups of women who smoked, used vitamins, used prescription drugs, or were alcohol users. In this study aspirin use was found to be associated with hypospadia (3.5 odds ratio) and OC use with pes cavus. Judging from surveys by Gunnarskog and Kallan (1993) and Isacsson, Wasserman, and Bergman (1995), drug overdose during pregnancy does not necessarily carry a substantial teratogenic risk. In 70 infants whose mothers had taken an accidental or intentional overdose of psychoactive drugs, no congenital malformation was observed.

Table 10.4. *Psychotropic drugs and hormones associated with anomalies following first trimester exposure*

Drug	Documented malformations
Phenytoin	Microcephaly, facial clefts
Valproic acid	Neural tube defects, fetal valproate syndrome
Carbamazepine	Spinal defects
Lithium carbonate	Cardiovascular malformations; Ebstein's anomaly
Benzodiazepines	Oral clefts
	Withdrawal: "floppy " infant syndrome (tremors, apneic spells, hypotonia)
Tricyclic antidepressants	Withdrawal: tachycardia, respiratory distress, heart failure
Antipsychotic drugs	Withdrawal: sedation followed by motor excitement, jaundice, tremor, poor sucking reflexes
Hormones	
Diethylstilbestrol	Vaginal adenosis and adenocarcinoma
17 Beta-estradiol	Vaginal and urinary tract lesions
Progestogens	Masculinization
17-Methyltestosterone	Masculinization

Antiepileptic drugs

The newer antiepileptic drugs (AEDs) have recently been proven effective as psychotropic compounds for controlling bipolar mood disorders. Moreover, the FDA has now approved divalproex sodium (Depakote) for the prevention of migraine headaches. Therefore, observations that antiepileptic drugs (in particular, phenytoin and valproic acid) have high teratogenic potential (higher than lithium use) are crucial. Malformations were present in 7 percent of infants born to mothers with epilepsy compared to 1.36 percent of infants in the general population. Phenobarbital in combination with phenytoin was more teratogenic than phenobarbital alone (Dravet et al., 1992). Lindhout et al. (1992) compared changes in prescription patterns over a 10-year period. Whereas 10 percent of 151 live-born infants, exposed to phenytoin between 1972 and 1979, had congenital heart defects, facial clefts, and/or dysmorphism with mental retardation, this rate was 7.6 percent in infants whose mothers had received monotherapy with valproate and carbamazepine, spinal defects being more prominent. At 1 year of age the children had more minor anomalies than unexposed children. Recently, a fetal valproate syndrome, consisting of a distinctive facial appearance, sometimes accompanied by a neural tube defect, heart disease, cleft lip or palate, genitourinary malformations, or limb defects has been described (Clayton-Smith and Donnai, 1995). Folic acid administration is thought to reduce the risk. Because these studies were conducted in women with epilepsy, not in psychiatric patients, some have argued that the findings cannot be generalized because epilepsy may impart a risk for malformations independent of drug use.

Benzodiazepine use

In the 1970s a Finnish study (Saxen and Saxen, 1975) and a Norwegian study (Aarskog, 1975) reported an association between BZD use and oral clefts. In the late 1980s a Swedish report that described 7 children with dysmorphism and mental retardation born to mothers who used high doses of BZDs regularly during pregnancy again alarmed clinicians because BZDs are the drugs most commonly used in pregnancy (Laegreid et al., 1987). Subsequent studies confirmed impaired intrauterine growth and a high rate of craniofacial abnormalities in 17 infants born to mothers who used BZDs in therapeutic doses throughout pregnancy compared to 29 infants whose mothers did not use drugs (Laegreid, Hagberg, and Lundberg, 1992). A delay in mental development of up to 18 months was observed, albeit the children by then had caught up on their physical development. If BZDs are used for a short time in low doses during the first trimester, even in an overdose, no adverse effects have been found. The risk increases again with late third trimester exposure including delivery, which has been found associated with the "floppy infant" syndrome, a BZD withdrawal syndrome including tremors, apneic spells, and hypo- or hypertonia (McElhatton, 1994). Pregnant women on BZDs should be gradually withdrawn over a 1-month period. Intravenous diazepam (30 mg) during labor has been associated with apneic spells, hypotonia, and temporary loss of heartbeat and therefore ought to be avoided (Shannon et al., 1972; Cree, Meyer, and Hailey, 1973).

Lithium

Shortly after the introduction of lithium, Schou's group in Denmark founded an international register of lithium babies (Schou et al., 1973). Initial studies suggested an increased risk of stillbirths and a 400-fold rise in the risk of cardiovascular abnormalities, especially Ebstein's anomaly (a downward displacement of the tricuspid valve into the right ventricle) with first trimester exposure to lithium (Nora, Nora, and Toews, 1974; Weinstein and Goldfield, 1975). Newer studies (Edmonds and Oakley, 1990; Zalzstein et al., 1990), reviewed by Cohen, Friedman, Jefferson, Johnson, and Weiner (1994), suggest a lower risk, from 10- to 20-fold (0.1%, or 1:1000). Other malformations involve the central nervous system and external ears (Troutman, 1979). Babies born to lithium-treated mothers without signs of malformation had no increased frequency of mental or physical abnormalities at 5 years of age in a follow-up study by Schou (1976). Lithium easily crosses the placenta, so lithium toxicity has been seen even at plasma levels below the therapeutic range (Linden and Rich, 1983). Neonatal signs of lithium intoxication include hypotonia, lethargy, hypothermia, poor suckling reflex, jaundice, and reversible neonatal goiter (Karlsson, Lindstedt, and Lundberg, 1975). To protect the fetus, lithium ought to be discontinued a week before delivery. Given the risk for anomalies, lithium ought to be avoided during the first trimester. Considering that valproic acid and CBZ carry their own risk of teratogenicity, unfortunately no safe alternatives to lithium are currently available.

Alcohol

Most women decrease alcohol consumption during pregnancy or give up alcohol altogether, yet 18.8 percent continue to drink alcohol (National Institute on Drug Abuse, 1994). White women and women with 16 or more years of education and those with income of $40,000 or more are more likely to drink during pregnancy (Kleber, 1996). Drinking while pregnant increases the risk of miscarriage, fetal death, and by more than 50 percent, death during the infant's first year (Harlap and Shiono, 1980). Heavy drinking early in pregnancy can lead to physical malformations, characteristic of the fetal alcohol syndrome (FAS): gestational and/or postnatal growth retardation, facial malformations, a small head size, and central nervous system abnormalities with behavioral and cognitive deficits (Clarren and Smith, 1978). About 6 percent of alcoholic women have a child with FAS. Apparently genetic factors are involved in the development of FAS (Streissguth and Dehaene, 1993). Rates of the fetal alcohol syndrome have increased dramatically from 1:10,000 live births in 1979 to 6.7:10,000 live births in 1993 (Kleber, 1996). Drinking in the third trimester of pregnancy may retard the baby's weight gain and overall growth (Day et al., 1989). Alcohol use is one of the most common causes of mental retardation, with 5 percent of all congenital anomalies being attributed to alcohol (Sokol, Miller, and Reed, 1980). Predictors of prenatal alcohol consumption are presence of depressive symptoms, low pregnancy support, and prepregnancy drinking of more than one drink per day (Hanson, Streissguth, and Smith, 1978; Zuckerman et al., 1989). Women who are at risk for heavy alcohol abuse can be screened with the CAGE questions: Have you ever *cut* down on drinking? Have you been *annoyed* by criticism of drinking? Have you felt *guilty* over drinking? Have you used alcohol as an *eye* opener in the morning? (Sokol, 1989). If one of the questions is positive, a more thorough evaluation, and in most cases, a referral to an alcohol treatment program becomes necessary, because abstinent women have significantly fewer infants with low birth weights and signs of the FAS.

Nicotine

Smoking during pregnancy increases the risk of miscarriage, low-birth-weight babies, and perinatal deaths. The risk of sudden infant death syndrome (SIDS) is five times greater for infants born to mothers who smoke during the second trimester of pregnancy compared to those who have never smoked (Klonoff-Cohen et al., 1995). Many women continue to smoke in order to avoid weight gain during pregnancy and are not aware that exposure from even half a pack of cigarettes has been related to lower scores on intelligence tests (Fried, 1993). Giving up smoking lengthens the time of pregnancy and reduces the chance of complications (Li et al., 1993).

Antidepressant drugs

Tricyclic antidepressants. Although their safe use in pregnancy has not been established, exposure to the tricyclic drugs, imipramine and amitriptyline, does not result in a greater than normal risk of malformations, even when taken during the first trimester. Four retrospective studies reviewing 200 cases of intrauterine tricyclic exposure (Scanlon, 1969; Crombie, Pinsent, and Fleming, 1972; Sims, 1972; Heinonen, Slone, and Shapiro, 1977) reported no or a moderately higher incidence of congenital malformations. The validity of these studies is limited by the retrospective design and the small number of mothers who continued to take tricyclic drugs in pregnancy. However, two prospective studies support these conclusions; in the first no abnormalities were observed in the offspring of 74 women taking tricyclics, albeit the risk of miscarriage was doubled (Pastuszak, Schick-Boschetto, and Zuber, 1993). In the second study, the European Network of Teratology Information Services (Arnon et al., 1996) collected prospective data on 689 pregnancies, over 90 percent exposed to tricyclic or nontricyclic antidepressants during the first trimester. Among the liveborn babies 97 percent were morphologically normal. Elective termination of pregnancy occurred in 18 percent of mothers on multidrug therapy as opposed to 10 percent of mothers on single-drug therapy. An increase in neonatal problems was associated with chronic multidrug therapy near term. In addition, Ware and DeVane (1990) reported continuous imipramine use in two women who delivered healthy infants. A fetal tricyclic (imipramine, amitriptyline, chlormipramine) withdrawal syndrome has been described, which consists of seizures, tachypnea, irritability, and difficulty feeding as well as anticholinergic effects, bladder distention, and gastrointestinal motility changes (Webster, 1973; Breyer-Pfaff et al., 1995). These withdrawal symptoms can be avoided by tapering the dose 5–10 days before delivery.

Nulman et al. (1997) conducted a postnatal follow-up of children born to 80 mothers exposed to tricyclic drugs and 55 children whose mothers had taken fluoxetine during pregnancy and compared them to the offspring of 84 mothers who had not taken drugs known to affect the fetus adversely. No significant differences between the groups were found in mean global IQ values, language development, and behavioral development at ages 16 to 86 months.

Monoamine oxidase inhibitors. Monoamine oxidase inhibitors (MAOIs) have not been studied, but given the irreversible MAO enzyme inhibition with phenelzine or tranylcypromine sulfate, irreversible MAOIs would be expected to increase the risk for severe hypertension with all its complications.

Selective serotonin reuptake inhibitors. An increased risk (1.9 odds ratio) for miscarriages (12–13 percent in women on drugs vs. 6.8 percent in women not on drugs) characterizes the use of SSRIs and tricyclic antidepressants during the first trimester (Pastuszak, Schick-Boschetto, and Zuber, 1993). This prospective study enrolled 128 pregnant women exposed to fluoxetine during the first trimester (mean daily maternal dose: 25.8 mg) who contacted one of four teratogen information services. There were no differences in the rates (1–3 percent) of major birth defects when live births exposed to fluoxetine were compared to nonteratogenic controls and to women on tricyclics. Another prospective study (Chambers et al., 1996), which compared 228 women who had called the California Teratogen Information Service because they were taking fluoxetine to 254 women who had called with questions about drugs not considered teratogenic, found similar rates (5.5 percent and 4.0 percent, respectively) of major malformations. More newborns exposed to fluoxetine (15.5 percent) had minor structural anomalies than babies of mothers not exposed (6.5 percent). Babies exposed to fluoxetine up to term had a threefold higher rate of prematurity and poor neonatal adaptation, and they had lower birth weights and lengths, whereas babies exposed during the first trimester did not differ from normal controls. This study did not screen for coexisting illnesses. For sertraline, U.S. and worldwide case reports mention two cases of reduction deformity (undeveloped fingers on one or both hands), although no causal relationship could be determined. Even if pharmaceutical companies advise careful precautions, they are not always successful in avoiding exposure of pregnant women. For example, during phase II and phase III studies with venlafaxine, five cases of first-trimester exposure (dose unknown) occurred. Apparently healthy babies were born. Rare spontaneous reports of congenital malformations following venlafaxine exposure, one involving a full-term infant with craniofacial defect and "abnormal eyelids," have been received (Wyeth-Ayerst, 1996). Amantadine used to treat extrapyramidal side effects and more recently to enhance dopaminergic transmission in treatment resistant depressions (Bouckoms and Mangini, 1993) has been associated with organ dysgenesis in animals (Hirsh and Swartz, 1980) and in one infant with cardiovascular malformation (Nora, Nora, and Way, 1975).

Antipsychotics

Exposure to phenothiazines or butyrophenones during human embryonic development has led to conflicting reports, ranging from no adverse outcome to doubling the risk for fetal malformations (Edlund and Craig, 1984). Sobel (1960) found similar rates of fetal deaths or anomalies in the offspring of schizophrenic women with and without exposure to chlorpromazine, yet the rates were twice as high as those in the general population. A French follow-up of nearly 12,000 live births of the offspring of 350 women who took phenothiazines during the first trimester found a marked increase (odds ratio 2.1) in fetal central nervous system malformations, microcephaly, and septal and limb defects (Rumeau-Roquette, Goujard, and Heul, 1977). In this study exposure to chlorpromazine, a phenothiazine with a three-carbon aliphatic side chain, conferred the greater risk, whereas phenothiazines with the two-carbon side chain, such as piperazine, did not enhance the risk. A prospective study by Slone et al. (1977) in which 1,300 mothers were exposed to phenothiazines found a lower increase in risk with a trend for more cardiac malformations with first-trimester exposure (odds ratio 1.13). Very little is known about in utero exposure to high-potency antipsychotics, such as haloperidol, which are less likely to cause hypotension with the risk for uteroplacental insufficiency. Exposure to haloperidol has been associated with phocomelia, although other factors might have contributed (Kopelman, McCullar, and Heggeness, 1975). High-potency neuroleptics are said to carry a lower risk of congenital malformations than do low-potency neuroleptics such as chlorpromazine. Placental transfer of risperidone has been documented in rat pups with increased rates of pup deaths and stillbirth at three to six times the human dose. Agenesis of the corpus callosum has been reported for one infant exposed to risperidone in utero (Janssen Pharmaceutica product information).

Phenothiazines in low doses are still given as antinauseants or antiemetics. Since a neonatal phenothiazine withdrawal syndrome has been reported, a 5- to 10-day washout period before delivery is advisable. Anticholinergic effects can cause tachyarrhythmia, and dopaminergic effects can result in extrapyramidal symptoms in the infant, which can persist for 6–9 months (Levy and Wisniewski, 1974).

Psychotropic drug use during lactation

Women in the developed countries have returned to breast-feeding, recognizing its emotional and nutritional benefits to the infant. The fervor with which nursing is currently supported has created conflicts for women who require medication to function as mothers and in their work.

Table 10.5 lists the principal components in human milk. All drugs are excreted into breast milk and bioavailable to the infant (American Academy of Pediatrics Committee on Drugs 1989; Pons, Rey, and Matheson, 1994). Because the dose of the drug transferred to the infant depends on the plasma concentra-

Table 10.5. *Percentage composition of human milk (400–600 ml/day)*

Water	88
Lactose	7
Lipids	3.8
Protein	0.9

- Diffusion is the primary transport mechanism.
- Concentration depends on free drug; due to low milk protein, drug protein binding is low.
- The pH 7.1 is lower than maternal plasma and therefore creates a gradient for increased diffusion of weak ionized bases into milk.

tion and volume, higher drug doses and more frequent feedings will increase drug exposure. Weighing the infant before and after nursing is a good measure of intake (Infante et al., 1991). For drugs with a short half-life, the drug exposure can be minimized by planning nursing periods just before drug ingestion and by pumping breast milk before drug ingestion for feeding the infant later. Altshuler et al. (1995) studied 8 samples of breast milk in 2 nursing mothers and found the lowest levels 1–2 hours before and the highest 5–9 hours following drug ingestion, but the study did not include measurements of metabolites.

Milk to maternal plasma drug concentration ratios (*M/P*) are used as an index of the extent of drug excretion in milk and can be estimated as follows:

$$C_{m \, = \, Cp \, \times \, M/P}$$

where C_m = drug concentration in milk and C_p = drug concentration in maternal plasma at the time of feeding. Ito and Koren (1994) have amended this index to include the drug's clearance as an important factor in determining the exposure level in the infant.

The amount of a drug with a long half-life and one or more active metabolites that gets transferred during lactation is more difficult to determine (Begg, Atkinson, and Duffull, 1992). Misri and Sivertz (1991) have argued that even though the drug concentrations in breast milk might be negligible, brain concentrations can be 10- to 30-fold greater than serum concentrations. Drug sampling in breast milk (tricyclics and SSRIs) on similar doses revealed widely differing levels of drug and metabolite concentration in maternal serum and breast milk, and rarely detected drug in the baby's serum (Wisner and Perel, 1991). Other recent studies have identified measurable quantities of imipramine, desipramine, and amitriptyline in breast milk (O'Brien, 1974; Sovner and Orsulak, 1979; Bader and Newman, 1980; Breyer-Pfaff et al., 1995).

Mothers taking oral contraceptives can breast-feed safely (Shenfield and Griffin, 1991). Lithium is contraindicated, because one third to one half of maternal plasma levels have been measured in the infant's plasma and the classical signs of lithium toxicity have been reported in newborns (Schou et al., 1973; Sykes, Quarrie, and Alexander, 1976. Antipsychotic drugs would be contraindicated, not only because infants become too drowsy and lethargic to nurse but also because concentrations have been reported to be much higher in milk than in maternal plasma (Uhlir and Ryznar, 1973). Occasional use of low doses of drugs is probably compatible with breast-feeding (Murray and Seger, 1994). Nursing is clearly not advisable if long-term drug administration is required, especially not for drugs with a long elimination half-life, such as some BZDs and fluoxetine. If the mother takes drugs, the baby's plasma ought to be sampled at 1 and 2 weeks. If any drug is detected, nursing should be discontinued. If no drug is found, it must be kept in mind that the sensitivity of the assay may be too low.

Sex-related differences in treatment response and side effect profile

Placebo response. Another reason physicians overdispense drugs to women is based on the belief that women are more often placebo responders than men. This view is unsupported by data. To our knowledge there are virtually no studies on gender differences in the placebo response. In fact, early on, Trouton (1957) reported that women were not more likely than men to receive relief from a placebo. A recent analysis (unpublished) of the placebo response in 144 men and 215 women with panic attacks based on the Cross-National Collaborative Panic Study (1992) conducted by E. Uhlenhuth and M. Hearron found remarkably similar reductions in panic attacks and phobic symptoms in men and women in response to 8 weeks of placebo administration.

Reimherr, Ward, and Byerly (1989) evaluated the overall effect of gender and clinical symptoms on the placebo response by pooling data from 7 placebo-controlled clinical trials of antidepressant drugs. Females with a single episode of depression had the highest (66.7 percent) therapeutic response to placebo, and females with recurrent episodes had the lowest (13.3 percent) response. The presence of somatic anxiety and psychomotor retardation predicted a low placebo response. In a controlled placebo study on circadian rhythms, more women than men exhibited a temperature rhythm that was desynchronized from 24 hours and had a tau less than 24 hours. Placebo administration obliterated this gender-related difference and normalized desynchronized rhythms of left- and right-hand grip strength, yet the latter only in men (Reinberg et al., 1994).

Nocebo response. Sex-related nocebo effects, adverse effects from placebo administration, have not been much investigated either. A large-scale phase I study reported adverse events in 19 percent of healthy volunteers. Complaints were more frequent after repeated dosing (28 percent) and in elderly subjects (26 percent) (Rosenzweig, Broheir, and Zipfel, 1993). Nocebo effects can be frankly toxic; for instance, angioneurotic edema has resulted from placebo therapy (Wolf and Pinsky, 1954).

Adverse drug reactions

Adverse drug reactions are any noxious unintended and undesired effects of a drug that occur at the dose used in man or woman for treatment, diagnosis, or prophylaxis. Few studies have been published on the frequency and nature of adverse drug reactions. The following factors have been shown to increase the frequency of adverse drug reactions: age over 50, female sex, previous history of allergies, and reactions to drugs. Thus, postmenopausal women seem to have the highest incidence of adverse drug reactions. Depending upon the definition, 7–20 percent show definite and up to 36 percent of all patients show probable adverse reactions to drugs. In studies by Green and Krueger (1963), Hurwitz (1969), Stewart and Kluff (1974), and Domecq et al. (1980), women have been reported to experience more adverse drug reactions, in particular gastrointestinal disturbances and an increase in cutaneous allergic reactions. Gelenberg et al. (1977) and Jaffe and Zisook (1978) reported that hyperprolactinemia and galactorrhea associated with amoxapine therapy occurred more often in women, an effect well documented for antipsychotic drugs (Hussain, Harinath, and Murphy, 1972). In Ellinwood's study (1984) women off contraceptives were found to have significantly more psychomotor impairment than women on contraceptives, supporting the notion that diazepam was absorbed more quickly, leading to higher peak levels in the absence of hormones. Factors that make females more susceptible than males to adverse drug reactions are not known; they might be related to lack of estrogens and to the fact that women receive more drugs than men (Domecq et al., 1980). However, women do not have more fatal reactions to drugs (Bottiger, Furhoff, and Holmberg, 1979).

Gender differences in therapeutic efficacy

Basic science research has shown that estrogens modulate several of the neurotransmitter systems implicated in psychiatric disorders: They downregulate beta-adrenergic and serotonin receptors, they have cholinergic trophic effects, and they show dopamine antagonist activity.

Antipsychotic drugs. Estrogens appear to influence the clearance and metabolism of antipsychotic drugs, because many investigators have observed that women reach higher plasma levels of antipsychotic drugs than men with the same drug dose (Seeman, 1983; D'Mello and McNeil, 1990; Simpson et al., 1990). In a drug trial with Fluspirilene, a depot antipsychotic not marketed in the United States, in which doses were titrated to clinical improvement, Chouinard, Annable, and Steinberg (1986) found that women of similar weights and ages required about half the dose required by men. This finding that young women show greater improvement than young men on equivalent doses has been attributed to the antidopaminergic properties of estrogen (Fields and Gordon, 1982; Seeman, 1996), although complementary, sedative, effects of progesterone or progesterone metabolites, which block GABA receptors (Majewska and Schwartz, 1987), may be involved. Since some of these studies did not control for smoking, contraceptive use, and concurrent medications, better controlled fixed-dose studies with measurements of estradiol and progesterone as well as drug plasma levels might shed more light on the factors mediating sex-related differences.

Gender differences in the incidence of side effects add support to the antidopaminergic theory of estrogen. Studies (Chouinard et al., 1980; Smith and Dunn, 1979) suggest a higher incidence and greater severity of tardive dyskinesia in older women and young and old men compared to premenopausal women. Morgenstern, Glazer, and Doucette (1996) described a positive relationship between right-hand preference and tardive dyskinesia that was stronger in men than in women.

Antidepressant drugs. There is scant experimental support for the theory that estrogens are directly involved in the etiology of depressive symptoms. A placebo-controlled study by Klaiber et al. (1979) of large doses of estrogen (15–25 mg) given for 3 months that showed improvement in treatment-resistant depressed pre- and postmenopausal women has not been replicated to our knowledge. Some of the earliest clinical trials investigating antidepressant drug response analyzed the data for sex effects. In a sample of moderately depressed outpatients, females tended to drop out more frequently on drugs and males on placebo. Males reported side effects when on drug and females when on drug or placebo; also, male depressives had a more robust treatment response to imipramine (Rickels, 1965). In 1974 Raskin published an analysis of sex and age effects on drug (imipramine, chlorpromazine, diazepam vs. placebo) response following 3 weeks of in-hospital treatment. In this study age-dependent gender effects were observed. In women under 40 years cognitive disturbances responded best to placebo. The sedative effects of chlorpromazine reduced hostility, whereas imipramine increased hostility scores. Women over 40 had greater cognitive difficulties at baseline, which responded significantly better than in younger women to imipramine but responded poorly to placebo or chlorpromazine. Men under 40 had a negative placebo response when they were compared to men on chlorpromazine as opposed to the male diazepam comparison group, who had a positive placebo response. Older men responded better to drug treatment than younger men, and when all groups were compared older women improved the least.

In recent investigations women responded better to phenelzine than men (Raskin, 1974; Davidson and Pelton, 1986), and in a study of patients with chronic depression, men responded better to imipramine and less well to sertraline, whereas women did somewhat better on sertraline than they did on imipramine (Schatzberg et al., 1995). There is also evidence that subtle gender differences exist in the clinical phenomenology of depression. In a survey of psychopathology among state hospital patients, women displayed significantly more withdrawal and retardation than men (Pokorny and Overall, 1970). A recent factor analysis of depressive symptoms among urban teenagers tends to support these observations: The first factor for male students reflected symptoms of "anger and tension," the second "school problems," whereas for female students "sadness with irritation" and "lethargy" emerged as the first and second factors, respectively (Casper, Belanoff, and Offer, 1996). Katz et al. (1993) found on videotape ratings of depressed inpatients after drug washout that in depressed women anxiety was highly related to motor retardation, whereas in depressed men anxiety was related to hostility. The findings suggest that depressed mood and anxiety may lead to deactivation and apathy in women and activation in men and that drugs might affect these symptoms differentially. Future treatment response studies will need to control for age and menstrual status (young women frequently report worsening of depressive symptoms premenstrually) and for comorbidity (see Chapter Four). Recent findings that thought disturbances might be inversely related to estrogen levels (Riecher-Roessler and Haefner, 1993) might be another vantage point for research.

The use of drugs in the elderly

About a third of all prescriptions in the United States are written for patients 65 years or older, even though these comprise at most 12 percent of the population. Pharmacokinetic changes in elderly patients are related to changes in body composition and in the function of pharmacokinetically important organs. A decrease in gastric acid secretion and in mucosal absorptive surface of the small bowel by about 30 percent and a decrease in mesentery blood flow by about 40 percent can have an effect on drug absorption. The distribution of drugs changes as well because the percentage of total body fat increases. Therefore, for lipid-soluble drugs (most psychotropic medications fall into this category) the V_d relative to body weight is increased. Plasma concentration of albumin decreases frequently with aging, so drugs that are bound to plasma albumin can be affected. Alpha 1-acid glycoprotein, a plasma protein that binds basic drugs, is not diminished with aging.

On the other hand, because cardiac output and blood flow to the kidneys and liver can decrease by about 30–40 percent with aging and glomular filtration may be reduced by as much as 50 percent, the clearance of most drugs is diminished (Ochs, Greenblatt, and Otten, 1981; Ho et al., 1985; Rugstad et al., 1986). This means that drugs with a long elimination half-life – for instance, diazepam – tend to accumulate in the elderly, leading to sedation with the risk for falls and bone fractures (Ray et al., 1987). Age-related pharmacodynamic changes following administration of antianxiety agents or hypnotic drugs tend to produce greater degrees of depression in the elderly than in younger patients at the same plasma concentration. The hypotensive side effects of many psychotropic drugs also tend to be more pronounced in the elderly owing to reduced functioning of adrenergic receptor reflexes. Overall reduced clearance and lower drug binding in the elderly outweigh the lower drug uptake. This means in practice that lower doses of anxiolytic, antidepressant, or hypnotic drugs are indicated with advancing age.

Conclusion

In this overview of psychopharmacologic issues relevant to women, several areas merit attention. The tendency of physicians more often to prescribe medication to women than to men may not meet women's expectations or their needs. The "placebo effect" of the personal contact with the physician on symptom presentation is well documented and may well be worth an evaluation before drugs are prescribed. The wide therapeutic index characteristic of psychoactive drugs suggests that the study of factors contributing to interindividual variance is important. Nonetheless, despite evidence that estrogens modulate the function of CYP enzymes and reduce the activity of alcohol-metabolizing enzyme systems, the effect, size, and clinical implications of sex-related pharmacokinetic and pharmacodynamic changes are not well quantified, perhaps with the exception of lower antipsychotic dose requirements for women during their reproductive years. The effect seems to be significant for age, in that older patients generally require less medication. The more frequent psychotropic drug use in women can potentiate clinically significant drug–drug interactions. Women also have less tolerance for the psychological and physiologic effects of alcohol and nicotine.

Maternal drug use during pregnancy and lactation is another area in which more research is urgently needed. Data on maternal health and prenatal drug use, outcome of pregnancy, birth weight, perinatal and neonatal complications, and presence or absence of birth defects, which underlie our estimates for teratogenic risk, have relied on voluntary reports or retrospective case studies and only recently on prospective studies that have recruited women enrolled in drug registries and teratogen information services. These sources will remain important for the collection of data on the safety:risk ratio for drugs in pregnancy, because for ethical reasons drug safety or efficacy studies are unlikely to be conducted in pregnant women. The studies show that even psychotropic drugs with no documented teratogenic effects appear to increase the risk for miscarriage. Significant malformations have been associated with first-trimester exposure to valproic acid, CBZ, and lithium, and despite the much lower risk associated with other psychotropic drugs, it seems prudent to avoid all psychotropic drugs during the first trimester of pregnancy. To the extent that drug use during lactation is just beginning to be studied systematically, breast-feeding ought to be avoided if psychoactive drugs, in particular those with a long half-life, are required for long-term treatment. Investigations into sex-related differences in treatment response point to behavioral differences (i.e., women tend to display withdrawal and retardation when depressed and anxious) as well as to a protective action of estrogen in psychotic illness; both observations might have implications for drug treatement. Finally, this overview provides ample evidence from research to justify further exploration into hormonal influences in psychopharmacology.

CHAPTER 11

INTERVENTION TRIALS CONCERNED WITH DISEASE PREVENTION IN WOMEN

JENNIFER L. KELSEY

AND ROBERT MARCUS

Until recently most large randomized trials to test the effectiveness of methods of reducing risk for disease occurrence and mortality were conducted among men. Examples are trials of cholesterol-lowering drugs, antihypertensive medications, and aspirin and beta carotene. It has become apparent that trials in women are also needed, for several reasons: The results of studies in men cannot necessarily be generalized to women, to some extent different prophylactic agents are available to men and women, and the relative importance of some diseases differs between men and women. Several prophylactic trials in women have been started in recent years. However, some of the trials are quite controversial.

   This chapter describes and critically reviews some major prophylactic trials that have been recently initiated among women in the United States, including the Postmenopausal Estrogen/Progestin Interventions (PEPI) Trial of the effects of several hormone replacement therapy regimens on predictors of coronary heart disease, the Women's Health Initiative of long-term effects of a low-fat dietary pattern, hormone replacement therapy, and calcium/vitamin D supplements on the incidence of several diseases, the Heart Estrogen/progestin Replacement Study (HERS) of hormone replacement therapy to prevent recurrence of coronary heart disease, the Breast Cancer Prevention Trial of the chemotherapeutic agent tamoxifen to reduce the risk of breast cancer, the

Women's Health Study of aspirin, beta carotene, and vitamin E as protective agents against coronary heart disease and cancer, and a small pilot study to explore whether use of luteinizing hormone–releasing hormone agonists combined with other hormones can reduce the incidence of female cancers. We also briefly describe some smaller trials of agents to prevent osteoporosis, as trials in this area have been undertaken among women for several decades. Finally, we briefly mention the Nurses Health Study, which although not a randomized trial, has provided an enormous amount of information on risk factors for diseases in women. Because several of the trials described in this chapter are concerned with hormone replacement therapy, we begin with a discussion of what had previously been learned about risks and benefits and why it was felt that randomized trials were needed. The rationale for other agents being tested in the various trials is discussed as the trials are presented.

Hormone replacement therapy: Background

Under provisions of the Food, Drug and Cosmetics Act of 1938, conjugated estrogens were approved for marketing in the United States in 1942. The approved estrogens were a mixture of active estrogens obtained from the urine of pregnant horses. Conjugated estrogens were approved initially because they satisfied the requirement of being safe for their intended use in the treatment of menopausal symptoms, vaginitis, and amenorrhea. In 1962, it became necessary to show efficacy as well as safety. The Food and Drug Administration (FDA) declared a group of estrogen products to have satisfied this additional requirement, and to be "probably effective" for selected cases of osteoporosis. In 1986, on the basis of the results of two randomized trials (Genant et al., 1982; Lindsay et al., 1984) the FDA upgraded the status of estrogen to "effective" for use in postmenopausal osteoporosis. Although several of the trials discussed in this chapter focus on potential protective actions of hormone replacement against cardiovascular disease, the FDA has not approved estrogen use for this purpose. Manufacturers of hormone replacement therapy may not discuss or distribute promotional materials concerning cardioprotective effects. The FDA has taken the position that epidemiologic evidence supporting such effects is not sufficient to warrant approval.

Hormone replacement therapy achieved wide popularity in North America during the 1950s, fueled largely by the notion that, in addition to preventing menopausal symptoms, estrogen would permit women to be forever young. During that era, the great majority of women who received estrogen were prescribed conjugated estrogens (Premarin). Until recently, this single regimen has accounted for about 70 percent of all oral estrogen replacement use in the United States (Kennedy, 1985).

Use of oral estrogen rapidly increased from the early 1960s to the mid-1970s (Kennedy, 1980). Most of the prescriptions were intended for short-term use, primarily to counteract symptoms of vasomotor motor instability. In the mid-1970s, evidence began to accumulate that continuous administration of estrogen was associated with an increased risk for endometrial hyperplasia and cancer (Smith et al., 1975; Ziel and Finkle, 1975). Public acceptance of estrogen precipitously declined over the next 5 years and then increased again (Kennedy, 1980, 1985). Over the past 20 years, a number of strategies have been introduced to protect the uterus while providing estrogen sufficiency. These regimens include the use of progestins, most often medroxyprogesterone acetate, either as part of an intermittent cyclic regimen (e.g., 5–10 mg/day for 12 days each month) or a continuous regimen (e.g., 2.5 mg/day without interruption) along with estrogen. Use of progestins increased rapidly starting around 1980 (Kennedy, 1985).

During the past 20 years, three important threads of inquiry began to dominate discussions of postmenopausal estrogen: use of estrogen to stabilize bone mass and protect against osteoporotic fractures; the possible impact of estrogen on breast cancer risk; and the possible effect of estrogen on risk for coronary heart disease. The protective effect of estrogen replacement on loss of bone mass is well established (Grady et al., 1992), whereas the possible effect of estrogen on breast cancer risk derives primarily from the belief that breast cancer is a hormone-dependent tumor (Pike et al., 1993) and from some epidemiologic studies which suggest that long-term use of estrogen or of estrogen plus progestin may somewhat increase the risk for breast cancer (Grady et al., 1992).

The effect of estrogen replacement on risk for coronary heart disease, which is the leading cause of death in women, has been of particular interest. Compelling evidence from observational epidemiologic studies has indicated a substantial protective effect of estrogen replacement on the risk for cardiovascular morbidity and mortality (Grady et al., 1992). The basis for this effect is not certain, but it appears that estrogen produces beneficial changes in circulating lipoproteins known to affect coronary heart disease (Bush et al., 1987; Lobo, 1991; Walsh et al., 1991). Specifically, estrogen replacement increases the circulating concentrations of high-density lipoprotein (HDL) cholesterol, which is strongly inversely associated with risk for coronary heart disease in women, and lowers the concentration of low-density lipoprotein (LDL) cholesterol, which is an independent predictor of some importance in women. The changes in HDL cholesterol may account for half of the overall effect of estrogen in reducing cardiovascular disease mortality (Bush et al., 1987). Progestins suppress the beneficial changes of estrogen alone on HDL cholesterol (Tikkanen et al., 1986; Lobo, 1991; Lobo et al., 1994). Therefore, when practice standards dictated inclusion of progestins for uterine protection, concern was voiced that this modification of therapy might negate the beneficial effects of estrogen alone. This concern was instrumental in formulating the PEPI Trial.

The Postmenopausal Estrogen/Progestin Interventions Trial

The PEPI Trial was designed to determine the effects of unopposed estrogen and of three combined estrogen/progestin regimens on several coronary heart disease risk factors, including HDL cholesterol, fibrinogen, insulin, and blood pressure in postmenopausal women of ages 45–64 years (Writing Group for the PEPI Trial, 1995). When the concept of conducting such a trial was first proposed in the mid-1980s, it was understood that any study aimed at clinical endpoints, such as incidence of coronary events or mortality, would necessitate recruiting thousands of women for long-term follow-up and would therefore require an enormous investment of resources. Little institutional support was forthcoming for this sort of investment, so predictors of coronary heart disease, rather than coronary heart disease itself, were the endpoints. The primary endpoints listed earlier were generally accepted as being independent predictors of coronary heart disease, and the relationships between their levels and risk of coronary heart disease were well established. The trial was initiated by the National Institutes of Health and had a coordinating center at the Bowman Gray School of Medicine.

Between December 1989 and February 1991, seven clinical centers randomized 875 women, stratified by clinical center and hysterectomy status, to one of five groups: (1) placebo; (2) conjugated equine estrogen, 0.625 mg/day; (3) conjugated equine estrogen, 0.625 mg/day, plus medroxyprogesterone acetate, 10 mg/day, for 12 days of the 28-day cycle; (4) conjugated equine estrogen, 0.625 mg/day, plus medroxyprogesterone acetate, 2.5 mg/day; and (5) conjugated equine estrogen, 0.625 mg/day, plus micronized progesterone, 200 mg/day, for 12 days of each 28-day cycle. Women were scheduled to be seen at 3, 6, and 12 months after randomization during the first year and every 6 months thereafter for a total of 3 years. Physical examination, mammography, and endometrial biopsy were performed annually.

The main results were analyzed by the intention-to-treat principle. That is, women were considered to be in the group to which they had been randomized regardless of their compliance. Thus, differences among groups would be likely to be greater than reported if all women had stayed on their original treatment assignment for the duration of the study. Overall, about 80 percent of hysterectomized women and 75 percent of women with a uterus had pill counts exceeding 80 percent compliance at their 36-month visit.

Over the 3 years of the trial, HDL cholesterol decreased slightly in the placebo group (decrease of 1.2 mg/dl), increased in the two groups taking estrogen plus medroxyprogesterone acetate (increases of 1.2 to 1.6 mg/dl), and increased more in the groups taking conjugated estrogen plus cyclic micronized progesterone (increase of 4.1 mg/dl) and taking conjugated estrogen alone (increase of 5.6 mg/dl). Compared with placebo, all of the active treatments were associated with decreases in mean LDL cholesterol and increases in triglyceride. Mean fibrinogen level increased more in the placebo groups than in any active treatment group. Systolic blood pressure increased and postchallenge insulin levels decreased during the 3 years, but treatment assignment did not influence these changes. Compared with the other active treatments, unopposed estrogen was associated with a greatly increased risk of adenomatous or atypical hyperplasia (34 vs. 1 percent) and of hysterectomy (6 vs. 1 percent).

Because evidence suggests that HDL cholesterol is the most important predictor of coronary heart disease in women, the results regarding this lipoprotein are of particular interest. Women randomized to estrogen alone or to estrogen in combination with micronized progestin had the largest increases in HDL cholesterol, so these compounds would be expected to have the most favorable effect on incidence of coronary heart disease. However, the high proportion of women developing endometrial hyperplasia among those using estrogen alone is a major drawback. Thus, in this trial, conjugated estrogen with cyclic micronized progestin had the most favorable effect on HDL cholesterol combined with lack of excess risk for endometrial hyperplasia. Micronized progestin is not readily available in this country, and its long-term effects have not been well studied in other trials.

In regard to the effects of hormone replacement on bone, the PEPI Trial clearly showed that unopposed estrogen had a favorable effect on bone mineral density in the lumbar spine, resulting in about a 5 percent increase over 3 years, and about a 2.5 percent increase in the hip (Marcus et al., 1995). Over 95 percent of women who received 0.625 mg of conjugated estrogen per day maintained bone mass at the spine, although some showed loss at the hip. In addition, PEPI results indicated that addition of a progestin to the treatment schedule had no perceptible effect on bone density.

Women in all treatment groups gained weight. Mean weight gain was greatest in women assigned to placebo and least in those taking unopposed estrogen. The PEPI Trial has provided much useful information for women trying to decide whether to use hormone replacement therapy and which regimen to use. Because women were randomized to the various treatment groups, this study adds substantially to the body of evidence from observational studies indicating that hormone replacement therapy reduces the risk of coronary heart disease and that the association is not merely attributable to a tendency for healthier people to use hormone replacement. The magnitudes of the changes in HDL levels associated with use of estrogen alone or estrogen with micronized progestin suggest that the risk for coronary heart disease would be reduced by 20 to 25 percent among these women. The increase in HDL cholesterol and decrease in fibrinogen levels compared to placebo suggest that estrogen has both a long-term beneficial effect and an immediate effect, in turn indicating that the greatest degree of protection will be achieved in long-term current users. On the other hand, the finding of a 10 percent per year incidence of adenomatous or atypical endometrial hyperplasia among women in the estrogen-alone group provides strong evidence that women electing to take this regimen need to be under annual endometrial surveillance.

Limitations of this study include its reliance on intermediate endpoints, that is, on predictors of coronary heart disease rather than on coronary heart disease itself, and its relatively short period of follow-up. Thus, this trial allows only rough estimates of the magnitude of the decreased risk for coronary heart disease incidence or mortality in the various groups or of other long-term risks and benefits such as osteoporotic fractures. Premarin was the only type of estrogen used in this trial; the effects of other types of estrogen or estrogens administered transdermally cannot be evaluated from this study. Also, the study had small numbers of racial and ethnic minorities, so the results cannot necessarily be generalized to them. Thus, although the PEPI Trial was considerably less expensive than the large trials described later and provided a great deal of useful information, it leaves unanswered some key questions that can be answered only by larger trials of longer duration.

The Women's Health Initiative

The Women's Health Initiative is the largest and most expensive research study ever funded by the National Institutes of Health. Its overall goals are to test means of reducing the risk for cardiovascular disease, breast cancer, colorectal cancer, and osteoporotic fractures in women. It was planned that it include a randomized trial, an observational study, and a community prevention study. Because the randomized trial has received most of the attention to date, only this component is reviewed here. The randomized trial is to include 63,000 women between the ages of 50 and 79 years of diverse racial/ethnic groups and socioeconomic classes. It has three branches that will test hypotheses concerning (1) dietary modification, (2) hormone replacement, and (3) calcium/vitamin D. Its large sample size is needed primarily to test the hypothesis that dietary modification can reduce the incidence of breast cancer. The Women's Health Initiative was initially proposed in 1991 by the then director-designate of the National Institutes of Health, Bernadine Healey, and received considerable support from the Congressional Caucus on Women's Issues. The study is funded by the U.S. Congress as a separate line item in the budget of the National Institutes of Health. The coordinating center is at the University of Washington. Recruitment began in 16 Vanguard Clinical Centers in the fall of 1993 and in 24 additional clinical centers in early 1995 (Rossouw et al., 1995).

Dietary modification branch

The primary hypotheses to be tested in the dietary modification branch of the Women's Health Initiative are that a low-fat dietary pattern reduces the risks of breast cancer and colon cancer. A secondary hypothesis is that a low-fat dietary pattern reduces the risk of coronary heart disease.

Evidence that a diet high in fat increases the risk for breast cancer comes mainly from comparisons of breast cancer incidence rates in countries with high and low per capita fat consumption, studies of migrants from one country to another, and animal studies. However, since there are many other differences between these countries other than their fat consumption, because migrants change many lifestyle characteristics other than just their dietary habits, and because results from animal studies cannot necessarily be generalized to humans, such evidence can be considered only suggestive. Epidemiologic case-control studies at most suggest a weak association between fat consumption in individuals and risk of breast cancer, and most cohort studies show no association. In fact, a recent meta-analysis of cohort studies of the relationship between dietary fat intake during adulthood and breast cancer found no association (Hunter et al., 1996). Moreover, it is has been hypothesized that if a high-fat diet is involved in the etiology of breast cancer, it may be fat intake early in life rather than in adulthood that is important. Another consideration is that some evidence suggests that antioxidant vitamins protect against breast cancer, and because diets high in fat tend to be low in antioxidant vitamins, it is difficult to distinguish which, if either, of these dietary constituents might be important (Hunter and Willett, 1993).

Evidence is strong, however, that people who have diets high in meat, protein, and fat have an elevated risk of colon cancer and that persons with diets high in vegetables and fibers are at reduced risk (Potter et al., 1993). It is uncertain which of these foods are important, because people who eat large quantities of meat, protein, and fat tend to consume relatively small quantities of vegetables and fibers. However, this general dietary pattern does appear to be related to colon cancer risk.

It is generally agreed that a diet low in fat, saturated fat, and cholesterol lowers total cholesterol and LDL cholesterol levels, both of which are risk factors for coronary heart disease. A diet low in fat may also reduce HDL cholesterol (Institute of Medicine Committee to Review the NIH Women's Health Initiative, 1993), however, and, as mentioned earlier, a high HDL cholesterol level protects against coronary heart disease, especially in women (Castelli, 1988; Bass et al., 1993). Thus, the net effect of the low-fat dietary pattern on coronary heart disease incidence in women is not certain.

Forty-eight thousand women are to be enrolled in this branch of the trial, with 40 percent in the intervention group and 60 percent in the control group. The goal for women in the intervention group is to attain a low-fat dietary pattern consisting of (1) total fat no more than 20 percent of daily calories, (2) saturated fats less than 7 percent of daily calories, (3) at least five daily servings of fruits and vegetables, and (4) at least six daily servings of grain products. Both control and intervention groups are being provided with a standard packet of health promotion materials, including information on a healthy diet. Several other techniques are being used to try to persuade the intervention group to reach and maintain a low-fat dietary pattern, including group meetings with a nutritionist and self-monitoring tools. The average intervention period is anticipated to be 9 years.

Although reductions in risk of breast and colon cancers are certainly worthy goals, several major reservations have been expressed about initiating such a large trial at this time (Institute of Medicine Committee to Review the NIH Women's Health Initiative, 1993). First, as noted earlier, there is at most only weak evidence that a diet high in fat increases the risk for breast cancer or that a diet high in fruits and vegetables decreases breast cancer risk (Hunter and Willett, 1993). If there is any effect, it is likely to be small. Thus, it does not seem worth such an enormous investment to test a regimen that is unlikely to have much impact on the incidence of breast cancer. Meanwhile, the objective to test the hypothesis that a low-fat dietary pattern reduces the risk for colon cancer does not seem worthwhile because the evidence from observational studies is already so strong (Potter et al., 1993) that further study does not seem of high priority. Another secondary objective, that is, to test the hypothesis that a low-fat dietary pattern reduces the risk of coronary heart disease in women, may in fact need study, but it would be more cost effective to focus on women at higher risk for coronary heart disease in order to reduce the size of the cohort. Another concern is that if a change in risk is seen for breast cancer, colon cancer, or coronary heart disease, it will not be possible to attribute it to any one specific factor such as fat, vegetables, or even weight loss. In addition, a continued trend toward decreasing dietary fat consumption in the United States may make it difficult to detect a small association with breast cancer. Assumptions about recruitment, retention, and adherence were generally believed to have been overly optimistic, especially in regard to the many older women and minority women who are to be in the trial. However, early experience in the trial suggests that recruitment and compliance are quite good. Finally, despite the high cost of the study, most investigators experienced with large prevention trials believe that the Women's Health Initiative is severely underfunded for what it proposes to accomplish.

Hormone replacement branch

The original primary aim of the hormone replacement branch of the Women's Health Initiative was to test the hypotheses that estrogen replacement therapy with progestin and estrogen replacement therapy alone reduce the risk of coronary heart disease. Secondary hypotheses were that estrogen replacement therapy with progestin and estrogen replacement therapy alone reduce the risk of osteoporotic fractures and increase the risk of breast cancer.

As mentioned earlier, almost all observational studies report that estrogen replacement therapy reduces the risk for coronary heart disease, but there is concern that a tendency for healthier women to use estrogen replacement therapy may have exaggerated the apparent beneficial effect. At the time the Women's Health Initiative started, results from the PEPI Trial had not been reported, but small randomized trials had shown that estrogen replacement therapy affects HDL and LDL cholesterol levels in directions that would be expected to reduce risk for coronary heart disease (Lobo, 1991; Walsh et al., 1991). The effects of progestin and estrogen replacement therapy are less certain because this combination of hormones has not been in use for so long. Evidence indicates that progestin and estrogen therapy decreases loss of bone mass and that the beneficial effects of progestin and estrogen on lipoprotein levels may be less than those of estrogen alone (Tikkanen et al., 1986; Lobo et al.,

1994). Insufficient data are available to reach conclusions about the effect of progestin and estrogen replacement therapy on risk of breast cancer.

Twenty-five thousand women are to be included in the hormone replacement branch. Women without a uterus are randomized to either (1) conjugated equine estrogen alone (0.625 mg/day) or (2) placebo. Initially, it was intended that women with a uterus be randomized to one of three groups: (1) conjugated equine estrogen alone (0.625 mg/day), (2) conjugated equine estrogen (0.625 mg/day) plus continuous low-dose progestin (2.5 mg/day), and (3) placebo. Although women with a uterus were at first randomized to one of these three groups, when the results of the PEPI Trial were published, indicating that a relatively high proportion of the women on estrogen alone had to be taken off it because of endometrial bleeding, the women in this group were switched to the estrogen-plus-progestin group.

The hormone replacement branch of the Women's Health Initiative is likely to produce some new knowledge. Gaining information on major risks and benefits of estrogen plus continuous low-dose progestin among women of various ages and racial/ethnic groups is particularly important. Valuable data will be obtained on adverse side effects such as uterine bleeding in women of various ages and on hypothesized beneficial effects such as on memory. However, given the tremendous expense and large size of the trial, it is unfortunate that several questions about its design have arisen. One major question is why this trial started before the results from the PEPI Trial were published, because the PEPI findings caused major changes in the hormone replacement branch shortly after its inception. A second issue is why only one regimen, conjugated estrogen with continuous low-dose progestin, is being tested. Because the optimal dose of progestin is not clear at this time, since other forms of estrogen could be tested and since micronized progestin with estrogen might turn out to be the regimen of choice, it is unfortunate that other forms and combinations of hormone replacement are not being tested in this trial. This trial will provide little information to assist women in deciding which of several possible regimens will be optimal for them. Third, if the primary aim is indeed to determine whether hormone replacement therapy affects the incidence of coronary heart disease, it would seem much more cost effective if women at low risk for coronary heart disease were not included in this branch. Finally, as new information about risks and benefits emerges from other ongoing studies, women who have been randomized may wish to switch from their assigned treatment status. In addition, recruitment for this branch of the trial has been much more difficult than anticipated, since many women already have decided that they do or do not wish to use some form of hormone replacement. Such women do not wish to be randomized.

Calcium/vitamin D supplementation branch

The primary hypothesis to be tested in the calcium/vitamin D supplementation branch of the Women's Health Initiative is that this supplementation reduces the risk of hip fracture. Secondary aims are that supplementation reduces the risk of other fractures and of colorectal cancer.

Evidence from randomized trials indicates that use of calcium supplementation somewhat retards bone loss (Cumming, 1990). Bone mass is a moderately strong predictor of hip fracture. Results from observational studies are inconsistent as to whether calcium intake affects hip fracture risk. However, a recent randomized trial in France (Chapuy et al., 1992) showed substantial reduction in fracture incidence among elderly women taking supplemental calcium with vitamin D. It is not clear from available evidence whether the addition of vitamin D to calcium supplements enhances any protection afforded by calcium alone against bone loss. In addition, evidence is inconsistent as to whether supplemental calcium and/or vitamin D protects against colorectal cancer (Potter et al., 1993).

Women in the dietary modification and hormone replacement branches of the Women's Health Initiative are invited at their 1-year anniversary to join the calcium/vitamin D supplementation branch as well. It is expected that 45,000 women will participate. Half of the participants are randomized to a regimen of calcium carbonate plus vitamin D and half are randomized to placebo.

This branch of the trial is perhaps the least expensive and least controversial, because it is unlikely that the supplementation will have adverse effects, and it may be able to shed more light on long-term effects of this supplementation specifically on fracture risk in women of different ages. Also, it may be able to provide some indication as to whether simultaneous administration of hormone replacement therapy enhances any effect of calcium/vitamin D. It is unfortunate, however, that this trial was not designed to shed light on the relative effectiveness of calcium alone compared to calcium plus vitamin D. Also, recruitment has been slower than expected.

Heart Estrogen/Progestin Replacement Study

The primary objective of HERS is to determine whether hormone replacement therapy is associated with a reduced risk for fatal coronary heart disease and nonfatal and fatal myocardial infarction among women with an intact uterus who have already been diagnosed with coronary heart disease. Secondary objectives include examining the effects of hormone replacement therapy on a variety of other outcomes in this group, including other cardiovascular changes, cancer, osteoporotic fractures, uterine bleeding, and symptomatic side effects. The coordinating center is at the University of California, San Francisco. The study is funded by Wyeth-Ayerst pharmaceutical company.

HERS is a double blind randomized trial started in 1992. It includes 2,763 postmenopausal women up to the age of 79 years who have been randomized in equal numbers either to a daily pill containing 0.625 mg Premarin plus 2.5 mg medroxyprogesterone acetate or to placebo. Eighteen centers in the United States have enrolled women. Annual follow-up of these women, which is to last for 5 years, includes cardiovascular and gynecologic examinations, electrocardiogram, mammography, and a questionnaire concerned with a variety of symptoms.

HERS should be able to address the question of whether hormone replacement therapy protects against recurrence of coronary heart disease, not just predictors of it, among women with diagnosed coronary heart disease. In addition, because coronary heart disease occurs in virtually all adult women to at least some extent, even if not clinically apparent, one could conjecture that the results from this study will apply to the general population of women as well. However, one cannot be certain of this. Unfortunately, only one type of hormone replacement regimen is being tested, so that this study will not be able to help women decide which particular regimen to use. Nevertheless, the study will provide valuable information to women with coronary heart disease and will probably be of help to women in the general population as well. This information will be provided in a much shorter period of time and at a much lower cost than other studies based on much larger numbers of women not at particularly high risk for coronary heart disease.

The Breast Cancer Prevention Trial

Tamoxifen, when used as a chemotherapeutic agent in women with breast cancer, has been shown to reduce the incidence of contralateral breast tumors and to delay breast cancer recurrence (Early Breast Cancer Trialists' Collaborative Group, 1992). Compared to other chemotherapeutic agents, serious side effects and adverse reactions have been reported to be rare (Nayfield et al., 1991; National Surgical Adjuvant Breast and Bowel Project [NSABP], 1992; Powles, 1992). Because of these characteristics, tamoxifen is now being considered as a possible chemopreventive agent to reduce the risk of developing breast cancer in healthy women. Some trials of tamoxifen in breast cancer patients have suggested a protective effect against myocardial infarction (Rutqvist and Mattsson,

1993; McDonald et al., 1995), probably because of favorable effects on serum lipid profile (Love et al., 1994). A favorable effect on bone mass has also been noted in postmenopausal women (Love et al., 1992).

The Breast Cancer Prevention Trial, initiated by the National Institutes of Health and with a coordinating center at the University of Pittsburgh, is a randomized, double blind placebo-controlled trial to test the efficacy of tamoxifen in the prevention of breast cancer. It was begun in 1992 in 250 centers in the United States and Canada. A secondary aim of this trial is to determine whether tamoxifen reduces the incidence of cardiovascular diseases. Eligible women are those who are at least 35 years of age and whose risk of breast cancer is at least as high as that of an average 60-year-old woman in the United States. Expressed differently, women are eligible for the trial if their risk for breast cancer over a 5-year period exceeds 1.7 percent. For the first 12,000 entrants into the trial, the level of risk is on average twice this minimum (Ford and Johnson, 1996). It is planned to recruit 16,000 women, of whom half will receive tamoxifen at a dose of 20 mg/day for at least 5 years and half will receive a placebo. Recruitment was to have been completed during the first 2 years, but has been slower than expected and was halted briefly in 1994. As of early 1996, 12,000 women had been recruited. At randomization, about one third were in the age group 35–49 years, one fourth were 50–59 years of age, and 40 percent were 60 years of age or older. About 80 percent have at least one first-degree relative with breast cancer (Ford and Johnson, 1996). Because of the relatively high average risk for breast cancer among the participants, the power to detect differences is greater than it otherwise would be.

Several serious concerns about the Breast Cancer Prevention Trial have arisen. First, before this trial began it would have seemed advisable to conduct a pilot study among smaller numbers of healthy women before undertaking such a large trial. A pilot study might have suggested unexpected side effects and have provided an idea of the degree of compliance to be expected. No such pilot study was undertaken. Second, tamoxifen is not risk free. Tamoxifen is associated with an increased risk of endometrial cancer and pulmonary embolism in cancer patients and may increase the risk of stomach and colon cancers and of retinopathy and other ocular conditions as well (Bush and Helzlsouer, 1993; DeGregorio et al., 1995; Rutqvist et al., 1995). The endometrial cancers associated with tamoxifen use tend to be of a particularly aggressive type (DeGregorio et al., 1995). The possibility that tamoxifen induces liver tumors is also a concern (Bush and Helzlsouer, 1993; DeGregorio et al., 1995). It has therefore been questioned whether large numbers of apparently healthy women should be exposed to a potentially toxic drug in order possibly to prevent a rare event. Third, breast cancer patients taking tamoxifen often experience vasomotor symptoms such as hot flashes (Bush and Helzlsouer, 1993) which are troublesome enough that compliance may be a problem. Healthy women have even less incentive to continue taking a medication that makes them uncomfortable for several years. Among women in the trial for 3 years, noncompliance (defined as discontinuation of protocol therapy for other than a protocol-specific reason) is about 33 percent, a figure only somewhat larger than the 27 percent anticipated when the study was planned (Ford, L., personal communication). Fourth, the risk–benefit equation to be used in assessing the results of the trial has been questioned because it equates events that have different implications for health and ignores certain adverse outcomes completely (Bush and Helzlsouer, 1993). Fifth, the advisability of including premenopausal women has been questioned by many people because available evidence indicates that the effects of tamoxifen on risk for breast cancer, coronary heart disease, and osteoporosis may differ in premenopausal and postmenopausal women (DeGregorio et al., 1995; Love, 1995). Failure to monitor bone mass in all premenopausal women, if not all women in the trial, would appear to be unconscionable because evidence suggests that tamoxifen has an unfavorable effect on bone mass in premenopausal women (Powles et al., 1996). Finally, there is concern that tamoxifen may actually stimulate breast tumor growth in some patients (DeGregorio et al., 1995). In both premenopausal and postmenopausal breast cancer patients who initially respond to tamoxifen but who later develop resistance, the breast tumors in some instances appear dependent on tamoxifen for growth. There have also been reports of new primary breast cancers years after tamoxifen has been discontinued. In particular, a higher-than-expected incidence of estrogen-receptor-negative contralateral breast tumors following tamoxifen treatment has been reported (Rutqvist et al., 1991; DeGregorio et al., 1995).

The Women's Health Study

The Women's Health Study was planned as a randomized trial of the benefits and risks of low-dose aspirin, beta carotene, and vitamin E on cardiovascular disease and cancer (Buring and Hennekens, 1994). It was initiated by investigators at Harvard University and is funded by the National Institutes of Health.

Several lines of evidence have suggested that low-dose aspirin might reduce the risk of coronary heart disease (Buring and Hennekens, 1994). Low-dose aspirin irreversibly inhibits the tendency of platelets to aggregate, thus preventing the formation of clots or thrombi. Randomized trials in both men and women have shown that among patients with cardiovascular disease, aspirin reduces the subsequent risk of myocardial infarction, stroke, and vascular death. In 1982 the Physicians' Health Study, a large randomized double blind placebo-controlled trial of the primary prevention of cardiovascular disease in apparently healthy male physicians was begun to test the effects of aspirin and beta carotene taken every other day on the incidence of cancer and cardiovascular disease. In 1988 the aspirin component of the Physicians' Health Study was terminated prematurely because of the finding of a substantially reduced risk of a first myocardial infarction among those assigned aspirin (Steering Committee of the Physicians' Health Study Research Group, 1989). However, the mortality rate from all cardiovascular causes was almost identical among those assigned and not assigned aspirin, and the rate of moderate to severe or fatal hemorrhagic stroke, based on small numbers, was higher among the aspirin users. Thus, decisions about aspirin use even among men are not entirely clear-cut.

The need for a study of aspirin use among women arose from several considerations (Buring and Hennekens, 1994). A major limitation of the Physician's Health Study was that it included only men, so any recommendation about use of aspirin in women must be extrapolated from men. Observational studies of the effect of aspirin on cardiovascular disease risk in women have produced inconsistent results. Moreover, women have lower rates of myocardial infarction than men but similar rates of strokes. Thus, the net balance of risks and benefits may be different in women and men.

Antioxidants such as beta carotene and vitamin E have been suggested by some epidemiologic and laboratory studies as agents that might reduce the incidence of cardiovascular disease and cancer (Greenwald et al., 1995; Rich-Edwards et al., 1995). It has been hypothesized that antioxidant vitamins scavenge free radicals and excited oxygen molecules and thereby prevent damage to DNA that can lead to cancer. In regard to cardiovascular disease, it has been proposed that antioxidant vitamins might inhibit the oxidation of LDL cholesterol into an especially artherogenic form and that they also preserve endothelial function (Hennekens, Buring, and Peto, 1994). However, foods such as fruits and vegetables with high levels of beta carotene and vitamin E are also rich in other potential cancer inhibitory substances. Thus, whether supplementation with these specific agents (as opposed to other constituents of fruits and vegetables) will reduce risk for cancer (and cardiovascular disease) is unknown. Because any effect of antioxidants is likely to be on the order of only a 20–30 percent reduction in risk (Hennekens and Buring, 1994), and because people with diets high in fruits and vegetables tend to have healthy lifestyles in other respects (Serdula et al., 1996), it is difficult to reach conclusions without randomized trials.

Accordingly, the Women's Health Study was started in 1991 (Buring and Hennekens, 1994). The study population of 40,000 apparently healthy women of age 45 years and older is being recruited from nurses, physicians, dentists, and other health professionals. The trial is using a two-by-two-by-two factorial design whereby women are randomized to eight combinations of placebo, aspirin, beta carotene, and vitamin E. The use of health professionals introduces various efficiencies into the study. Specifically, other studies have found that many members of these groups are willing to provide accurate and complete information over long periods of time. Because of the quality of the information supplied by health professionals, the trial can be conducted entirely by mail at a greatly reduced cost compared to other large trials. However, because coronary heart disease is less common in women than men, a large study population is needed.

In January 1996, the beta carotene arm of the trial was stopped because results from two other trials suggested an increased risk for lung cancer among people (mostly men) taking supplemental beta carotene (Alpha-Tocopherol, Beta Carotene Cancer Prevention Study Group, 1994; Greenwald, P., personal communication). Two other trials, nevertheless, have not found an increased risk (Greenwald, P., personal communication). Two recent reports from randomized trials suggest either no change in risk for cardiovascular disease mortality among men and women (Greenberg et al., 1996) or a slight increase in risk for angina pectoris among men (Rapola et al., 1996) in the group assigned to take beta carotene compared to those assigned to take placebo.

In general, the Women's Health Study is a cost-effective way of testing hypotheses regarding aspirin and certain nutritional supplements in women, although some might question the representativeness of the study population on which it is based.

Pilot study to assess prevention through the use of luteinizing hormone–releasing hormone agonists

Use of oral contraceptives is known to reduce the risk of ovarian and endometrial cancers and may increase the risk for breast cancer in young women (Kelsey and Whittemore, 1994). Pike et al. (1989) at the University of Southern California have proposed using luteinizing hormone–releasing hormone agonists as a contraceptive agent. Such an agent would not only inhibit ovulation, it would eliminate ovarian estrogen and progesterone production and possibly reduce the risk of certain cancers. Pike et al. propose that such a regimen would reduce the risk for ovarian cancer (because of the suppression of ovulation) and endometrial cancer (because of low estrogen exposure) and would also reduce risk for breast cancer (because of reduced exposure to estrogen and progesterone). These authors predict that if taken for 5 years, this regimen would reduce breast cancer risk by 38 percent, and if taken for 15 years might reduce breast cancer risk by 80 percent.

However, when used in a small pilot study, this regimen was found to be associated with adverse effects such as hot flashes, bone loss, and probably an increased risk for cardiovascular disease because of an increase in LDL cholesterol levels (Spicer et al., 1994). Therefore, estrogen was added at a low dose so as to reduce the occurrence of hot flashes and produce a beneficial lipid profile while retaining most of the hypothesized beneficial effects on breast cancer risk. Periodic progestin was also added so as to minimize the risk of endometrial hyperplasia or cancer associated with estrogen alone. A small amount of testosterone was added to replace that normally produced by the ovary in order to reduce further the risk of bone loss.

These regimens have been tested over a 2-year period in a small group of premenopausal women at very high risk of breast cancer. Beneficial changes were seen on mammograms (Spicer et al., 1993), and few side effects were observed (Spicer et al., 1994). Further evaluation of the regimen is being carried out.

Although this regimen is based on current understanding of the biology of these cancers, current understanding is quite conjectural. So much is not known about the etiology of these cancers and about other risks and benefits of this compound that its use must be considered experimental. Limiting its use at this time to small numbers of high-risk women is sensible. Love (1994) has pointed out that the regimen may be more appropriate for women in their forties than for younger women because these women would not need to take the contraceptives for as long a period of time and because the effects on fertility are uncertain.

Trials of agents to prevent and retard osteoporosis

This chapter began with the statement that most randomized trials to test methods of reducing risk for disease occurrence and mortality had been conducted among men. Osteoporosis constitutes a notable exception. Although osteoporosis clearly affects men, it has traditionally been viewed as a woman's disease. This view reflects not only higher incidence of osteoporosis in women than men but also the fact that osteoporotic fractures primarily afflict older people, two out of three of whom are women.

Estrogen

It is remarkable that studies presented to the Food and Drug Administration to secure approval for estrogen as an osteoporosis treatment reflect a total experience of just a few hundred women. Nonetheless, there is no longer any doubt that sustained administration of conjugated estrogens to menopausal women conserves bone (Lindsay, 1993). Such conservation should theoretically protect against osteoporotic fractures, and, indeed, epidemiologic studies support the view that long-term estrogen replacement does afford women such protection. On the other hand, questions persist about optimizing the therapeutic schedule, including the type, dose, and mode of estrogen administration. Other questions concern the age at which treatment should begin, its duration, and the consequence of adding progestins to the treatment regimen. Most of these questions have been addressed by small, short-term, and, too frequently, nonrandomized trials.

To date, adequate information regarding the skeletal response to other estrogens or treatment schedules has not been developed using placebo-controlled, randomized clinical trials. However, it appears from less rigorously controlled studies that similar results can be expected regardless of the estrogen preparation or mode of administration, so long as circulating estradiol concentrations of about 60 pg/ml are achieved. Published studies generally assess the dose of hormone necessary for a treatment group to show conservation of bone mass relative to a placebo group. They have rarely had adequate power to compare one dose of hormone with another, nor has it been possible to determine anything beyond *group* responses. It would be desirable also to know what proportion of patients can be expected to respond to any given dose. Finally, with few exceptions, conclusions regarding minimum effective dose reflect the experience at only one skeletal site, the lumbar spine.

The level of uncertainty for these questions grows considerably when the endpoint is fracture rather than bone mass. Most published evidence for the antifracture efficacy of estrogen comes from observational epidemiologic studies rather than randomized trials (Cauley et al., 1995). Current industry-sponsored trials aimed at showing antifracture benefits of other agents have needed to enroll several thousand osteoporotic women for at least 3 years of observation. This has simply not been done with estrogen, and given that estrogen is already approved therapy, it is unlikely that such a study will ever be funded by industry. The Women's Health Initiative may provide some relevant data, at least with regard to conjugated estrogen with continuous low-dose progestin.

Bisphosphonates

These antiresorptive compounds have been enthusiastically received as important advances in osteoporosis therapy. Essentially all major trials have been conducted in women. Trials of bisphosphonates have been well designed, randomized, and placebo controlled. Attention has been given to the adequacy of statistical power. Nonetheless, initial studies using etidronate (Didronel) did not have sufficient power to address antifracture efficacy in a definitive manner (Watts et al., 1990), resulting in failure of this drug to receive FDA approval. Data from trials with alendronate (Fosamax) (Liberman et al., 1995) show a 48 percent reduction in the number of women who experience new vertebral fractures compared to placebo, as well as a decrease in the progression of previous vertebral deformity and loss of height. Alendronate promoted increases in bone mass (greater than 8 percent at the lumbar spine after 3 years) that exceeded predictions based solely on its actions as an antiresorbing agent. The manufacturer, Merck & Co., is nearing completion of a massive study, the multicenter Fracture Intervention Trial (FIT), in which more than 6,000 women are enrolled for 3 years of randomized treatment with alendronate, 10 mg/day, or placebo. This study was designed to have power to detect differences in vertebral as well as nonvertebral fractures.

Although alendronate represents a major advance in osteoporosis therapy, many questions remain unanswered by the studies reported to date. Should alendronate be given together with estrogen, or only in estrogen-deplete women? How long should therapy continue? What is the consequence of stopping treatment? A number of clinical trials are currently in progress that address these issues.

Calcitonin

This peptide hormone is approved for prevention and treatment of osteoporosis. Calcitonin abruptly slows bone resorption and conserves bone mass. Its effects on bone dissipate rapidly when treatment stops. Its pharmacodynamic profile is well understood, and it is reasonably safe. Trials aimed at fracture endpoints have generally been small and often poorly conducted. Patient acceptance of calcitonin has been limited because it was given by injection, but a nasal-spray formulation recently received FDA approval. This formulation was evaluated in a well-conceived and well-executed clinical trial (Overgaard et al., 1992), which showed maintenance of bone mass. This 2-year trial tested multiple doses of drug; no individual treatment arm had sufficient power to detect a change in fracture incidence, but when all calcitonin groups were combined, reductions in both vertebral and nonvertebral fracture were statistically significant.

Fluoride

In contrast to the agents described earlier, sodium fluoride is capable of stimulating massive increases in spinal bone mineral density in at least some patients. Although fluoride has been studied for several decades, only recently has any attempt been made to conduct properly controlled clinical trials. In two trials sponsored by the National Institutes of Health (Riggs et al., 1990; Kleerekoper et al., 1991) fluoride substantially increased lumbar spine density but achieved no fracture benefit. Most experts agree that the reason for this failure was the very high dose of fluoride that was employed (75 mg/day) and the rapidity with which it was absorbed at high levels. Most recently, Pak et al. (1994) reported the results of a clinical trial of a slow-release sodium fluoride preparation, in which the dose was only 25 mg, twice daily, and did not seem to achieve peak concentrations that are of clinical concern. Fluoride was given cyclically for 2 years, and even though the study was relatively small, it was associated with an impressive and statistically significant reduction in vertebral fractures. Other clinical trials of fluoride at the same or similar doses are currently under way.

Calcium/vitamin D

Many small, short-term trials attest to the ability of supplemental calcium to slow the rate of bone loss in postmenopausal women (Cumming, 1990), although the protection is not nearly so great as with estrogen. These studies have not had large enough numbers to consider fractures as endpoints. Questions have remained, however, about the effectiveness of calcium at older ages. After about 60 years of age, many people no longer adapt readily to low calcium intakes. Chapuy et al. (1992) reported results of a randomized trial of tricalcium phosphate (1.2 g elemental calcium) plus a small amount of vitamin D (800 IU vitamin D_3) in over 3,000 elderly French women (average age 84 years) who were residents of sheltered-living communities. Compared to placebo, significant reductions of about 30 percent were observed in fracture incidence within a few months of initiating treatment, an effect that has persisted over 4 years of follow-up and that was associated with significant reductions in total mortality. If confirmed, this study provides an example of a simple, safe, and inexpensive intervention that could exert a profound influence on morbidity and mortality in frail elderly women.

Observational study: The Nurses' Health Study

The single study that has probably provided the most information about risk factors for disease in women is not a randomized trial but a study of exposures and diseases as they are naturally occurring in the population (i.e., an observational study). The Nurses' Health Study was started in 1976, when questionnaires were sent to all married female registered nurses born between 1921 and 1947 and living in 11 states of the United States. It was initiated by investigators from Harvard University and is funded by the National Institutes of Health. Nurses were selected for this cohort not because of any particular occupational exposure but because it was believed that their cooperation would be high and that they could report disease occurrence with a high degree of accuracy. Some 121,700 nurses responded to the initial questionnaire, which covered known and suspected risk factors for cancer and coronary heart disease such as height, weight, smoking habits, use of estrogen replacement therapy, and use of oral contraceptives. A follow-up questionnaire is mailed to cohort members every 2 years to update information on possible risk factor exposure and to determine whether major medical events have occurred. New areas of interest, such as a dietary history, have been added to the questionnaire.

Numerous publications have resulted from this study concerning such exposures as oral contraceptives, hormone replacement therapy, cigarette smoking, alcohol consumption, diet, and use of hair dyes and such conditions as cancers, coronary heart disease, and hip fracture. Examples of recent findings from the Nurses' Health Study are an inverse association between height and coronary heart disease (Rich-Edwards et al., 1995), a reduction in risk for colorectal cancer among women who had frequently used aspirin (Giovannucci et al., 1995), an increased risk for breast cancer among women who were currently using hormone replacement therapy (Colditz et al., 1995), and a lack of association between selenium levels in toenail clippings and cancer (Garland et al., 1995). Following such a large cohort over so many years might be prohibitively expensive, except that most of the information is collected through a questionnaire sent through the mail. Studies of the validity and reliability of selected items of information have in general shown the quality of the data to be good (Colditz et al., 1986). Nurses are one of the few groups that can be expected to provide medical information in a relatively accurate manner. Concerns about the cohort include the possibility that nurses are not representative of the general population of women in respect to the associations being studied and that the study is observational, not randomized. Thus, it is sometimes uncertain whether the associations between certain exposures and diseases are causal or whether women with these exposures have other characteristics that are responsible for their higher (or lower) risk of disease. Nevertheless, the advantages of the Nurses' Health Study have far outweighed these limitations, and a study of a new group of nurses has now begun.

Conclusion

In view of the various strengths and weaknesses of these trials, it is not surprising that much divergence of opinion exists as to their relative overall merits. What some people consider important advantages or major limitations of a trial, others do not. Designing each of these trials has of necessity involved trade-offs regarding what questions can be addressed, at what cost and at what risk.

Perhaps the most controversial issue is whether the possible side effects of the prophylactic agents being tested outweigh the hypothesized benefits. This is of particular concern in the Breast Cancer Prevention Trial and the trial of luteinizing hormone–releasing hormone agonists. In the latter trial, only small numbers of women at very high risk of breast cancer are being included, but in the Breast Cancer Prevention Trial, large numbers of healthy women are being exposed to a potentially toxic agent. The most serious questions have been raised about the use of tamoxifen as a prophylactic agent in premenopausal women, in whom the risks and benefits are likely to be quite different from those in postmenopausal women.

Another controversial characteristic of these trials is cost. The PEPI Trial, for instance, was relatively inexpensive and quick, but it used intermediate endpoints (i.e., predictors of coronary heart disease) rather than morbidity and mortality endpoints. Nevertheless, many feel that the results of the PEPI Trial, together with results of epidemiologic studies without randomization but with morbidity and mortality endpoints, already provide very strong evidence of a cardioprotective effect of hormone replacement therapy. Opinions differ as to whether a larger, longer, and very expensive trial such as the Women's Health Initiative, which is based on more representative groups of women and on morbidity and mortality endpoints, is necessary to provide definitive answers about long-term effects of both hormone replacement therapy and a healthy diet. Opinions also differ as to whether it is worthwhile investing a large amount of money to detect what is likely to be a relatively small effect, if any, of a low-fat diet.

The HERS trial is able to use a smaller sample size than the Women's Health Initiative because it includes women at very high risk for coronary heart disease (i.e., women who already had coronary heart disease diagnosed). Its results should be very useful to this subgroup of women, but whether the results can be generalized to presumably healthy women is uncertain. The Women's Health Study cohort consists of medical professionals. Use of this cohort saves considerable money because the study can be conducted almost entirely through the mail. However, the question of generalizability may again arise, although it is difficult to understand why results in this group would not be applicable to most other healthy women.

Another problem with trials of long duration, such as the Women's Health Initiative, is that results will not be available for many years, and in the meantime many women will be making decisions, particularly about hormone replacement regimens. Also, during the course of the Women's Health Initiative, new knowledge will become available that changes practice. This trend has already been illustrated by the decision to stop the estrogen arm of the trial because of the side effects of estrogen alone reported in the PEPI Trial. It is possible that new regimens, such as estrogen with micronized progestin, may become regimens of choice in the future, yet it is too late to include them in the trial. Trends over time in dietary consumption in the population may substantially decrease the power of a study to detect differences between groups. Nevertheless, if disease occurrence and mortality are the endpoints of greatest interest, trials of long duration are necessary, and if one wants to be reasonably certain that results can be generalized to various subgroups of the population, broad inclusion criteria must be used.

Also debatable is whether it is worth testing only one regimen, such as one type of hormone replacement therapy versus placebo, when there are several other potential regimens to be tested. The same concern applies to the calcium/vitamin D supplementation branch of the Women's Health Initiative, because a critical question at this time is whether calcium plus vitamin D is more effective than calcium alone in retarding loss of bone mass and decreasing the risk for osteoporotic fractures.

In summary, considerable knowledge about important women's health issues will undoubtedly be gained from these trials. However, a great deal of money will be expended acquiring this knowledge, and several key questions will remain unanswered. Some of the trials involve risks. Only time will tell whether the considerable monetary investment and risks to the participants have been worthwhile. Since all of these trials have been started, the question of whether they should have been initiated in the first place is now moot. However, it is hoped that (1) the data will be collected carefully and analyzed wisely so that as much information as possible can be gleaned from these trials, and (2) if during the course of any of these trials the risks of a given agent clearly outweigh the benefits or if new knowledge becomes available suggesting the wisdom of another course of action, appropriate changes in protocol, including possibly cessation of an entire trial in some or all women, will be accomplished.

References

Aarskog, D. (1975). Association between maternal intake of diazepam and oral clefts [Letter]. *Lancet*, 2, 921.

Abbott, R. D., Donahue, R. P., Kannel, W. B., and Wilson, P. W. (1988). The impact of diabetes on survival following myocardial infarction in men versus women: The Framingham Study. *JAMA*, 260, 3456–3460.

Abe, T., Furuhashi, N., Yoshiro, U., et al. (1976). Correlation between climacteric symptoms and serum levels of estrogen, progesterone, FSH and LH. *Am J Obstet Gynecol*, 129, 65–67.

Adams, J., and Wacher, A. (1968). Specific changes in the glycoprotein components of seromucoid in pregnancy. *Clin Chim Acta*, 21, 155–157.

Adams, M. R., Williams, J. K., Clarkson, T. B., and Jayo, M. J. (1991). Effects of oestrogens and progestogens on coronary atherosclerosis and osteoporosis of monkeys. *Baillieres Clin Obstet Gynaecol*, 519–534.

Adams, R. D., and DeLong, G. R. (1986). Thyroid diseases: Disorders that cause thyrotoxicosis. The neuromuscular system and brain. In S. H. Ingbar and L. E. Braverman (Eds.), *The Thyroid* (pp. 1168–1180). Philadelphia: J. B. Lippincott.

Ades, P. A., Waldmann, M. L., Polk, A. D., and Coflesky, J. T. (1992). Referral patterns and exercise response in the rehabilitation of female coronary patients ages 62 years. *Am J Cardiol*, 69, 1422–1425.

Adler, N., and Matthews, K. (1994). Health psychology: Why do some people get sick and some stay well? *Annu Rev Psychol*, 45, 229–259.

Adriaanse, R., Brabant, G., Endert, E., and Wiersinga, W. M. (1993). Pulsatile thyrotropin release in patients with untreated pituitary disease. *J Clin Endocrinol Metab*, 77, 205–209.

Aguilera, G., Wynn, P. C., Harwood, J. P., et al. (1986). Receptor-mediated actions of corticotropin-releasing factor in pituitary gland and nervous system. *Neuroendocrinology*, 43, 79–88.

Ahima, R. S., Lawson, A. N., Osei, S. Y., and Harlan, R. E. (1992). Sexual dimorphism in regulation of type II corticosteroid receptor immunoreactivity in the rat hippocampus. *Endocrinology*, 131, 1409–1416.

Alder, E. M., Cook, A., Davidson, P., West, C., and Bancroft, J. (1986). Hormones, mood and sex in lactating women. *Br J Psychol*, 148, 74–79.

Alder, E. M., and Cox, J. L. (1983). Breast feeding and post-natal depression. *J Psychosom Res*, 27, 139–144.

Alexander, G. E., Delong, M. R., and Strick, P. L. (1986). Parallel organization of functionally segregated circuits linking basal ganglia and cortex. *Annu Rev Neurosci*, 9, 357–81.

Aldridge, A., Bailey, J., and Neims, A. (1981). The disposition of caffeine during and after pregnancy. *Semin Perinatol*, 5, 310–314.

Allen, L. S., Hines, M., Shryne, J. E., and Gorski, R. A. (1989). Two sexually dimorphic cell groups in the human brain. *J Neurosci*, 9, 497–506.

Allen, M. T., Stoney, C. M., Owens, J. F., and Matthews, K. A. (1993). Hemodynamic adjustments to laboratory stress: The influence of gender and personality. *Psychosom Med*, 55, 505–517.

Alpha-Tocopherol, Beta Carotene Cancer Prevention Study Group. (1994). The effect of vitamin E and beta carotene on the incidence of lung cancer and other cancers in male smokers. *N Engl J Med*, 330, 1029–1035.

Altemus, M., Hetherington, M., Kennedy, B., Licinio, J, and Gold, P. (1996). Thyroid function in bulimia nervosa. *J Psychoneuroendocrinol*, 21, 249–261.

Alter, C., Plecovitz, D., Axelrod, A., et al. (1996). Identification of PTSD in cancer survivors. *Psychosomatics*, 37, 137–143.

Altshuler, L., Burt, V., McMullen, M., and Hendrick, V. (1995). Breastfeeding and sertraline: A 24-hour analysis. *J Clin Psychiatry*, 56, 243–245.

Altshuler, L. L., Cohen, L., Szuba, M. P., et al. (1996). Pharmacologic management of psychiatric illness during pregnancy: Dilemmas and guidelines. *Am J Psychiatry*, 153, 592–606.

Alvarez, L., Dimas, C., Castro, A., et al. (1972). Growth hormone in malnutrition. *J Clin Endocrinol Metab*, 34, 400–409.

American Academy of Pediatrics Committee on Drugs. (1989). Transfer of drugs and other chemicals into human milk. *Pediatrics*, 84, 924–936.

American Heart Association. (1996). *Heart and stroke facts: 1996. Statistical Supplement.* Dallas, TX: American Heart Association.

American Psychiatric Association. (1987). *Diagnostic and statistical manual of mental disorders* (DSM-IIIR). Washington: American Psychiatric Press.

American Psychiatric Association. (1994). *Diagnostic and statistical manual of mental disorders*, 4th ed. Washington: American Psychiatric Press.

Amsterdam, J. D., Maislin, G., Winokur, A., et al. (1988). The oCRH test before and after clinical recovery from depression. *J Affect Disord*, 14, 213–222.

Amsterdam, J. D., Marinelli, D. L., Arger, P., and Winokur, A. (1987). Assessment of adrenal gland volume by computed tomography in depressed patients and healthy volunteers: A pilot study. *Psychiatry Res*, 21, 189–197.

Amsterdam, J. D., Winokur, A., Abelman, E., Lucki, I., and Rickels, K. (1983). Cosyntropin (ACTH) stimulation test in depressed patients and healthy subjects. *Am J Psychiatry*, 140, 907–909.

Anandatheerthavarada, H., Williams, J., and Wecker, L. (1993). The chronic administration of nicotine induces cytochrome P_{450} in rat brain. *J Neurochem*, 60, 1941–1944.

Anastos, K., Charney, P., Charon, R. A., et al. (1991). Hypertension in women: What is really known? *Ann Intern Med*, 155(4), 287–293.

Andersen, A. (1990). *Males with eating disorders*. New York: Brunner/Mazel.

Andersen, B. L. (1993). Predicting sexual and psychologic morbidity and improving the quality of life for women with gynecologic cancer. *Cancer*, 71, 1678–1690.

Angermeyer, M. C., and Kuhn, L. (1988). Gender differences in age at onset of schizophrenia: An overview. *Eur Arch Psychiatry Neurol Sci*, 237, 351–364.

Angold, A., and Costello, E. (1995). Developmental epidemiology. *Epidemiol Rev*, 17, 74–83.

Angold, A., and Worthman, C. W. (1993). Puberty onset of gender differences in rates of depression: A developmental, epidemiologic and neuroendocrine perspective. *J Affect Disord*, 29, 145–158.

Appels, A., and Mulder, P. (1988). Excess fatigue as a precursor of myocardial infarction. *Eur Heart J*, 9, 758–764.

Apter, D, and Vihko, R. (1977). Serum pregnenolone, progesterone, 17-hydroxyproges-terone, testosterone and 5 alpha-dihydrotestosterone during female puberty. *J Clin Endocrinol Metab*, 45, 1039–1048.

Arana, G. W., Baldessarini, R. J., and Orsteen, M. (1985). The dexamethasone suppression test for diagnosis and prognosis in psychiatry. *Arch Gen Psychiatry*, 42, 1193–1204.

Arana, G. W., and Mossman, D. (1988). The DST and depression: Approaches to the use of a laboratory test in psychiatry. *Neurol Clin,* 6, 21–39.

Arana, G. W., Santos, A. B., Laraia, M. T., et al. (1994). Dexamethasone for the treatment of depression: A randomized, placebo-controlled, double-blind trial. *Am J Psychiatry*, 152, 265–270.

Arason, A., Barkardottir, R. B., and Egllsson, V. (1993). Linkage analysis of chromosome 17q markers and breast-ovarian cancer in Icelandic families, and possible relationship to prostatic cancer. *Am J Hum Genet* 52, 711–717.

Arato, M., Banki, C. M., Bissette, G., and Nemeroff, C. B. (1989). Elevated CSF CRF in suicide victims. *Biol Psychiatry*, 25, 355–359.

Arato, M., Banki, C. M., Nemeroff, C. B., and Bissette, B. (1986). Hypothalamic-pituitary-adrenal axis and suicide. *Ann NY Acad Sci*, 487, 263–270.

Arnetz, B. B., Wasserman, J., Petrini, B., et al. (1987). Immune function in unemployed women. *Psychosom Med,* 19, 3–12.

Arnon, J., Rodriguez-Pinilla, E., Schaefer, C., Pexieder, T., et al. (1996). The outcome of pregnancy in 689 women exposed to therapeutic doses of antidepressants. A collaborative study of the European Network of Teratology Information Services (ENTIS). *Reprod Toxicol*, 10, 285–294.

Arriza, J. L., Weinberger, C., Cerelli, G., et al. (1987). Cloning of human mineralocorticoid receptor complementary DNA: Structural and functional kinship with the glucocorticoid receptor. *Science*, 237, 268–275.

Ashby, C. R., Carr, L. A., Cook, C. L., et al. (1990). Alteration of 5-HT uptake by plasma fractions in the premenstrual syndrome. *J Neural Trans Gen Sect*, 79, 41–50.

Ashby, C. R., Carr, L. A., Cook, C. L., Steptoe, M. M., Franks, D. D. (1988). Alteration of platelet serotonergic mechanisms and monoamine oxidase activity in premenstrual syndrome. *Biol Psychiatry*, 24, 225–233.

Atterwill, C. K., Bunn, S. J., Atkinson, D. J., Smith, S. L., and Heal, D. J. (1984). Effects of thyroid status on presynaptic alpha-2 adrenoreceptor function and beta-adrenoreceptor binding in the rat brain. *J Neural Transm*, 59, 43–55.

Auchus, R., J., and Fuqua, S. A. (1994). Hormone-nuclear receptor interactions in health and disease. The oestrogen receptor. *Baillieres Clin Endocrinol Metab*, 8, 433–449.

Austin, M. A. (1989). Plasma triglycerides and risk factors for coronary heart disease: The epidemiologic evidence and beyond. *Am J Epidemiol*, 129, 249–259.

Axelson, D. A., Doraiswamy, P. M., Boyko, O. B., et al. (1992). In vivo assessment of pituitary volume using MRI and systemic stereology: Relationship to dexamethasone suppression test results in patients with affective disorder. *Psychiatry Res*, 46, 63–70.

Ayanian, J. Z., and Epstein, A. M. (1991). Differences in the use of procedures between women and men hospitalized for coronary heart disease. *N Engl J Med*, 325, 221–225.

Aylward, M. (1973). Plasma tryptophan levels and mental depression in postmenopausal subjects: Effects of natural piperazine-oestrone sulphate. *IRCS Med Sci*, 1, 30–34.

Babb, P. (1995). Birth statistics 1993. *Popul Trends*, 79, 31–33.

Bachmann, A., Leiblum, S. R., Sandler, B., et al. (1993). Correlates of sexual desire in post-menopausal women. *Maturitas*, 7, 211–216.

Back, D., Grimmer, S., Orme, M., et al. (1988). Evaluation of Committee on Safety of Medicines yellow card reports on oral contraceptive–drug interactions with anticonvulsants and antibiotics. *Br J Clin Pharmacol*, 25, 527–532.

Backstrom, C. T., McNeilly, A. S., Leask, R. M., and Baird, D. T. (1982). Pulsatile secretion of LH, FSH, prolactin, oestradiol and progesterone during the human menstrual cycle. *Clin Endocrinol*, 17, 29–42.

Bacon, S., and McClintock, M. (1994). Multiple factors determine the sex ratio of post-partum-conceived Norway rat litters. *Physiol Behav*, 56, 359–366.

Bader, T., and Newman, K. (1980). Amitriptyline in human breast milk and nursing infant's serum. *Am J Psychiatry*, 137, 855–856.

Baird, D. T. (1978). Pulsatile secretion of LH and ovarian estradiol in the follicular phase of the sheep estrous cycle. *Biol Reprod*, 18, 359–364.

Ballinger, C. B. (1976). Subjective sleep disturbance at menopause. *J Psychosomatic Res*, 20, 509–513.

Ballinger, C. B. (1990). Psychiatric aspects of the menopause. *Br J Psychiatry*, 156, 773–787.

Ballinger, C. B., Browning, M. C., and Smith, A. H. (1987). Hormone profile and psychological symptoms in perimenopausal women. *Maturitas*, 9, 235–251.

Bancroft, J., Boyle, H., Warner, P., et al. (1987). The use of LHRH agonist, buserelin, in the long-term management of premenstrual syndromes. *Clin Endocrinol*, 27, 171–182.

Banki, C. B., Karmacsi, L., Bissette, G., and Nemeroff, C. B. (1992). CSF corticotropin-releasing hormone and somatostatin in major depression: Response to antidepressant treatment and relapse. *Eur Neuropsychopharmacol*, 2, 107–113.

Banki, C. M. (1975). Triiodothyromine treatment in depression [Abstract]. *Orv Hetil*, 116, 2543–2546.

Banki, C. M. (1977). Cerebrospinal fluid amine metabolites after combined amitriptyline-triiodothyronine treatment of depressed women. *Eur J Pharmacol*, 41, 311–315.

Banki, C. M., Bissette, G., Arato, M., and Nemeroff, C. B. (1988). Elevation of immunoreactive CSF TRH in depressed patients. *Am J Psychiatry*, 145, 1526–1531.

Banki, C. M., Bissette, G., Arato, M., O'Connor, L., and Nemeroff, C. B. (1987). Cerebrospinal fluid corticotropin-releasing factor-like immunoreactivity in depression and schizophrenia. *Amer J Psychiatry*, 144, 873–877.

Bardenstein, K. K., and McGlashan, T. H. (1990). Gender differences in affective, schizoaffective, and schizophrenic disorders. *Schizophr Res*, 3, 159–172.

Bardoni, B., Zanaria, E., Guiolo, S., et al. (1994). A dosage sensitive locus at chromosome Xp21 is involved in male to female sex reversal. *Nature Genet*, 7, 497–501.

Barr, J., and Skett, P. (1984). The role of cytochrome P-450, NADPH cytochrome P-450 reductase and lipids in sex differences in hepatic drug metabolism. *Br J Pharmacol*, 83, 396–408.

Barraclough, J., Pinder, P., Cruddas, M., et al. (1992). Life events and breast cancer prognosis. *Br J Med*, 304, 1078–1081.

Barrett-Connor, E. (1994). Heart disease in women. *Fertil Steril*, 62, (Suppl. 2, No. 6), 1275–1325.

Barrett-Conner, E., and Dritz-Silverstein, D. (1993). Estrogen replacement therapy and cognitive function in older women. *JAMA*, 269, 2637–2641.

Bartalena, L., Pellegrini, L., Meschi, M., et al. (1990). Evaluation of thyroid function in patients with rapid-cycling and non-rapid-cycling bipolar disorder. *Psychiatry Res*, 34, 13–17.

Bartalena, L., Placidi, G. F., Martino, E., et al. (1990). Nocturnal serum thyrotropin (TSH) surge and the TSH response to TSH-releasing hormone: Dissociated behavior in untreated depressives. *J Clin Endocrinol Metab*, 71, 650–655.

Bartrop, R. W., Lazarus, L., Luckherst, E., et al. (1977). Depressed lymphocyte function after bereavement. *Lancet*, 1, 834–836.

Bass, K. M., Newschaffer, C. J., Klag, M. J., and Bush, T. L. (1993). Plasma lipoprotein levels as predictors of cardiovascular death in women. *Arch Intern Med*, 153, 2209–2216.

Bast, R. C., Jr. (1993). Perspectives on the future of cancer markers. *Clin Chem*, 39, 2444–2451.

Bauer, M. S., Droba, M., and Whybrow, P. C. (1987). Disorders of the thyroid and parathyroid. In C. B. Nemeroff and P. T. Loosen (Eds.), *Handbook of clinical psychoneuroendocrinology* (pp. 41–70). New York: Guilford Press.

Bauer, M. S., and Whybrow, P. C. (1988). Thyroid hormones and the central nervous system in affective illness: Interactions that may have clinical significance. *Integrative Psychiatry*, 6, 75–100.

Bauer, M. S., and Whybrow, P. C. (1990). Rapid cycling bipolar affective disorder. II. Treatment of refractory rapid cycling with high-dose levothyroxine: A preliminary study. *Arch Gen Psychiatry*, 47, 435–440.

Bauer, M. S., Whybrow, P. C., and Winokur, A. (1990). Rapid cycling bipolar affective disorder. I. Association with grade I hypothyroidism. *Arch Gen Psychiatry*, 47, 427–432.

Baum, A., and Grunberg, N. E. (1991). Gender, stress and health. *Health Psychol*, 10, 80–85.

Baumgartner, A., Bauer, M., and Hellweg, R. (1994). Treatment of intractable non–rapid cycling bipolar affective disorder with high-dose thyroxine: An open clinical trial. *Neuropsychopharmacology*, 10, 183–189.

Baumgartner, A., Graf, K. J., Kurten, I., and Meinhold, H. (1988). The hypothalamic-pituitary-thyroid axis in psychiatric patients and healthy subjects: Parts 1–4. *Psychiatry Res*, 24, 271–332.

Beach, F. (1975). Behavioral endocrinology: An emerging discipline. *Am Sci*, 63, 178–187.

Beck, D., Casper, R. and Anderson, A. (1996). Truly late onset of eating disorders: A study of 11 cases averaging 60 years of age at presentation. *Int J Eating Disord*, 20, 389–395.

Beckman, L. J. (1994). Treatment needs of women with alcohol problems. *Alcohol Health Res World*, 18, 206–211.

Bedard, P. L. P., Langelier, J., Dankova, A., et al. (1979). Estrogens, progesterone and the extrapyramidal system. In L. J. Poirer, T. L. Sourkes, and P. J. Bedard (Eds.), *Advances in neurology*, vol. 24. New York: Raven Press.

Begg, E., Atkinson, H., and Duffull, S. (1992). Prospective evaluation of a model for the prediction of milk: plasma drug concentrations from physicochemical characteristics. *Br J Clin Pharmacol*, 33, 501–505.

Bell, I. R. (1994). Somatization disorder: Health care costs in the decade of the brain. *Biol Psychiatry*, 35, 81–83.

Bell, R. (1985). *Holy anorexia*. Chicago: University of Chicago Press.

Ben-Eliyahu, S., Yirmiya, R., Liebeskind, J. C., et al. (1991). Stress increases metastatic spread of a mammary tumor in rats: Evidence for mediation by the immune system. *Brain Behav Immun*, 5, 193–205.

Berger, C. P., and Presser, B. (1994). Alprazolam in the treatment of two samples of patients with late luteal phase dysphoric disorder: A double blind, placebo controlled study. *Obstet Gynecol*, 84, 379–385.

Berelowitz, M., Szabo, M., Frohman, L., et al. (1981). Somatomedin-C mediates growth hormone negative feedback by effects on both the hypothalamus and the pituitary. *Science*, 212, 1279–1281.

Berkman, L. F., Leo-Summers, L., and Horwitz, R. I. (1992). Emotional support and survival after myocardial infarction. *Ann Intern Med*, 117, 1003–1009.

Berkman, L. F., Vaccarino, V., and Seeman, T. (1993). Gender differences in cardiovascular morbidity and mortality: The contribution of social networks and support. *Ann Behav Med*, 15, 112–118.

Bermudez, F., Surks, M., and Oppenheimer, J. (1975). High incidence of decreased serum triiodothyronine concentration in patients with nonthyroidal disease. *J Clin Endocrinol Metab*, 41, 27–40.

Berrino, F., Muti, P., Micheli, A., et al. (1996). Serum sex hormone levels after menopause and subsequent breast cancer. *J Natl Cancer Inst*, 88, 291–296.

Besedovsky, H. O., del Rey, A., Sorkin, E., and Dinarello, C. A. (1986). Immunoregulatory feedback between interleukin-1 and glucocorticoid hormones. *Science*, 233, 652–654.

Best, N. R., Rees, M. P., Barlow, D. H., and Cowen, P. J. (1992). Effect of estradiol implant on noradrenergic function and mood in menopausal subjects. *Psychoneuroendocrinology*, 17, 87–93.

Beumont, P., Burrows, G., and Casper, R. (Eds.). (1987). *Handbook of eating disorders. Part 1: Anorexia and bulimia nervosa*. Amsterdam: Elsevier.

Beaumont, P., Friessen, H., Gelder, M., and Kolakowska, T. (1974). Plasma prolactin and luteinizing hormone levels. *Psychol Med*, 4, 219–221.

Bickel, M. (1975). Binding of chlorpromazine and imipramine to red cells, albumin, lipoproteins and other blood components. *J Pharm Pharmacol*, 27, 733–738.

Bickell, N. A., Pieper, K. S., Lee, K. L., and Mark, D. B. (1992). Referral patterns for coronary heart disease treatment: Gender bias or good clinical judgment? *Ann Intern Med*, 116, 791–797.

Biegon, A. (1990). Effects of steroid hormones on the serotonergic system. In Whitaker-Azmidea, P. M., and Peroutka, S. J. (Eds.), *The neuropharmacology of serotonin.* New York Academy of Sciences, 600, 427–431.

Biegon, A., and McEwen, B. S. (1982). Modulation by estradiol of serotonin receptors in brain. *J Neurosci,* 2, 199–205.

Biegon, A., Reches, A., Snyder, L., and McEwen, B. S. (1983). Serotonergic and noradrenergic receptors in the rat brain: Modulation by chronic exposure to ovarian hormones. *Life Sci,* 32, 2015–2021.

Blair, S. N., Kohl, H. W., and Barlow, C. E. (1993). Physical activity, physical fitness and mortality in women: Do women need to be active? *J Am Coll Nutr,* 12, 368–371.

Blair, S. N., Kohl, H. W., Paffenbarger, R. S., et al. (1989). Physical fitness and all-cause mortality: A prospective study of healthy men and women. *JAMA,* 262, 2395–2401.

Blanchard, B. A., and Glick, S. D. (1995). Sex differences in mesolimbic dopamine responses to ethanol and relationship to ethanol intake in rats. In M. Galanter (Ed.), *Recent developments in alcoholism,* vol. 12: *Women and alcoholism* (pp. 231–241). New York: Plenum Press.

Bland, R. C., Orn, H., and Newman, S. C. (1988). Lifetime prevalence of psychiatric disorders in Edmonton. *Acta Psychiatr Scand Suppl,* 33, 24–32.

Blehar, M. C., and Oren, D. A. (1995). Women's increased vulnerability to mood disorders: Integrating psychobiology and epidemiology. *Depression,* 3, 3–12.

Blinder, B. J., Freeman, D. M. A., and Stunkard, A. J. (1970). Behavior therapy of anorexia nervosa: Effectiveness of activity as a reenforcer of weight gain. *Am J Psychiatry,* 126, 1093–1098.

Bluthé, R., and Dantzer, R. (1990). Social recognition does not involve vasopressinergic neurotransmission in female rats. *Brain Res,* 535, 301–304.

Board, F., Wadeson, R., and Persky, H. (1957). Depressive affect and endocrine functions. *Arch Neurol Psychiatry,* 78, 612–620.

Boccardo, F., Guarneri, D., Rubagotti, A., et al. (1984). Endocrine effects of tamoxifen in postmenopausal breast cancer patients. *Tumori,* 70, 61–68.

Bocchetta, A., Bernardi, F., Pedditzi, M., et al. (1991). Thyroid abnormalities during lithium treatment. *Acta Psychiatr Scand,* 83, 193–198.

Boccuzzi, G., Aragno, M., Brignardello, E., et al. (1992). Opposite effects of dehydroepiandrosterone on the growth of 7,12-dimethylbenz(a)anthracene-induced rat mammary carcinomas. *Anticancer Res,* 12, 1479–1483.

Bologa, M., Tang, B., Klein, J., Tesoro, A., and Koren, G. (1991). Pregnancy-induced changes in drug metabolism in epileptic women. *J Pharmacol Exp Ther,* 257, 735–740.

Bommer, M., Eversmann, T., Pickardt, R., Leonhardt, A., Naber, D. (1990). Psychopathological and neuropsychological symptoms in patients with subclinical and remitted hyperthyroidism. *Klin Wochenschr,* 68, 552–558.

Bonati, M., Bortolus, R., Marchetti, F., Romano, M., and Tognoni, G. (1990). Drug use in pregnancy: An overview of epidemiological (drug utilization) studies. *Eur J Clin Pharmacol,* 38, 325–358.

Bonica, J. J. (1990). Evolution and current status of pain programs. *J Pain Symptom Management,* 5, 368–374.

Bonnier, P., Romain, S., Giacalone, P. L., et al. (1995). Clinical and biologic prognostic factors in breast cancer diagnosed during postmenopausal hormone replacement therapy. *Obstet Gynecol*, 85, 11–17.

Boogaard, M. A. (1984). Rehabilitation of the female patient after myocardial infarction. *Nursing Clin North Am*, 19, 433–444.

Booth-Kewley, S., and Friedman, H. S. (1987). Psychological predictors of heart disease: A quantitative review. *Psychol Bull*, 101, 343–362.

Boring, C. C., Spuires, T. S., Tong, T., and Montgomery, S. (1994). Cancer statistics. *CA Cancer J Clin*, 44, 7–26.

Bottiger, L. E., Furhoff, A. K., and Holmberg, L. (1979). Fatal reactions to drugs. *Acta Scand*, 205, 451–456.

Bouckoms, A., and Mangini, L. (1993). Pergolide: An antidepressant adjuvant for mood disorders? *Psychopharmacol Bull*, 29, 207–211.

Bovbjerg, D. H., and Valdimarsdottir, H. (1993). Familial cancer, emotional distress, and low natural cytotoxic activity in healthy women. *Ann Oncol*, 4, 745–752.

Bowen, D. J., Henderson, M. M., Iverson, D., Burrows, E., Henry, J., and Foreyt, J. (1994). Reducing dietary fat: Understanding the success of the women's health trial. *Cancer Prevention Int*, 1, 21–30.

Bowlby, J. (1982). *Attachment*, 2nd ed., vol. 1. New York: Basic Books.

Boyar, R., and Bradlow, H. (1977). Studies of testosterone metabolism in anorexia nervosa. In R. Vigersky (Ed.), *Anorexia nervosa* (pp. 271–276). New York: Raven Press.

Boyar, R., Hellman, L., and Roffwarg, H. (1977). Cortisol secretion and metabolism in anorexia nervosa. *N Engl J Med*, 296, 190–193.

Boyar, R., Katz, J., and Finkelstein, J. (1974). Anorexia nervosa: Immaturity of the 24-hour luteinizing hormone secretory pattern. *N Engl J Med*, 291, 861–865.

Boyce, P. M., and Todd, A. L. (1992). Increased risk of postnatal depression after emergency caesarean section. *Med J Australia*, 157, 172–174.

Bradford, R. H., Downton, M., Chremos, A. N., et al. (1993). Efficacy and tolerability of Lovastatin in 3,390 women with moderate hypercholesterolemia. *Ann Intern Med*, 118, 850–855.

Brady, K. T., and Anton, R. F. (1989). The thyroid axis and desipramine treatment in depression. *Biol Psychiatry*, 25, 703–709.

Braftos, O., and Haug, J. (1966). Puerperal disorders in manic depressive females. *Acta Psychiatr Scand*, 42, 285–294.

Brambilla, F., Maggioni, M., Ferrari, E., Scarone, S., and Catalano, M. (1990). Tonic and dynamic gonadotropin secretion in depressive and normothymic phases of affective disorders. *Psychiatry Res*, 32, 299–239.

Brasel, J. (1976). Hormonal changes during adolescence: A selected review of literature. In J. Mckigney and H. Munro (Eds.), *Nutrient requirements in adolescence*. Cambridge, MA: MIT Press.

Braverman, J., and Roux, J. F. (1978). Screening for the patient at risk for postpartum depression. *Obstet Gynecol*, 52, 731–736.

Breedlove, S. M. (1994). Sexual differentiation of the nervous system. *Annu Rev Psychol*, 45, 389–418.

Breitbart, W. (1992). Psychotropic adjuvant analgesics for cancer pain. *Psychooncology*, 1, 133–145.

Bremner, J. D., Randall, P., Scott, T. M., et al. (1995). MRI-based measurement of hippocampal volume in patients with combat-related posttraumatic stress disorder. *Am J Psychiatry*, 152, 973–981.

Breslau, N., Schultz, L., and Peterson, E. (1995). Sex differences in depression: A role for preexisting anxiety. *Psychiatry Res*, 58, 1–12.

Brezinka, V. E., and Padmos, I. (1994). Coronary heart disease risk factors in women. *Eur Heart J*, 15(11), 1571–1584.

Breyer-Pfaff, U., Nill, K., Entenmann, K., and Gaertner, H. (1995). Secretion of amitriptyline and metabolites into breast milk [letter]. *Am J Psychiatry*, 152, 812–813.

Bridges, R. (1984). A quantitative analysis of the roles of dosage, sequence and duration of estradiol and progesterone exposure in regulation of maternal behavior in the rat. *Endocrinology*, 114, 930–940.

Briggs, J., McBride, L., Hagino, O., Brown, W., and Bauer, M. (1993). Screening depressives for causative medical illness; the example of thyroid testing: II. Hypothesis testing in ambulatory depressives. *Depression*, 1, 220–224.

Bringer, J., Hedon, B., and Jaffiol, C. (1985). Influence of the frequency of gonadotropin-releasing hormone (GnRH) admission on ovulatory responses in women with anovulation. *Fertil Steril*, 44, 42–48.

Briscoe, M. (1982). *Sex differences in psychological well-being*. Cambridge, UK: Cambridge University Press.

Briscoe, M. E. (1987). Why do people go to the doctor? Sex differences in the correlates of GP consultation. *Soc Sci Med*, 25, 507–513.

Brockington, I. F., Kelly, A., Hall, P., and Deakin, W. (1988). Premenstrual relapse of puerperal psychosis. *J Affect Disord*, 14, 287–292.

Brown, C. S., Ling, F. W., Andersen, R. N., et al. (1994). Efficacy of depot leuprolide in premenstrual syndrome: Effect of symptom severity and type in a controlled trial. *Obstet Gynecol*, 84, 779–786.

Brown, J., Ye, H., Bronson, R., Dikkes, P., and Greenberg, M. (1996). A defect in nurturing in mice lacking the immediate early gene *fosB*. *Cell*, 86, 297–309.

Brown, L. L., Tomarken, A. J., Orth, D. N., et al. (1996). Individual differences in repressive-defensiveness predict basal salivary cortisol levels. *J Pers Soc Psychol*, 70, 362–371.

Brown, W. A., Sirota, A. D., Niaura, R., and Engebretson, T. O. (1993). Endocrine correlates of sadness and elation. *Psychosom Med*, 55, 458–467.

Browne, J. L., Rice, J. L., Evans, D. L., and Prange, A. J., Jr. (1990). Triiodothyronine augmentation of the antidepressant effect of the nontricyclic antidepressant trazodone. *J Nerv Ment Dis*, 178, 598–599.

Bruch, H. (1974). *Eating disorders: Obesity, anorexia nervosa and the person within*. London: Routledge Kegan Paul.

Bruera, E., Macmillan, K., Kuehn, N., and Miller, M. J. (1992). Circadian distribution of extra doses of narcotic analgesics in patients with cancer pain: A preliminary report. *Pain*, 49, 311–314.

Bruera, E., Miller, M. J., Macmillan, K., and Kuehn, N. (1992). Neuropsychological effects of methylphenidate in patients receiving a continuous infusion of narcotics for cancer pain. *Pain*, 48, 163–166.

Bryant-Waugh, R., Hankins, M., Shafran, R., Lask, B., and Fosson, A. (1996). A prospective follow-up of children with anorexia nervosa. *J Youth Adolesc*, 25, 431–437.

Bryant-Waugh, R., Knibbs, J., Fosson, A., Kaminski, Z., and Lask, B. (1988). Long-term follow-up of patients with early onset anorexia nervosa. *Arch Dis Child*, 63, 5–9.

Buchanan, C., Eccles, J., and Becker, J. (1992). Are adolescents the victims of raging hormones? Evidence for activational effects of hormones on moods and behavior at adolescence. *Psychol Bull*, 111, 62–107.

Buist, A., Norman, T. R., and Dennerstein, L. (1990). Breastfeeding and the use of psychotropic medication: A review. *J Affect Disord*, 19, 197–206.

Bukberg, J., Penman, D., and Holland, J. C. (1984). Depression in hospitalized cancer patients. *Psychosom Med*, 28, 530–539.

Bungay, G. T., Vessey, M. P., and McPherson, C. K. (1950). Study of symptoms in middle life with special reference to menopause. *Br J Med*, 2, 181–189.

Burger, J., Horwitz, S. M., Forsyth, B. W., et al. (1993). Psychological sequelae of medical complications during pregnancy. *Pediatrics*, 91, 566–571.

Buring, J. E., and Hennekens, C. H. (1994). Randomized trials of primary prevention of cardiovascular disease in women. An investigator's view. *Ann Epidemiol*, 4, 111–114.

Burish, T. G., and Jenkins, R. A. (1992). Effectiveness of biofeedback and relaxation training in reducing the side effects of cancer chemotherapy. *Health Psychol*, 11, 17–23.

Burns, J. W., and Katkin, E. S. (1993). Psychological, situational, and gender predictors of cardiovascular reactivity to stress: A multivariate approach. *J Behav Med*, 16, 445–465.

Bush, T. L., Barrett-Connor, E., Cowan, L. D., et al. (1987). Cardiovascular mortality and noncontraceptive use of estrogen in women: Results from the Lipid Research Clinics Program Follow-Up Study. *Circulation*, 75, 1102–1109.

Bush, T. L., Fried L. P., and Barrett-Connor, E. (1988). Cholesterol, lipoproteins, and coronary heart disease in women. *Clin Chem*, 34, B60–B70.

Bush, T. L., and Helzlsouer, K. J., et al. (1993). Tamoxifen for the primary prevention of breast cancer: A review and critique of the concept and trial. *Epidemiol Rev*, 15, 233–243.

Butler, M., Lang, N., and Young, J. (1992). Determination of CYP1A2 and NAT2 phenotypes in human populations by analysis of caffeine urinary metabolites. *Pharmacogenetics*, 2, 116–117.

Buttolph, M. L., and Holland, A. (1990). Obsessive compulsive disorder and childbirth. In M. Jenike, L. Baer, and W. Minchiello (Eds.), *Obsessive compulsive disorders: Theory and management* (pp. 89–95). Chicago: Yearbook Publications.

Cafferata, G., Kasper, J., and Bernstein, A. (1983). Family roles, structure, and stressors in relation to sex differences in obtaining psychotropic drugs. *J Health Soc Behav*, 24, 132–143.

Cahill, G. J., Herrera, M., Morgan, A., et al. (1966). Hormone-fuel interrelationships during fasting. *J Clin Invest*, 45, 1751–1769.

Calabrese, J. R., Gulledge, A. D., Hahn, K., et al. (1985). Autoimmune thyroiditis in manic-depressive patients treated with lithium. *Am J Psychiatry*, 142, 1318–1321.

Canino, G. J., Bird, H. J., Shrout, P. E., et al. (1987). The prevalence of specific psychiatric disorders in Puerto Rico. *Arch Gen Psychiatry*, 44, 727–735.

Cannistra, L. D., Balady, J., O'Malley, C. J., Weiner, D. A., and Ryan, T. J. (1992).

Comparison of the clinical profile and outcome of women and men in cardiac rehabilitation. *Am J Cardiol*, **69**, 1274–1279.

Caraco, Y., Zylber-Katz, E., Berry, E., and Levy, M. (1995). Caffeine pharmacokinetics in obesity and following significant weight reduction. *Int J Obes Related Metab Disord*, **19**, 234–239.

Carney, R. M., Rich, M. W., Freedland, K. E., et al. (1988). Major depressive disorder predicts cardiac events in patients with coronary artery disease. *Psychosom Med*, **50**, 627–633.

Carpenter, W., and Bunney, W. (1971). Adrenal cortical activity in depressive illness. *Am J Psychiatry*, **128**, 31–40.

Carr, B. R., Parker, C. R., Jr., Madeen, J. D., MacDonald, P. C., and Porter, J. C. (1981). Maternal plasma adrenocorticotropin and cortisol relationships throughout human pregnancy. *Am J Obstet Gynecol*, **139**, 416–422.

Carroll, B. J. (1968). Pituitary-adrenal function in depression. *Lancet*, **556**, 1373–1374.

Carroll, B. J. (1982). Use of the dexamethasone suppression test in depression. *J Clin Psychiatry*, **43**, 44–50.

Carter, C., Williams, J., Witt, D., and Insel, T. (1992). Oxytocin and social bonding. Reprinted from *Oxytocin in maternal, sexual and social behaviors*. *Ann N Y Acad Sci*, **652**, 204–211.

Carter, J. H., and Carter, H. W., (1988). Adrenal regulation of mammary tumorigenesis in female Sprague-Dawley rats: Histopathology of mammary tumors. *Cancer Res*, **48**, 3808–3815.

Case, R. B., Moss, A. J., Case, N., McDermott, M., and Eberly, S. (1992). Living alone after myocardial infarction: Impact on prognosis. *JAMA*, **267**, 514–519.

Casper, R. (1982). Treatment principles in anorexia nervosa. *Adolesc Psychiatry*, **10**, 431–454.

Casper, R. (1983). On the emergence of bulimia nervosa as a syndrome: A historical view. *Int J Eating Disord*, **2**, 3–16.

Casper, R. (1986). Pharmacologic and psychologic treatments of anorexia nervosa and bulimia nervosa. In E. Ferrari and F. Brambilla (Eds.), *Disorders of eating behavior—a psychoneuroendocrine approach* (pp. 287–294). Elmsford, NY: Pergamon Press.

Casper, R. (1990a). The dilemma of homonymous symptoms for evaluating comorbidity between affective disorders and eating disorders. In J. Maser and C. Cloninger (Eds.), *Comorbidity of mood and anxiety disorder* (pp. 253–269). Washington, DC, and London: American Psychiatric Press.

Casper, R. (1990b). Personality features of women with good outcome from restricting anorexia nervosa. *Psychosom Med*, **52**, 156–170.

Casper, R. (1991). Outpatient treatment for anorexia nervosa: What are its indications? In B. Beitman and G. Klerman (Eds.), *Integrating pharmacotherapy and psychotherapy* (pp. 395–408). Washington, DC: American Psychiatric Press.

Casper, R. (1995a). Eating disturbances and eating disorders in childhood. In F. Bloom and D. Kupfer (Eds.), *Psychopharmacology: The fourth generation of progress* (pp. 1675–1683). New York: Raven Press.

Casper, R. (1995b). Fear of fatness and eating disorders in childhood and early adolescence. In L. Cheung (Ed.), *Child health through nutrition and physical activity*. Champaign, IL: Human Kinetics Publishers.

Casper, R. (1996) Introduction to special issue. *J Youth Adolesc*, **25**, 413–418.

Casper, R., Belanoff, J., and Offer, D. (1996). Gender differences, but no racial group differences, in self-reported psychiatric symptoms in adolescents. *J Am Acad Child Adolesc Psychiatry*, 35, 500–508.

Casper, R., Chatterton, R. J., and Davis, M. (1979). Alterations in serum cortisol and its binding characteristics in anorexia nervosa. *J Clin Endocrinol Metab*, 49, 406–411.

Casper, R., and Davis, J. (1977). On the course of anorexia nervosa. *Am J Psychiatry*, 134, 974–978.

Casper, R., Davis, J., and Pandey, G. (1977). The effect of the nutritional status and weight changes on hypothalamic function tests in anorexia nervosa. In R. Vigersky (Ed.), *Anorexia nervosa* (pp. 137–149). New York: Raven Press.

Casper, R., Eckert, E., Halmi, K., Goldberg, S., and Davis, J. (1980). Bulimia: Its incidence and clinical significance in patients with anorexia nervosa. *Arch Gen Psychiatry*, 37, 1030–1035.

Casper, R., and Frohman, L. (1982). Delayed TSH release in anorexia nervosa following injection of thyrotropin-releasing hormone (TRH). *Psychoneuroendocrinology*, 7, 59–68.

Casper, R., Halmi, K., Goldberg, S., Eckert, E., and Davis, J. (1979). Disturbances in body image estimation as related to other characteristics and outcome measures in anorexia nervosa. *Br J Psychiatry*, 134, 60–66.

Casper, R., Hedeker, D., and McClough, J. (1992). Personality dimensions in eating disorders and their relevance for subtyping. *J Am Acad Child Adolesc Psychiatry*, 31, 830–840.

Casper, R., and Heller, W. (1991). "La douce indifférence" and mood in anorexia nervosa: Neuropsychological correlates. *Prog Neuropsychopharmacol Biol Psychiatry*, 15, 15–23.

Casper, R., and Jabine, L. (1996). An 8-year follow-up: Outcome from adolescent compared to adult onset anorexia nervosa. *J Youth Adolesc*, 25, 499–517.

Casper, R., Pandy, G., Jaspan, J., and Rubenstein, A. (1988). Hormone and metabolite plasma levels after oral glucose in bulimia and healthy controls. *Biol Psychiatry*, 24, 663–674.

Casper, R., Schoeller, D., Kushner, R., Hnilicka, J., and Gold, S. (1991). Total daily energy expenditure and activity level in anorexia nervosa. *Am J Clin Nutr*, 53, 1143–1150.

Castelli, W. P. (1988). Cardiovascular disease in women. *Am J Obstet Gynecol*, 158, 1553–1560.

Castle, D. J., and Murray, R. M. (1991). The neurodevelopmental basis of sex differences in schizophrenia. *Psychol Med*, 21, 565–575.

Castiglione-Gertsch, M., Johnsen, C., Goldhirsch, A., et al. (1994). The International (Ludwig) Breast Cancer Study Group Trials I–IV: 15 years' follow-up. *Ann Oncol*, 5, 717–724.

Cathcart, C. K., Jones, S. E., Pumroy, C. S., et al. (1993). Clinical recognition and management of depression in node negative breast cancer patients treated with tamoxifen. *Breast Cancer Res Treat*, 27, 277–281.

Cauley, J. A., LaPorte, R. E., Kuller, L. H., Bates, M., and Sandler, R. B. (1983). Menopausal estrogen use, high density lipoprotein subfractions and liver function. *Atherosclerosis*, 49, 31–39.

Cauley, J. A., Seeley, D. G., Enstrud, K, et al. for the Study of Osteoporotic Fractures

Research Group. (1995). Estrogen replacement therapy and fractures in older women. *Ann Intern Med*, 122, 9–16.

Cavalca, G. G., Covezzi, E., and Boncinelli, A. (1974). Clinical experiences with the combination of thyroid extract and tricyclics in the treatment of depressed patients. *Riv Sper Freniat Med Leg Alienazioni Ment*, 98, 271–300.

Cella, D. F., Mahon, S. M., and Donovan, M. I. (1990). Cancer recurrence as a traumatic event. *Behav Med*, 16, 15–22.

Chakravarti, S., Collins, W. P., Thom, J., et al. (1979). Relation between plasma hormone profiles, symptoms and response to oestrogen treatment in women approaching the menopause. *Br Med J*, i, 983–985.

Challis, G. B., Stam, H. J. (1992). A longitudinal study of the development of anticipatory nausea and vomiting in cancer chemotherapy patients: The role of absorption and autonomic perception. *Health Psychol*, 11, 181–189.

Chamberlain, S., Hahn, P., Casson, P., and Reid, R. (1990). Effect of menstrual cycle phase and oral contraceptive use on serum lithium levels after a loading dose of lithium in normal women. *Am J Psychiatry*, 147, 907–909.

Chambers, C. D., Johnson, K. A., Dick, L. M., Felix, R. J., and Jones, K. L. (1996). Birth outcomes in pregnant women taking fluoxetine. *N Engl J Med*, 335, 1010–1015.

Chang, S. S., and Renshaw, D. C. (1986). Psychosis and pregnancy. *Comp Ther*, 12, 36–41.

Chapuy, M. C., Arlot, M. E., Duboef, F., et al. (1992). Vitamin D_3 and calcium to prevent hip fractures in elderly women. *N Engl J Med*, 327, 1637–1642.

Chesney, M. A. (1993). Social isolation, depression, and heart disease: Research on women broaden the agenda. *Psychosom Med*, 55, 434–435.

Chess, S., and Thomas, A. (1968). *Temperament in clinical practice.* New York: Guilford Press.

Cheymol, G. (1993). Clinical pharmacokinetics of drugs in obesity. An update. *Clin Pharmacokinet*, 25, 103–114.

Cho, J. T., Bone, S., Dunner, D. L., Colt, E., and Fieve, R. R. (1979). The effect of lithium treatment on thyroid function in patients with primary affective disorder. *Am J Psychiatry*, 136, 115–116.

Chorot, P., and Sandin, B. (1994). Life events and stress reactivity as predictors of cancer, coronary heart disease and anxiety disorders. *Int J Psychosom*, 41, 34–40.

Chouinard, G., Annable, L., and Steinberg, S. (1986). A controlled clinical trial of fluspirilene, a long-acting injectable neuroleptic, in schizophrenic patients with acute exacerbation. *J Clin Psychopharmacol*, 6, 21–26.

Chouinard, G., Jones, B., Annable, L., and Ross-Chouinard, A. (1980). Sex differences and tardive dyskinesia [Letter]. *Am J Psychiatry*, 137, 507.

Ciraulo, D., Shader, R., Greenblatt, D., and Creelman, W. (Eds.). (1995). *Drug interactions in psychiatry*, 2nd ed. Baltimore: Williams & Wilkins.

Clarke, I. J., and Cummins, J. T. (1982). The temporal relationship between gonadotropin releasing hormone (GnRH) and luteinizing hormone (LH) secretion in ovariectomized ewes. *Endocrinology*, 111, 1737–1739.

Clarren, S., and Smith, L. (1978). The fetal alcohol syndrome. *N Engl J Med*, 298, 1063–1067.

Clayton-Smith, J., and Donnai, D. (1995). Fetal valproate syndrome. *J Med Genet*, 32, 724–727.

Claus, E. B., Risch, N., and Thompson, W. D. (1994). Autosomal dominant inheritance of early-onset breast cancer. *Cancer*, 73, 643–651.

Cleary, P. D., Mechanic, D., and Greenly, J. R. (1982). Sex differences in medical care utilization: An empirical investigation. *J Health Soc Behav*, 23, 106–119.

Clevenger, C. V., Chang, W. P., Ngo, W., et al. (1995). Expression of prolactin and prolactin receptor in human breast carcinoma. Evidence for an autocrine/paracrine loop. *Am J Pathology*, 146, 695–705.

Clinical Society of London. (1888). Report on myxedema. *Trans Clin Soc London*, 21 (Suppl), 18–38.

Cloninger, C. R., Reich, T., and Wetzel, R. (1979). Alcoholism and affective disorders: Familial associations and genetic models. In D. W. Goodwin and C. K. Erickson (Eds.), *Alcoholism and affective disorders* (pp. 57–86). New York: SP Medical and Scientific Books.

Coe, C. L., Rosenberg, L. T., and Levine, S. (1988). Prolonged effect of psychological disturbance on macrophage chemiluminescence in the squirrel monkey. *Brain Behavior Immun*, 2, 151–160.

Cohen, I., Beyth, Y., Tepper, R., et al. (1996). Ovarian tumors in postmenopausal breast cancer patients treated with tamoxifen. *Gynecol Oncol*, 60, 54–58.

Cohen, L., Friedman, J., Jefferson, J., Johnson, E., and Weiner, M. (1994). A reevaluation of risk of in utero exposure to lithium. *JAMA*, 271, 146–150.

Cohen, L. S., Sichel, D. A., Dimmock, J. A., and Rosenbaum, J. F. (1994). Postpartum course in women with preexisting panic disorder. *J Clin Psychiatry*, 55, 289–292.

Cohen, L. S., Sichel, D. A., Robertson, L. H., Heckscher, E., and Rosenbaum, J. F. (1995). Postpartum prophylaxis for women with bipolar disorder. *Am J Psychiatry*, 152, 1641–1645.

Coiro, V., Volpi, R., Marchesi, C., et al. (1994). Lack of seasonal variation in abnormal TSH secretion in patients with seasonal affective disorder. *Biol Psychiatry*, 35, 36–41.

Colditz, G. A.,. Hankinson, S. E., Hunter, D. J., et al. (1995). The use of estrogens and progestins and the risk of breast cancer in postmenopausal women. *N Engl J Med*, 332, 1589–1593.

Colditz, G. A., Martin, P., Stampfer, M. J., et al. (1986). Validation of questionnaire information on risk factors and disease outcomes in a prospective cohort study of women. *Am J Epidemiol*, 123, 894–900.

Collaborative Group on Drug Use in Pregnancy. (1990). Drugs in pregnancy: A preliminary report of the International Collaborative Drug Utilization Study. *Pharm Weekbl*, 12, 75–78.

Collaborative Group on Drug Use in Pregnancy. (1991). An international survey on drug utilization during pregnancy. *Int J Risk Safety Med*, 2, 1–5.

Collaborative Group on Drug Use in Pregnancy. (1992). Medication during pregnancy: An intercontinental cooperative study. *Int J Gynecol Obstet*, 39, 185–196.

Collings, S., and King, M. (1994). Ten-year follow-up of 50 patients with bulimia nervosa. *Br J Psychiatry*, 164, 80–87.

Collins, N. L., Dunkel-Schetter, C., Lobel, M., and Scrimshaw, S. C. (1993). Social support in pregnancy: Psychosocial correlates of birth outcomes and postpartum depression. *J Pers Soc Psychol*, 65, 1243–1258.

Collins, P., Shay, J., Jiang, C., and Moss, J. (1994). Nitric oxide accounts for dose dependent estrogen-mediated coronary relaxation after acute estrogen withdrawal. *Circulation*, 90, 1964–1968.

Conrad, C., and Hamilton, J. (1986). Recurrent premenstrual decline in serum lithium concentration: Clinical correlates and treatment implications. *J Am Acad Child Adolesc Psychiatry*, 26, 852–853.

Coope, J. (1981). Is oestrogen therapy effective in the treatment of menopausal depression? *J R Coll Gen Pract*, 31, 134–140.

Coope, J., Thomson, J. M., and Poller, L. (1975). Effects of natural oestrogen replacement therapy on menopausal symptoms and blood clotting. *Br Med J*, 18, 139–143.

Cooper, C. L., and Faragher, E. B. (1993). Psychosocial stress and breast cancer: The interrelationship between stress events, coping strategies and personality. *Psychol Med*, 23, 653–662.

Cooper, D., Halpern, R., Wood, L., Levin, A., and Ridgeway, E. (1984). L-Thyroxine therapy in subclinical hypothyroidism. *Ann Intern Med*, 101, 18–24.

Cooper, P. J., and Murray, L. (1995). Course and recurrence of postnatal depression. Evidence for the specificity of the diagnostic concept. *Br J Psychiatry*, 166, 191–195.

Coppen, A., Whybrow, P. C., Noguera, R., Maggs, R., and Prange, A. J. J. (1972). The comparative antidepressant value of L-tryptophan and imipramine with and without attempted potentiation by liothyronine. *Arch Gen Psychiatry*, 26, 234–241.

Corner, G. (1965). The early history of the oestrogenic hormones. *J Endocrinol*, 31, iii–xvii.

Corney, R. H., Crowther, M. E., Everett, H., Howells, A., and Shepherd, J. H. (1993). Psychosexual dysfunction in women with gynaecological cancer following radical pelvic surgery. *Br J Obstet Gynaecol*, 100, 73–78.

Coronary Drug Project Research Group. (1973). The Coronary Drug Project: Findings leading to discontinuation of the 2.5 mg/day estrogen group. *JAMA*, 226, 652–657.

Correy, J., Newman, N., Collins, J., et al. (1994). Use of prescription drugs in the first trimester and congenital malformations. *Aust NZ J Obstetr Gynecol*, 31, 340–344.

Cowdry, R. W., Wehr, T. A., Zis, A. P., and Goodwin, F. K. (1983). Thyroid abnormalities associated with rapid-cycling bipolar illness. *Arch Gen Psychiatry*, 40, 414–420.

Cowley, D. S., and Roy-Byrne, P. P. (1989). Panic disorder during pregnancy. *J Psychosom Obstet Gynecol*, 10, 193–210.

Coyne, J. S., Kessler, R. C., Tal, M., et al. (1987). Living with a depressed person. *J Consult Clin Psychol*, 55, 347–352.

Craft, S., Gourovitch, M. L., Dowton, S. B., Swanson, J. M., and Bonforte, S. (1992). Lateralized deficits in visual attention in males with developmental dopamine depletion. *Neuropsychologia*, 30, 341–351.

Cramer, O. W., Hutchinson, G. B., Welch, W. R., et al. (1983). Determinants of ovarian cancer risk. I. Reproductive experiences and family history. *J Natl Cancer Inst*, 71, 711–716.

Cree, J., Meyer, J., and Hailey, D. (1973). Diazepam in labour: Its metabolism and effect on the clinical condition and thermogenesis of the newborn. *Br Med J*, 4, 251–255.

Crisp, A. (1970). Reported birth weights and growth rates in a group of patients with primary anorexia nervosa (weight phobia). *J Psychosom Res*, 14, 23–50.

Crisp, A., Blendis, L., and Pawan, G. (1968). Aspects of fat metabolism in anorexia nervosa. *Metabolism*, 17, 1109–1118.

Crombie, D., Pinsent, R., and Fleming, D. (1972). Imipramine in pregnancy. *Br Med J*, 1, 745.

Cross-National Collaborative Panic Study, Second Phase Investigators. (1992). Drug treatment of panic disorder: Comparative efficacy of alprazolam, imipramine, and placebo. *Br J Psychiatry*, 160, 191–202.

Crow, T. J., Ball, J., Bloom, S. R., et al. (1989). Schizophrenia as an anomaly of development of cerebral asymmetry: A postmortem study and a proposal concerning the genetic basis of the disease. *Arch Gen Psychiatry*, 46, 1145–1150.

Crow, T. J., DeLisi, L. E., Lofthouse, R., et al. (1994). An examination of linkage of schizophrenia and schizoaffective disorder to the pseudoautosomal region (Xp22.3). *Br J Psychiatry*, 164, 159–164.

Crown, S. (1949). Notes on an experimental study of intellectual deterioration. *Br Med J*, 2, 684–685.

Cruickshank, D. J., Haites, N., Anderson, S., et al. (1992). The multidisciplinary management of a family with epithelial ovarian cancer. *Br J Obstet Gynaecol*, 99, 226–231.

Cumming, R. G. (1990). Calcium intake and bone mass: A quantitative review of the evidence. *Calcif Tissue Int*, 47, 194–201.

Cunnick, J. E., Cohen, S., Rabin, B. S., et al. (1991). Alterations in specific antibody production due to rank and social instability. *Brain Behav Immun*, 5, 357–369.

D'Mello, D., and McNeil, J. (1990). Sex differences in bipolar affective disorder: Neuroleptic dosage variance. *Comp Psychiatry*, 31, 80–83.

Dalton, K. (1980). *Depression after childbirth*. Oxford: Oxford University Press.

Dantzer, R., and Kelley, K. W. (1989). Stress and immunity: An integrated view of relationships between the brain and the immune system. *Life Sci*, 44, 1995–2008.

Dantzer, R., Koob, G., Bluthe, R., and Le Moal, M. (1988). Septal vasopressin modulates social memory in male rats. *Brain Res*, 457, 143–147.

Datz, F., Christian, P., and Moore, J. (1987). Gender-related differences in gastric emptying. *J Nucl Med*, 28, 1204–1207.

Davidson, J., and Pelton, S. (1986). Forms of atypical depression and their response to antidepressant drugs. *Psychiatr Res*, 17, 87–95.

Davidson, J. R. T., Krishnan, K. R. R., Charles, H. C., et al. (1993). Magnetic resonance spectroscopy in social phobia: Preliminary findings. *J Clin Psychiatry*, 54, 19–25.

Davidson, K. M., and Ritson, E. B. (1993). The relationship between alcohol dependence and depression. *Alcohol Alcohol*, 28, 147–155.

Davis, S. R., McCloud, P., Strauss, B. U., and Burger, H. (1995). Testosterone enhances estradiol's effects on postmenopausal bone density and sexuality. *Maturitas*, 21, 227–236.

Davison, J., Davison, M., and Hay, D. (1970). Gastric emptying time in late pregnancy and labour. *J Obstet Gynaecol Br Commonw*, 77, 37–41.

Dawson, D. A., and Grant, B. F. (1993). Gender effects in diagnosing alcohol abuse and dependence. *J Clin Psychol*, 49, 298–307.

Day, N., Jaspere, D., Richardson, G., et al. (1989). Perinatal exposure to alcohol: Effect on infant growth and morphologic characteristics. *Pediatrics*, 84, 536–541.

Dean, M., Stock, B., and Patterson, R. (1980). Serum protein binding of drugs during and after pregnancy in humans. *Clin Pharmacol Ther*, 28, 253–261.

DeBellis, M. D., Gold, P. W., Geracioti, T. D., Listwak, S., and Kling, M. A. (1993). Fluoxetine significantly reduces CSF CRH and AVP concentrations in patients with major depression. *Am J Psychiatry*, 150, 656–657.

Degner, L. F., and Sloan, J. A. (1992). Decision making during serious illness: What role do patients really want to play? *J Clin Epidemiol*, 45, 941–950.

DeGregorio, M. W., Maenpaa, J. U., and Wiebe, V. J. (1995). Tamoxifen for the prevention of breast cancer: No 12. *Important Adv Oncol*, 175–185.

Dekaban, A., and Sadowsky, D. (1978). Changes in brain weights during the span of human life: Relation of brain weights to body heights and body weights. *Ann Neurol*, 4, 345–356.

Demey-Ponsart, E., Foidart, J. M., Sulon, J., and Sodoyez, J. C. (1982). Serum CBG, free and total cortisol and circadian patterns of adrenal function in normal pregnancy. *J Steroid Biochem*, 16, 165–169.

Dennerstein, L., Brown, J. B., Gotts, G., et al. (1993). Menstrual cycle hormonal profiles of women with and without premenstrual syndrome. *J Psychosom Obstet Gynaecol*, 14, 259–268.

Dennerstein, L., and Burrows, G. (1986). Psychological effects of progestogens in the post-menopausal years. *Maturitas*, 8, 101–106.

Derogatis, L. R., Abeloff, M. D., and Melisaratos, N. (1979). Psychological coping mechanisms and survival time in metastatic breast cancer. *JAMA*, 242, 1504–1508.

Derogatis, L. R., Morrow, G. R., Fetting, J., et al. (1983). The prevalence of psychiatric disorders among cancer patients. *JAMA*, 249, 751–757.

Deter, L., and Herzog, W. (1994). Anorexia nervosa in a long-term perspective: Results of the Heidelberg-Mannheim Study. *Psychosom Med*, 56, 20–27.

DeVane, C. (1994). Pharmacokinetics of the newer antidepressants: Clinical relevance. *Am J Med*, 97, 13S–23S.

Dewhurst, K. E., El Kabir, D. J., Exley, D., et al. (1968). Blood levels of TSH, protein-bound iodine, and cortisol in schizophrenia and affective states. *Lancet*, 2, 1160–1162.

Dhar, V., and Murphy, G. E. (1990). Double blind randomized crossover trial of luteal phase estrogens (premarin) in the premenstrual syndrome (PMS). *Psychoneuroendocrinology*, 15, 489–493.

Diamond, M. C. (1991). Hormonal effects on the development of cerebral lateralization. *Psychoneuroendocrinology*, 16, 121–129.

Dick, C. L., Bland, R. C., and Newman, S. C. (1994). Epidemiology of psychiatric disorders in Edmonton. Panic disorder. *Acta Psychiatr Scand*, 376, 45–53.

Dills, W. L., Jr. (1993). Nutritional and physiological consequences of tumour glycolysis. *Parasitology*, 107, S177–S186.

DiLorenzo, T. A., Jacobsen, P. B., Bovbjerg, D. H., et al. (1995). Sources of anticipatory emotional distress in women receiving chemotherapy for breast cancer. *Ann Oncol*, 6, 705–711.

Dimsdale, J. E. (1993). Coronary heart disease in women: Personality and stress-induced biological responses. *Ann Behav Med*, 15, 119–123.

DiPaolo, T., Poyet, P., and Labrie, F. (1981). Effect of chronic estradiol and haloperidol treatment on striatal dopamine receptors. *Eur J Pharmacol*, 73, 105–106.

Ditkoff, E. C., Crary, W. G., Cristo, M., and Lobo, R. A. (1991). Estrogen improves psychological function in asymptomatic postmenopausal women. *Obstet Gynecol*, 78, 991–995.

Divoll, M., Greenblatt, D., Harmatz, J., and Shader, R. (1981). Effect of age and gender on disposition of temazepam. *J Pharm Sci*, 70, 1104–1107.

Dobbin, J. P., Harth, M., McCain, G. A., et al. (1991). Cytokine production and lymphocyte transformation during stress. *Brain Behav Immun*, 5, 339–348.

Doering, P., and Stewart, R. (1978). The extent and character of drug consumption during pregnancy. *JAMA*, 239, 843–846.

Doerr, P., Fichter, M., and Pirke, K. (1980). Relationship between weight gain and hypothalamic pituitary adrenal function in patients with anorexia nervosa. *J Steroid Biochem*, 13, 529–537.

Domecq, C., Naranjo, C., Ruiz, I., and Busto, U. (1980). Sex-related variations in the frequency and characteristics of adverse drug reactions. *Int J Clin Pharm Ther Toxicol*, 18, 362–366.

Doraiswamy, P. M., Krishnan, K. R., Figiel, G. S., et al. (1990). A brain magnetic resonance imaging study of pituitary gland morphology in anorexia nervosa and bulimia. *Biol Psychiatry*, 28, 110–116.

Doraiwswamy, P. M., Potts, J. M., Axelson, D. A., et al. (1992). MR assessment of pituitary gland morphology in healthy volunteers: Age- and gender-related differences. *Am J Neuroradiol*, 13, 1295–1299.

Dorce, V. A., Palermo-Neto, J. (1992). Lithium effects on estrogen-induced dopaminergic supersensitivity in rats. *Brain Res Bull*, 29, 239–241.

Dorian, B., Garfinkel, P., Brown, G., et al. (1982). Aberrations in lymphocyte subpopulations and function during psychological stress. *Clin Exp Immunol*, 50, 132–138.

Dowlatshahi, D., and Paykel, E. S. (1990). Life events and social stress in puerperal psychoses: Absence of effect. *Psychol Med*, 20, 655–662.

Dratman, M. B., and Crutchfield, F. L. (1978). Synaptosomal [^{125}I]triiodothyronine after intravenous [^{125}I]thyroxine. *Am J Physiol*, 235(6): E638–E647.

Dratman, M. B., Crutchfield, F. L., Axelrod, J., Colburn, R. W., and Nguyen, T. (1976). Localisation of triiodothyronine in nerve ending fractions of rat brain. *Proc Natl Acad Sci USA*, 73, 941–944.

Dratman, M. B., Crutchfield, F. L., Gordon, J. T., and Jennings, A. S. (1983). Iodothyronine homeostasis in rat brain during hypo- and hyperthyroidism. *Am J Physiol*, 245, E185–E193.

Dratman, M. B., Futaesaku, Y., Crutchfield, F. L., et al. (1982). Iodine-125-labeled triiodothyronine in rat brain: Evidence for localization in discrete neural systems. *Science*, 215, 309–312.

Dravet, C., Julian, C., Legros, C., et al. (1992). Epilepsy, antiepileptic drugs and malformations in children of women with epilepsy: A French prospective cohort study. *Neurology*, 42, 75–82.

Driesen, N. R., and Raz, N. (1995). The influence of sex, age, and handedness on corpus callosum morphology: A meta-analysis. *Psychobiology*, 23, 240–247.

Drife, J. (1986). Breast development in puberty. *Ann N Y Acad Sci*, 464, 58–65.

Drucker, D., and McLaughlin, J. (1986). Adrenocortical dysfunction in acute medical illness. *Crit Care Med*, 14, 789–791.

Dunn, T., Ludwig, E., Slaughter, R., Camara, D., and Jusko, W. (1991). Pharmacokinetics and pharmacodynamics of methylprednisolone in obesity. *Clin Pharmacol Ther*, 49, 536–549.

Dunner, D. L., and Fieve, R. R. (1974). Clinical factors in lithium prophylaxis failure. *Arch Gen Psychiatry*, 30, 229–233.

Dworkin, R., and Adams, G. (1984). Pharmacotherapy of the chronic patient: Gender and diagnostic factors. *Community Men Health J*, 20, 253–261.

Eaker, E., Chesebro, J. H., Sacks, F. M., Wenger, N. K., Whisnant, J. P., and Winston, M. (1993). Special report: Cardiovascular disease in women. *Circulation*, 88, 1999–2209.

Eaker, E. D., Packard, B., and Thom, T. J. (1989). Epidemiology and risk factors for coronary heart disease in women. *Cardiovasc Clin*, 19, 129–145.

Eaker, E. D., Pinksy, J., and Castelli, W. P. (1992). Myocardial infarction and coronary death among women: Psychosocial predictors from a 20-year follow-up of women in the Framingham Study. *Am J Epidemiol*, 135, 854–864.

Earle, B. V. (1979). Thyroid hormone and tricyclic antidepressants in resistant depressions. *Am J Psychiatry*, 126, 1667–1669.

Early Breast Cancer Trialists' Collaborative Group. (1992). Systemic treatment of early breast cancer by hormonal, cytotoxic, or immune therapy. *Lancet*, 339, 1–15, 71–85.

Easton, D. F., Bishop, D. T., Ford, D., Crockford, G. P., and the Breast Cancer Linkage Consortium. (1993). Genetic linkage analysis in familial breast and ovarian cancer: Results from 214 families. *Am J Hum Genet*, 52, 678–701.

Eckert, E., Halmi, K., Marchi, P., Grove, W., and Crosby, R. (1995). Ten-year follow-up of anorexia nervosa: Clinical course and outcome. *Psychol Med*, 25, 143–156.

Edgar, L., Rosberger, Z., and Nowlis, D. (1992). Coping with cancer during the first year after diagnosis. *Cancer*, 69, 817–828.

Edlund, M., and Craig, T. (1984). Antipsychotic drug use and birth defects: An epidemiologic reassessment. *Compr Psychiatry*, 25, 32–37.

Edmonds, L., and Oakley, G. (1990). Ebstein's anomaly and maternal lithium exposure during pregnancy. *Teratology*, 41, 551–552.

Elks, M. L. (1993). Open trial of fluoxetine therapy for premenstrual syndrome. *South Med J*, 86, 503–507.

Ell, K., Nishimoto, R., Mediansky, L., et al. (1992). Social relations, social support and survival among patients with cancer. *J Psychosom Res*, 36, 531–541.

Ellinwood, E. J., Easler, M., Linnoila, M., et al. (1984). Effects of oral contraceptives on diazepam-induced psychomotor impairment. *Clin Pharmacol Ther*, 35, 360–366.

Elliott, B., and Huppert, F. (1991). In sickness and in health: Associations between physical and mental well-being, employment and parental status in a British nationwide sample of married women. *Psychol Med*, 21, 515–524.

Ellman, R., and Thomas, B. A. (1995). Is psychological well-being impaired in long-term survivors of breast cancer? *J Med Screening*, 2, 5–9.

Elster, A. D., Chen, M. Y. M., Williams, D. W., and Key, L. L. (1990). Pituitary gland: MR imaging of physiologic hypertrophy in adolescence. *Radiology*, 174, 681–685.

Elster, A. D., Sanders, T. G., Vines, F. S., and Chen, M. Y. M. (1991). Size and shape of the pituitary gland during pregnancy and post partum: Measurement with MR imaging. *Radiology*, 181, 531–535.

Emerson, C. H. (1991). Thyroid disease during and after pregnancy. In L. E. Braverman and R. D. Utiger (Eds.), *The thyroid*, (pp. 1263–1279). Philadelphia: J. B. Lippincott.

Endicott, J. (1993). The menstrual cycle and mood disorders. *J Affect Disord*, 29, 193–200.

Endicott, J., and Halbreich, U. (1982). Retrospective reports of premenstrual depressive symptoms: Factors affecting confirmation in daily ratings. *Psychopharmacol Bull*, 18, 109–112.

Erikson, E. (1963). *Childhood and society*, 2nd ed. New York: Norton.

Eriksson, E., Hedberg, M. A., Andersch, B., and Sunblad, C. (1995). The serotonin reuptake inhibitor paroxetine is superior to the noradrenergic reuptake inhibitor maprotiline in the treatment of premenstrual syndrome. *Neuropsychopharmacology*, 12, 167–176.

Eriksson, E., Lisjo, P., Sunblad, G., et al. (1990). Effects of clomipramine on premenstrual syndrome. *Acta Psychiatr Scand*, 81, 87–88.

Ernst, C., and Angst, J. (1992). The Zurich Study. XII. Sex differences in depression. Evidence from longitudinal epidemiological data. *Eur Arch Psychiatry and Clin Neurosci*, 241, 222–230.

Eskay, R. L., Grino, M., and Chen, H. T. (1990). Interleukins, signal transduction, and the immune system-mediated stress response. In J. C. Porter and D. Jezova (Eds.), *Circulating regulatory factors and neuroendocrine function* (pp. 331–343). New York: Plenum Press.

Etgen, A., and Karkanias, G. B. (1994). Estrogen regulation of noradrenergic signaling in the hypothalamus. *Psychoneuroendocrinology*, 19, 603–610.

Ettinger, B., Genant, H., and Cann, C. (1985). Long-term estrogen replacement therapy prevents bone loss and fractures. *Ann Intern Med*, 102, 319–324.

Evans, D. L., and Nemeroff, C. B. (1983a). The dexamethasone suppression test in mixed bipolar disorder. *Am J Psychiatry*, 140, 615–617.

Evans, D. L., and Nemeroff, C. B. (1983b). Use of dexamethasone suppression test using DSM III criteria on an inpatient psychiatric unit. *Biol Psychiatry*, 18, 505–511.

Ewart, C. K., and Kolodner, K. B. (1994). Negative affect, gender, and expressive style predict elevated ambulatory blood pressure in adolescents. *J Pers Soc Psychol*, 66(3), 596–605.

Eysenck, H. J. (1988). Personality, stress and cancer: Prediction and prophylaxis. *Br J Med Psychol*, 61, 57–75.

Fairburn, C., Marcus, M., and Wilson, G. T. (1993). Cognitive-behavioral therapy for binge eating and bulimia nervosa: A comprehensive treatment manual. In C. Fairburn and G. Wilson (Eds.), *Binge eating. Nature, assessment, and treatment* (pp. 361–419). New York: Guilford Press.

Fairburn, C., Norman, P., Welch, S. G., et al. (1995). A prospective study of outcome in bulimia nervosa and long-term effects of three psychological treatments. *Arch Gen Psychiatry*, 52, 304–312.

Fairburn, C., and Wilson, G. (Eds.). (1993). *Binge eating. Nature, assessment, and treatment*. New York: Guilford Press.

Faisal, M., Chiappelli, F., Ahmed. I. I., et al. (1989). Social confrontation "stress" in aggressive fish is associated with an endogenous opioid-mediated suppression of proliferative response to mitogens and nonspecific cytotoxicity. *Brain Behav Immun*, 3, 223–233.

Fallowfield, L., Hall, A., Maguire, G., and Baum, M. (1991). Psychological outcomes of different treatment policies in women with early breast cancer outside a clinical trial. *Br Med J*, 301, 575–580.

Farnham, A. M. (1887). Uterine disease as a factor in the production of insanity. *Alienist Neurologist*, 8, 532–547. Quoted in Schmidt, P. J., and Rubinow, D. R. 1991. Menopause-related affective disorders: A justification for further study. *Am J Psychiatry*, 148, 849.

Fava, G. A., Sonino, N., and Murphy, M. A. (1987). Major depression associated with endocrine disease. *Psychiatr Dev*, 5, 321–348.

Fawzy, F. I., Fawzy, N. W., Hyun, C. S., et al. (1993). Malignant melanoma: Effects of an early structured psychiatric intervention, coping, and affective state on recurrence and survival six years later. *Arch Gen Psychiatry*, 50, 681–689.

Fawzy, F. I., Kemeny, M. E., Fawzy, N. W., et al. (1990a). A structured psychiatric intervention for cancer patients: Changes over time in immunological measures. *Arch Gen Psychiatry*, 47, 720–725.

Fawzy, F. I., Kemeny, M. E., Fawzy, N. W., et al. (1990b). A structured psychiatric intervention for cancer patients II: Changes over time in immunological measures. *Arch Gen Psychiatry*, 47, 729–735.

Feighner, J. P., King, L. J., Schuckit, M. A., Croughan, J., and Briscoe, W. (1972). Hormonal potentiation of imipramine and ECT in primary depression. *Am J Psychiatry*, 128, 1230–1238.

Felton, B. J., Revenson, R. A., and Hintrichsen, G. A. (1984). Stress and coping in the explanation of psychological adjustment among chronically ill adults. *Soc Sci Med*, 18, 889–898.

Ferin, M., and Vande-Wiele, R. (1987). Endogenous opioid peptides and the control of the menstrual cycle. *Eur J Obstet Gynecol Reprod Biol*, 18, 365–373.

Ferrari, G. (1973). On some biological aspects of affective disorders. *Riv Sper Freniar Med Leg Aliazioni Ment*, 93, 1167–1175.

Ferrari, E., Foppa, S., Bossolo, P., et al. (1989). Melatonin and pituitary-gonadal function in disorders of eating behavior. *J Pineal Res*, 7, 115–124.

Ferrari, E., Fraschini, F., and Brambilla, F. (1990). Hormonal circadian rhythms in eating disorders. *Biol Psychiatry*, 27, 1007–1020.

Feski, A., Harris, B., Walker, R. F., Riad-Fahmy, D., and Newcombe, R. G. (1984). "Baby blues" and hormone levels in saliva. *J Affect Disord*, 6, 351–355

Fetting, J. H., Stefanek, M. E., Sheidler, V. R., et al. (1992). Noradrenergic activity in anticipatory nausea. *Psychosom Med*, 54, 641–647.

Fichter, M., and Pirke, K. (1984). Hypothalamic pituitary function in starving healthy subjects. In K. Pirke and D. Ploog (Eds.), *The psychobiology of anorexia nervosa* (pp. 124–135). Berlin/Heidelberg: Springer-Verlag.

Fielding, R. (1991). Depression and acute myocardial infarction: A review and reinterpretation. *Soc Sci Med*, 32, 1017–1027.

Fields, J., and Gordon, J. (1982). Estrogen inhibits the dopaminergic supersensitivity induced by neuroleptics. *Life Sci*, 30, 229–234.

Fillet, H., Weinreb, H., Cholst, I., et al. (1986). Observations in a preliminary open trial of estrogen therapy for senile dementia – Alzheimer's type. *Psychoneuroendocrinology*, 11, 332–345.

Fisher, D. A. (1986). Thyroid physiology in the perinatal period and during childhood.

In S. H. Ingbar and L. E. Braverman (Eds.), *The thyroid* (pp. 1387–1395). Philadelphia: J. B. Lippincott.

Fogel, R. (1993). New sources and new techniques for the study of secular trends in nutritional status, health, mortality and the process of aging. *Hist Meth*, 26, 5–43.

Folkman, J., Langer, R., Linhardt, R., et al. (1983). Angiogenesis inhibition and tumor regression caused by heparin or a heparin fragment in the presence of cortisone. *Science*, 221, 719–725.

Fong, Y., Moldawer, L. L., Shires, G. T., and Lowry, S. F. (1990). The biologic characteristics of cytokines and their implication in surgical injury. *Surg Gynecol Obstet*, 170, 363–378.

Ford, L. G., and Johnson, K. A. (In press). Tamoxifen Breast Cancer Prevention Trial – an update. In *Progress in clinical biological research*. New York: Wiley-Liss.

Ford, O., Easton, D. F., Bishop, D. T., Narod, S. A., Goidgar, D. E., and the Breast Cancer Linkage Consortium. (1994). Risks of cancer in BrCA1 – mutation carriers. *Lancet*, 343, 692–695.

Forsen, A. (1991). Psychosocial stress as a risk for breast cancer. *Psychother Psychosom*, 55, 176–185.

Fox B. H. (1989). Depressive symptoms and risk of cancer. *JAMA*, 262, 1231.

France, D., Urban, B., Krishnan, K. R. R., et al. (1988). CSF corticotropin-releasing factor-like immunoreactivity in chronic pain patients with and without major depression. *Biol Psychiatry*, 23, 86–88.

Fraser, S. C., Dobbs, H. J., Ebbs, S. R., et al. (1993). Combination or mild single agent chemotherapy for advanced breast cancer? CMF vs. epirubicin measuring quality of life. *Br J Cancer*, 67, 402–406.

Frasure-Smith, N., Lesperance, F., and Talajic, M. (1993). Depression following myocardial infarction. *JAMA*, 270, 1819–1825.

Frasure-Smith, N., Lesperance, F., and Talajic, M. (1995). The impact of negative emotions on prognosis following myocardial infarction: Is it more than depression? *Health Psychol*, 5, 388–398.

Freeman, E. W., Rickels, K., Sondheimer, S. J., et al. (1994). Nefazodone in the treatment of premenstrual syndrome: A preliminary study. *J Clin Psychopharmacol*, 14, 180–186.

Freeman, E. W., Rickels, K., Sondheimer, S. J., et al. (1995). A double blind trial of oral progesterone, alprazolam, and placebo in treatment of severe premenstrual syndrome. *JAMA*, 274, 51–57.

Freud, S. (1914 [1957]). *On narcissism: An introduction*, standard ed., vol. 14 (p. 73). London: Hogarth Press.

Frezza, L., di Padora, C., Pozzato, G., et al. (1990). High blood alcohol levels in women: The role of decreased gastric alcohol dehydrogenase activity and first pass metabolism. *N Engl J Med*, 322, 95–99.

Fried, P. (1993). Prenatal exposure to tobacco and marijuana: Effects during pregnancy, infancy, and early childhood. *Clin Obstet Gynecol*, 36, 319–337.

Friedman, G. D. (1994). Psychiatrically-diagnosed depression and subsequent cancer. *Cancer Epidemiol Biomarkers Prevention*, 3, 11–13.

Friedman, H. S., and Booth-Kewley, S. (1987). Personality, Type A behavior, and coronary heart disease: The role of emotional expression. *J Pers Soc Psychol*, 53, 783–792.

Friedman, H. S., Tucker, J. S., Tomlinson-Keasy, C., et al. (1993). Does childhood personality predict longevity? *J Pers Soc Psychol*, 65, 176–185.

Friedman, M., and Rosenman, R. H. (1959). Association of specific overt behavior pattern with blood and cardiovascular findings; blood cholesterol, blood clotting time, incidence of arcus senilis, and coronary artery disease. *JAMA*, 169, 1286–1296

Frisch, R. (1985). Fatness, menarche, and female fertility. *Perspect Biol Med*, 28, 611–633.

Frisch, R., and McArthur, J. (1974). Menstrual cycles: Fatness as a determinant of minimum weight for height necessary for their maintenance or onset. *Science*, 185, 949–951.

Fruchart J. C., Ailhaud, G., and Bard, J. M. (1993). Heterogeneity of high density lipoprotein particles. *Circulation*, 87 (Suppl 4): III22–III27

Fullerton, D., Swift, W., and Getto, C. (1986). Plasma immunoreactive beta-endorphin in bulimics. *Psychol Med*, 16, 59–63.

Gallion, H. H., and Bast, B. C., Jr. (1993). National Cancer Institute Conference on Investigational Strategies for Detection and Intervention in Early Ovarian Cancer. *Cancer Res*, 53, 3839–3842.

Gambert, S. R. (1991). Factors that control thyroid function: Environmental effects and physiologic variables. In L. E. Braverman and R. D. Utiger (Eds.), *The thyroid gland* (pp. 347–357). Philadelphia: J. B. Lippincott.

Ganz, P. A., Day, R., Ware, J. E., Jr., et al. (1995). Base-line quality-of-life assessment in the National Surgical Adjuvant Breast and Bowel Project Breast Cancer Prevention Trial. *J Natl Cancer Inst*, 87, 1372–1382.

Garbutt, J. C., Mayo, J. P., Jr., Gillette, G. M., Little, K. Y., and Mason, G. A. (1986). Lithium potentiation of tricyclic antidepressants following lack of T$_3$ potentiation. *Am J Psychiatry*, 143, 1038–1039.

Garfinkel, P., and Garner, D. (1982). *Anorexia nervosa: A multidimensional perspective.* New York: Brunner/Mazel.

Gargiulo, J., Brooks-Gunn, J., Attie, I., and Warren, M. (1987). Girls' dating behavior as a function of social context and maturation. *Dev Psychol*, 23, 730–737.

Garland, M., Morris, J. S., Stampfer, M. J., et al. (1995). Prospective study of toenail selenium levels and cancer among women. *J Natl Cancer Inst*, 87, 497–505.

Garn, S., LaVelle, M., Rosenberg, K., and Hawthorne, V. (1986). Maturational timing as a factor in female fatness and obesity. *Am J Clin Nutr*, 43, 879–883.

Garner, D. M., Olmstedt, M. P., Bohr, Y., and Garfinkel, P. E. (1982). The Eating Attitudes Test: Psychometric features and clinical correlates. *Psychol Med*, 12, 871–878.

Garvey, M. J., Tuason, V. B., Lumry, A. E., et al. (1983). Occurrence of depression in the postpartum state. *J Affect Disord*, 5, 97–101.

Gelber, R. D., Cole, B. F., Goldhirsch, A., et al. (1996). Adjuvant chemotherapy plus tamoxifen compared with tamoxifen alone for postmenopausal breast cancer: Meta-analysis of quality-adjusted survival. *Lancet*, 347, 1066–1071.

Gelenberg, A., Cooper, D., Doller, J., and Maloof, F. (1977). Galactorrhea and hyperprolactinemia associated with amoxapine therapy: Report of a case. *JAMA*, 242, 1900–1901.

Gellert, G. A., Maxwell, R. M., and Siegel, B. S. (1993). Survival of breast cancer patients receiving adjunctive psychosocial support therapy: A 10-year follow-up study. *J Clin Oncol*, 11, 66–69.

Genant, H. K., Christopher, C. E., Ettinger, B., and Gordan, G. S. (1982). Quantitative computed tomography of vertebral spongiosa: A sensitive method for detecting early bone loss after oophorectomy. *Ann Inter Med*, 97, 699–705.

George, D. T., Ladenheim, J. A., and Nutt, D. J. (1987). Effect of pregnancy on panic attacks. *Am J Psychol*, 144, 1078–1079.

Gerin, W., Milner, D., Chawla, S., and Pickering, T. G. (1995). Social support as a moderator of cardiovascular reactivity in women: A test of the direct effects and buffering hypotheses. *Psychosom Med*, 57, 16–22.

German, J., Simpson, J., Chaganti, R., et al. (1978). Genetically determined sex-reversal in 46, XY humans. *Science*, 202, 53–56.

Gerner, R., and Gwirtsman, H. (1981). Abnormalities of dexamethasone suppression test and urinary MHPG in anorexia nervosa. *Am J Psychiatry*, 138, 650–653.

Gewirtz, G. R., Malaspina, D., Hatterer, J. A., et al. (1988). Occult thyroid dysfunction in patients with refractory depression. *Am J Psychiatry*, 145, 1012–1014.

Geyer, S. (1992). Life events prior to manifestation of breast cancer: A limited prospective study covering eight years before diagnosis. *J Psychosom Res*, 35, 355–363.

Giani, C., Fierabracci, P., Bonacci, R., et al. (1996). Relationship between breast cancer and thyroid disease: Relevance of autoimmnune thyroid disorders in breast malignancy. *J Clin Endocrinol Metab*, 81, 990–994.

Gibbons, J. L., Gibson, J. G., and Maxwell, A. E. (1960). An endocrine study of depressive illness. *J Psychosom Res*, 5, 32–41.

Gibbons, J. L., and McHugh, P. R., (1962). Plasma cortisol in depressive illness. *J Psychiatr Res*, 1, 162–171.

Gillberg, I., Rastam, M., and Gillberg, C. (1994). Anorexia nervosa outcome: Six-year controlled longitudinal study of 51 cases including a population cohort. *J Am Acad Child Adolesc Psychiatry*, 33, 729–739.

Gilligan, D. M., Badar, D. M., Panza, J. A., Quyyumi, A. A., and Cannon R. O. (1994). Acute vascular effects of estrogen in postmenopausal women. *Circulation*, 90, 786–791.

Gilligan, D. M., Badar, D. M., Panza, J. A., Quyyumi, A. A., and Cannon R. O. (1995). Effects of estrogen replacement therapy on peripheral vasomotor function in postmenopausal women. *Am J Cardiol*, 75, 264–268.

Gilmore, D., Gal, J., Gerber, J., and Nies, A. (1992). Age and gender influence the stereoselective pharmacokinetics of propranolol. *J Pharmacol Exp Ther*, 261, 1181–1186.

Gilmore, D. H., Hawthorn, R. J., and Hart, D. M. (1985). Danazol for premenstrual syndrome: A preliminary report of a placebo-controlled double-blind study. *J Int Med Res*, 13, 129–130.

Giovannucci, E., Egan, K. M., Hunter, D. J., et al. (1995). Aspirin and the risk of colorectal cancer in women. *N Engl J Med*, 333, 609–614.

Girdler, S. S., Turner, J. R., Sherwood, A., and Light, K. C. (1990). Gender differences in blood pressure control during a variety of behavioral stressors. *Psychosom Med*, 52, 571–591.

Gitlin, M. J., Weiner, H., Fairbanks, L., Hershman, J. M., and Friedfeld, N. (1987). Failure of T_3 to potentiate tricyclic antidepressant response. *J Affect Disord*, 13, 267–272.

Giudicelli, J., and Tillement, J. (1977). Influence of sex on drug kinetics in man. *Clin Pharmacokinet*, 2, 157–166.

Gjerde, P. F., and Block, J. (1991). Preadolescent antecedents of depressive symptomatology at age 18: A prospective study. *J Youth Adolesc*, 20, 217–232.

Gjerris, A., Hammer, M., Vendsborg, P., Christensen, N. J., and Rafaelsen, O. J. (1985). Cerebrospinal fluid vasopressin – changes in depression. *Brit J Psychiatry*, 147, 696–701.

Glaser, R., Pearl, D. K., Kiecolt-Glaser, J. K., and Malarkey, W. B. (1994). Plasma cortisol levels and reactivation of latent Epstein-Barr virus in response to examination stress. *Psychoneuroendocrinology*, 19, 765–772.

Glaser, R., Rice, J., Speicher, C. E., et al. (1986). Stress depressed interferon production and natural killer cell activity in humans. *Behav Neurosci*, 100, 675–678.

Glickman, S., Frank, L., Licht, P., et al. (1992). Sexual differentiation of the female spotted hyena. One of nature's experiments. *Ann NY Acad Sci*, 662, 135–159.

Glover, V. (1992). Do biochemical factors play a part in postnatal depression? *Prog Neuropsychopharmacol Behav Psychiatry*, 16, 605–615.

Glover, V., Liddle, P., Taylor, A., Adams, D., and Sandler, M. (1994). Mild hypomania (the highs) can be a feature of the first postpartum week. Association with later depression. *Br J Psychiatry*, 164, 517–521.

Godwin, C. D., Greenberg, L. B., and Shukla, S. (1984). Predictive value of the dexamethasone suppression test in mania. *Am J Psychiatry*, 141, 1610–1612.

Gold, J. H., Severino, S. K. (1994). Premenstrual dysphorias: Myths and realities. Washington, DC: American Psychiatric Association Press.

Gold, M. S., Pottash, A. L. C., and Extein, I. (1981). Hypothyroidism and depression. *JAMA*, 245, 1919–1922.

Gold, M. S., Pottash, A. L. C., and Extein, I. (1982). "Symptomless" autoimmune thyroiditis in depression. *Psychiatr Res*, 6, 261–269.

Gold, P., Gwirtsman, H., and Avgerinos, P. (1986). Abnormal hypothalamic-pituitary-adrenal function in anorexia nervosa: Patholophysiologic mechanisms in underweight and weight-corrected patients. *N Engl J Med*, 314, 1335–1342.

Gold, P., Kaye, W., Robertson, G., and Ebert, M. (1983). Abnormalities in plasma and cerebrospinal-fluid arginine vasopressin in patients with anorexia nervosa. *N Engl J Med*, 308, 1117–1123.

Gold, P. W., Chrousos, G. P., Kellner, C., et al. (1984). Psychiatric implications of basic and clinical studies with corticotropin-releasing factor. *Am J Psychiatry*, 141, 619–627.

Gold, P. W., Goodwin, F. K., Wehr, T., and Rebar, R. (1977). Pituitary thyrotropin response to thyrotropin-releasing hormone in affective illness: Relationship to spinal fluid amine metabolities. *Am J Psychiatry*, 134, 1028–1031.

Gold, P. W., Loriaux, D. L., Roy, A., et al. (1986). Responses to corticotropin-releasing hormone in the hypercortisolism of depression and Cushing's disease. *N Engl J Med*, 314, 1329–1334.

Goldberg, J. A., Scott, R. N., Davidson, P. M., et al. (1992). Psychological morbidity in the first year after breast surgery. *Eur J Surg Oncol*, 18, 327–331.

Goldin, B., Adlercruety, H., Gorbach, S., et al. (1982). Estrogen excretion patterns and plasma levels in vegetarian and omnivorous women. *N Engl J Med*, 307, 1542–1547.

Golding, J. M., Rost, K., Kashner, T. M., and Smith, G. R. J. (1992). Family psychiatric history of patients with somatization disorder. *Psychiatr Med*, 10, 33–47.

Golding, J. M., Smith, S., and Kashner, F. M. (1991). Does somatization disorder occur in men? *Arch Gen Psychiatry*, 48, 231–235.

Goldstein, J., VanCauter, E., Linkowski, P., Vanhaelst, L., and Mendlewicz, J. (1980). Thyrotropin nycthohemeral pattern in primary depression: Differences between unipolar and bipolar women. *Life Sci*, 27, 1695–1703.

Goldstein, J. M. (1995a). Gender and the familial transmission of schizophrenia. In M. V. Seeman (Ed.), *Gender and psychopathology* (pp. 201–226). Washington, DC: American Psychiatric Association Press.

Goldstein, J. M. (1995b). The impact of gender on understanding the epidemiology of schizophrenia. In M. V. Seeman (Ed.), *Gender and psychopathology* (pp. 159–199). Washington, DC: American Psychiatric Association Press.

Gomberg, E. S. L. (1993a). Gender issues. In M. Galanter (Ed.), *Recent developments in alcoholism*, vol. II: *Ten years of progress* (pp. 95–107). New York: Plenum Press.

Gomberg, E. S. L. (1993b). Women and alcohol: Use and abuse. *J Nerv Ment Dis*, 181, 211–219.

Gomberg, E. S. L. (1994). Risk factors for drinking over a woman's life span. *Alcohol Health Res World*, 18, 220–227.

Goodwin, F. K., Prange, A. J. J., Post, R. M., Muscettola, G., and Lipton, M. A. (1982). Potentiation of antidepressant effect by L-triiodothyronine in tricyclic nonresponders. *Am J Psychiatry*, 139, 34–38.

Goodwin, S. J., Searles, R. P., and Tunk, K. S. (1982). Immunological responses of a healthy elderly population. *Clin Exp Immunol*, 48, 403–410.

Gordon, D. J., Knoke, J., and Probstfield, J. L. (1986). High-density lipoprotein cholesterol and coronary heart disease in hypercholesterolemic men: The Lipid Research Clinics Coronary Primary Prevention Trial. *Circulation*, 74, 1217–1225.

Gordon, T., Castelli, W. P., and Hjortland, M. C. (1977). Diabetes, blood lipids, and the role of obesity in CHD risk for women. The Framingham Study. *Ann Intern Med*, 87, 393–397.

Gorwood, P., Leboyer, M., Jay, M., Payan, C., and Feingold, J. (1995). Gender and age at onset in schizophrenia: Impact of family history. *Am J Psychiatry*, 152, 208–212.

Gould, E., Woolley, C. S., Frankfurt, M., and McEwen, B. S. (1990). Gonadal steroids regulate dendritic spine density in hippocampal pyramidal cells in adulthood. *J Neurosci*, 10, 1286–1291.

Grady, D., Rubin, S., Petitti, D. R., et al. (1992). Hormone therapy to prevent disease and prolong life in postmenopausal women. *Ann Intern Med*, 117, 1016–1037.

Graff-Low, K., Thoresen, C. E., Pattillo, J. R., King, A. C., and Jenkins, C. (1994). Anxiety, depression, and heart disease in women. *Int J Behav Med*, 1, 305–319.

Graham, P., and Rutter, M. (1973). Psychiatric disorder in the young adolescent: A follow-up study. *Proc R Soc Med*, 66, 1226–1229.

Green, D., and Krueger, R. (1963). Sex differences in drug effects. *Fed Proc*, 22, 543.

Green, L. A., and Ruffin, M. T. (1993). Differences in management of suspected myocardial infarction in men and women. *J Fam Prac*, 36, 389–393.

Greenberg, D. B., Sawicka, J., Eisenthal, S., and Rose, D. (1992). Fatigue syndrome due to localized radiation. *J Pain Symptom Management*, 7, 38–45.

Greenberg, E. R., Baron, J. A., Karagas, M. R., et al. (1996). Mortality associated with low plasma concentration of beta carotene and the effects of oral supplementation. *JAMA*, 275, 699–703.

Greenberg, P. E., Stiglin, L. E., Finkelstein, S. N., and Berndt, E. R. (1993). Depression: A neglected major illness. *J Clin Psychiatry*, 54, 419–424.

Greenblatt, D., Allen, M., Harmatz, J., and Shader, R. (1980). Diazepam disposition determinants. *Clin Pharmacol Ther*, 27, 301–312.

Greenblatt, D., Divoll, M., Abernethy, D., and Harmatz, J. (1982). Antipyrine kinetics in the elderly: Prediction of age-related changes on benzodiazepine oxidising capacity. *J Pharmacol Exp Ther*, 220, 120–126.

Greenblatt, D., Divoll, M., Abernethy, D., et al. (1989). Age and gender effects on chlordiazepoxide kinetics: Relation to antipyrine disposition. *Pharmacology*, 38, 327–334.

Greenwald, P., Kelloff, G., Burch-Whitman, C., and Kramer, B. S. (1995). Chemoprevention. *CA Cancer J Clin*, 45, 31–49.

Greer, S. (1991). Psychological response to cancer and survival. *Psychol Med*, 21, 43–49.

Greer, S., Moorey, S., Baruch, J. D. R., et al. (1992). Adjuvant psychological therapy for patients with cancer: A prospective randomized trial. *Br Med J*, 304, 675–680.

Gregoire, A. S., Kumar, R., Everett, B., Henderson, A., and Studd, J. W. (1996). Transdermal estrogen treatment of severe postpartum depression. *Lancet*, 347, 930–933.

Grossman, M., Kirsner, J., and Gillespie, I. (1963). Basal and histalog-stimulated gastric secretion in control subjects and in patients with peptic ulcer or gastric cancer. *Gastroenterology*, 45, 14–26.

Grover, S., Quinn, M. A., and Weideman, P. (1993). Patterns of inheritance of ovarian cancer. An analysis from an ovarian cancer screening program. *Cancer*, 72, 528–530.

Gruber, B. L., Hersh. S. P., Hall, N. R., et al. (1993). Immunological responses of breast cancer patients to behavioral interventions. *Biofeedback Self Regul*, 18, 1–22.

Grumbach, M., and Kaplan, S. (1990). The neuroendocrinology of human puberty: An ontogenetic perspective. In M. Grumbach, P. Sizonenko, and M. Albert (Eds.), *Control of the onset of puberty* (pp. 1–68). Baltimore: Williams & Wilkins.

Guidelines, A. P. A. P. (1993). Practice guidelines for eating disorders. *Am J Psychiatry*, 150, 208–228.

Gull, W. (1873 [1964]). Anorexia nervosa (apepsia hysterica, anorexia hysterica). In M. Kaufman and M. Heiman (Eds.), *Evolution of psychosomatic concepts* (pp. 132–188). New York: International Universities Press.

Gull, W. W. (1873). On a cretinoid state supervening in adult life in women. *Tran Clin Soc Lond*, 7, 180–185.

Gunnarskog, J., and Kallan, A. (1993). Drug intoxication during pregnancy: A study with central registries. *Reprod Toxicol*, 7, 117–121.

Gur, R. C., Gur, R. E., Obrist, W. D., et al. (1982). Sex and handedness differences in cerebral blood flow during rest and cognitive activity. *Science*, 217, 659–661.

Gur, R. C., Mozley, L. H., Mozley, D., et al. (1995). Sex differences in regional cerebral glucose metabolism during a resting state. *Science*, 267, 528–531.

Hackman, B. W., and Gallbraith, D. (1977). Six months' study of estrogen therapy with piperazine oestrone sulphate and its effects on memory. *Curr Med Res Opin*, 4, 21–27.

Häfner, H., Behrens, S., Devry, J., and Gattaz, W. F. (1991). An animal model for the effects of estradiol on dopamine-mediated behavior–implications for sex differences in schizophrenia. *Psychiatry Res*, 38, 125–134.

Häfner, H., Riecher-Rossler, A., An Der Heiden, W., et al. (1993). Generating and testing a causal explanation of the gender difference in age at first onset of schizophrenia. *Psychol Med*, 23, 925–940.

Haggerty, J. J., Jr., Evans, D. L., Golden, R. N., et al. (1990). The presence of antithyroid antibodies in patients with affective and nonaffective psychiatric disorders. *Biol Psychiatry*, 27, 51–60.

Haggerty, J. J., Jr., Evans, D. L., and Prange, A. J., Jr. (1986). Organic brain syndrome associated with marginal hypothyroidism. *Am J Psychiatry*, 143, 785–786.

Haggerty, J. J., Jr., Garbutt, J. C., Evans, D. L., et al. (1990). Subclinical hypothyroidism: A review of neuropsychiatric aspects. *Int J Psychiatry Med*, 20, 193–208.

Haggerty, J. J., Jr., and Prange, A. J., Jr. (1995). Borderline hypothyroidism and depression. *Annu Rev Med*, 46, 37–46.

Haggerty, J. J., Jr., Simon, J. S., Evans, D. L., and Nemeroff, C. B. (1987). Relationship of serum TSH concentration and antithyroid antibodies to diagnosis and DST response in psychiatric inpatients. *Am J Psychiatry*, 144, 1491–1493.

Haggerty, J. J., Jr., Stern, R. A., Mason, G. A., et al. (1993). Subclinical hypothyroidism: A modifiable risk factor for depression? *Am J Psychiatry*, 150, 508–510.

Hahn, P. M., Van Vugt, D. A., and Reid, R. L. (1995). A randomized placebo-controlled cross over trial of danazol for treatment of premenstrual syndrome. *Psychoneuroendocrinology*, 20, 193–209.

Halbreich, U., Asnis, G. M., Zumoff, B., Nathan, R. S., and Shindledecker, R. (1984). Effect of age and sex on cortisol secretion in depressives and normals. *Psychiatry Res*, 13, 221–229.

Halbreich, U., Endicott, J., Goldstein, S., and Nee, J. (1986). Premenstrual changes and changes in gonadal hormones. *Acta Psychiatr Scand*, 34, 576–586.

Halbreich, U., and Lumley, L. A. (1993). The multiple interactional biological processes that might lead to depression and gender differences in its appearance. *J Affect Disord*, 29, 159–173.

Halbreich, U., Rojansky, N., Palter, S., et al. (1994). Estrogen augments serotonergic activity in postmenopausal women. *Biol Psychiatry*, 37, 434–441.

Halbreich, U., and Tworek, H. (1993). Altered serotonergic activity in women with dysphoric premenstrual syndromes. *Intl J Psychiatry Med*, 23, 1–27.

Hall, J. M., Lee, M. K., Morrow, J., et al. (1990). Linkage of early onset breast cancer to chromosome 17q21. *Science*, 250, 1684–1689.

Halmi, K., Eckert, E., Marchi, P., et al. (1991). Comorbidity of psychiatric diagnoses in anorexia nervosa. *Arch Gen Psychiatry*, 48, 712–718.

Hambrecht, M., Maurer, K., and Häfner, H. (1993). Evidence for a gender bias in epidemiological studies of schizophrenia. *Schizophr Res*, 8, 223–231.

Hamill, P., Drizd, T., Johnson, C., et al. (1979). Physical growth: National Center for Health Statistics percentiles. *Am J Clin Nutr*, 32, 607–629.

Hamilton, J. A. (1989). Postpartum psychiatric syndromes. *Psychiatr Clin North Am*, 12, 89–103.

Hammarback, S., and Backstrom, T. (1988). Induced anovulation as treatment of premenstrual tension syndrome: A double-blind cross over study with GnRH-agonist versus placebo. *Acta Obstet Gynecol Scand*, 67, 159–166.

Hammarback, S., Backstrom, T., Host, J., von Scoultz, B., and Lyreias, S. (1985). Cyclical mood changes as in PMS during sequential estrogen-progesterone replacement therapy. *Acta Obstet Gynecol Scand*, 64, 393–397.

Hammarback, S., Damber, J. F., and Backstrom, T. (1989). Relationship between symptom severity and hormone changes in women with premenstrual syndrome. *J Clin Endocrinol Metab*, 68, 125–130.

Hannah, P., Adams, D., Lee, A., Glover, V., and Sandler, M. (1992). Links between early postpartum mood and post-natal depression. *Br J Psychiatry*, 160, 777–780.

Hanson, J., Streissguth, A., and Smith, D. (1978). The effects of moderate alcohol consumption during pregnancy on fetal growth and morphogenesis. *J Pediatr*, 92, 457–460.

Harlap, S., and Shiono, P. (1980). Alcohol, smoking and incidence of spontaneous abortions in the first and second trimesters. *Lancet*, 2, 173–176.

Harris, B., John, S., Fung, H., et al. (1989). The hormonal environment of post-natal depression. *Br J Psychiatry*, 154, 660–667.

Harris, B., Lovett, L., Newcombe, R. G., et al. (1994). Maternity blues and major endocrine changes: Cardiff puerperal mood and hormone study II. *Br Med J*, 308, 949–953.

Harris, R., Benet, L., and Schwartz, J. (1995). Gender effects in pharmacokinetics and pharmacodynamics [Review]. *Drugs*, 50, 222–239.

Harrison, W. M., Endicott, J., and Nee, J. (1990). Treatment of premenstrual dysphoria with alprazolam: A controlled study. *Arch Gen Psychiatry*, 47, 270–275.

Harrison, W. M., Endicott, I. J., and Rabkin, J. G. (1984). Treatment of premenstrual dysphoric changes: Clinical outcome and methodological implications. *Psychopharmacol Bull*, 20, 118–122.

Hartz, A., Barboriak, P., and Wong, A. (1979). The association of obesity with infertility and related menstrual abnormalities in women. *Int J Obesity*, 3, 57–73.

Harvey, I., and McGrath, G. (1988). Psychiatric morbidity in spouses of women admitted to a mother and baby unit. *Br J Psychiatry*, 152, 506–510.

Haskell, W. L., Alderman, E. L., Fair, J. M., et al. (1994). Effects of intensive multiple risk factor reduction on coronary atherosclerosis and clinical cardiac events in men and women with coronary artery disease. *Circulation*, 89, 975–990.

Hatotani, N., Nomura, J., Yamaguchi, T., and Kitayama, J. (1974). Clinical and experimental studies of the pathogenesis of depression. *Psychoneuroendocrinology*, 2, 115–130.

Haukkamaa, M. (1986). Contraception by Norplant subdermal capsules is not reliable in epileptic patients on anticonvulsant treatment. *Contraception*, 33, 559–565.

Havlik, R. J., Vukasin, A. P., and Ariyan, S. (1992). The impact of stress on the clinical presentation of melanoma. *Plast Reconstruct Surg*, 90, 57–61.

Hawton, K., and Goldacre, M. (1982). Hospital admissions for adverse effects of medicinal agents (mainly self-poisoning) among adolescents in the Oxford region. *Br J Psychiatry*, 140, 118–123.

Haynes, S. G., and Feinleib, M. (1980). Women, work and coronary heart disease: Prospective findings from the Framingham Heart Study. *Am J Public Health*, 70, 133–141.

Haynes, S. G., Feinleib, M., Levine, S., Scotch, N., and Kannel, W. B. (1978). The relationship of psychosocial factors to coronary heart disease in the Framingham Study. *Am J Epidemiol*, 107, 384–402.

Heidrich, A., Schleyer, M., Springler, H., et al. (1994). Postpartum blues: Relationship between non-protein bound steroid hormones in plasma and postpartum mood changes. *J Affect Disord*, 30, 93–98.

Heinonen, O., Slone, D., and Shapiro, S. (1977). *Birth defects and drugs in pregnancy*. Littleton, MA: Publishing Services Group.

Heller, W. (1993). Gender differences in depression: Perspectives from neuropsychology. *J Affect Disord*, 29, 129–143.

Helmer, D. C., Ragland, D. R., and Syme, S. L. (1991). Hostility and coronary artery disease. *Am J Epidemiol*, 133, 112–122.

Helmers, K. F., Krantz, D. S., Howell, R. H., et al. (1993). Hostility and myocardial ischemia in coronary artery disease patients: Evaluation by gender and ischemic index. *Psychosom Med*, 55, 29–36.

Helsing, K. J., Szklo, M., and Comstock, G. W. (1981). Factors associated with mortality after widowhood. *Am J Public Health*, 71, 802–809.

Helvacioglu, A., Yeoman, R. R., Hazleton, J. M., and Aksel (1993). Premenstrual syndrome and related hormonal changes. Long-acting gonadotropin releasing hormone agonist treatment. *J Repro Med*, 38, 864–871.

Helzer, J. E., Burnam, A., and McEvoy, L. T. (1991). Alcohol abuse and dependence. In L. N. Robins and D. A. Regier (Eds.), *Psychiatric disorders in America: The epidemiological catchment area study* (pp. 51–115). New York: Free Press.

Henderson, V. M., Paganini-Hill, A., Emanuel, C. K., Dunn, M. E., and Buckwalter, J. G. (1994). Estrogen replacement therapy in older women. Comparisons between Alzheimer's cases and nondemented control subjects. *Arch Neurol*, 51, 896–900.

Hennekens, C. H., and Buring, J. E. (1994). Contributions of observational evidence and clinical trials in cancer prevention. *Cancer Suppl*, 74, 2625–2629.

Hennekens, C. H., Buring, J. E., and Peto, R. (1994). Antioxidant vitamins – benefits not yet proved. *N Engl J Med*, 330, 1080–1081.

Hennekens, C. H., Buring, J. E., and Sandercock, P. (1989). Aspirin and other antiplatelet agents in the secondary and primary prevention of cardiovascular disease. *Circulation*, 80, 749–756.

Hermus, A. R. M. M., Pieters, G. F. F. M., Pes, J., et al. (1984). Differential effects of ovine and human corticotropin-releasing factor in human subjects. *Clin Endocrinol*, 21, 589–595.

Heroux, J. A., Grigoriades, D. E., and DeSouza, E. B. (1991). Age-related diseases in corticotropin-releasing factor receptors in rat brain and anterior pituitary gland. *Brain Res*, 542, 155–158.

Herpertz-Dahlmann, B., Wewetzer, C., Hennighausen, K., and Remschmidt, H. (1996). Outcome, psychosocial functioning and prognostic factors in adolescent anorexia nervosa, as determined by prospective follow-up assessment. *J Youth Adolesc*, 25.

Heuser, I., Wark, H. J., Keul, J., and Holsboer, F. (1991). Altered pituitary-adrenocortical function in elderly endurance athletes. *J Clin Endocrinol Metab*, 73, 485–488.

Hill, S. Y. (1995a). Mental and physical health consequences of alcohol use in women. In M. Galanter (Ed.), *Recent developments in alcoholism*, vol. 12: *Women and alcoholism* (pp. 181–197). New York: Plenum Press.

Hill, S. Y. (1995b). Vulnerability to alcoholism in women. Genetic and cultural factors. In M. Galanter (Ed.), *Recent developments in alcoholism*, vol. 12: *Women and alcoholism* (pp. 9–28). New York: Plenum Press.

Hines, M. (1982). Prenatal gonadal hormones and sex differences in human behavior. *Psychol Bull*, 92, 56–80.

Hines, M., and Green, R. (1991). Human hormonal and neural correlates of sex-typed behaviors. In A. Tasman and S. M. Goldfinger (Eds.), *American Psychiatric Press review of psychiatry* (pp. 536–555). Washington, DC: American Psychiatric Press.

Hirsh, M., and Swartz, M. (1980). Drug therapy: Antiviral agents. *N Engl J Med*, 302, 903–907.

Ho, P., Triggs, E., Bourne, D., and Heazelwood, V. (1985). The effects of age and sex on the disposition of acetylsalicylic acid and its metabolites. *Br J Clin Pharmacol*, 19, 675–684.

Hobfoll, S. E., Ritter, C., Lavin, J., Hulsizer, M. R., and Cameron, L. P. (1995). Depression prevalence and incidence among inner city pregnant and postpartum women. *J Consult Clin Psychol*, 63, 445–453.

Hoeflich, G., Kasper, S., Danos, P., and Schmidt, R. (1992). Thyroid hormones, body temperature, and antidepressant therapy. *Biol Psychiatry*, 31, 859–862.

Hogbin, B., Jenkins, V. A., and Parkin, A. J. (1992). Remembering "bad news" consultations: An evaluation of tape-recorded consultations. *Psychooncology*, 1, 147–154.

Holland, J. C. (1989). Anxiety and cancer: The patient and the family. *J Clin Psychiatry*, 50 (Suppl.), 20–25.

Holmes, M. C., Catt, K. J., and Aguilera, G. (1987). Involvement of vasopressin in the down-regulation of pituitary corticotropin-releasing factor in human subjects. *Clin Endocrinol*, 21, 589–595.

Holsboer, F., Gerken, A., von Bardeleben, U., et al. (1985). Relationship between pituitary responses to human corticotropin-releasing factor and thyrotropin-releasing hormone in depressives and normal controls. *Eur J Pharmacol*, 110, 153–154.

Holsboer, F., Von Bardeleben, U., Gerken, A., and Muler, D. (1984). Blunted corticotropin and normal cortisol response to human corticotropin-releasing factor in depression (Letter). *N Engl J Med*, 311, 1127.

Honjo, H., Ogino, Y., Naitoh, K., Wabe, M., and Kitawaki, J. (1995). In vivo effects of estrone sulphate on the CNS – senile dementia (Alzheimer type). *J Steroid Biochem*, 34, 521–525.

Hooper, W., and Qing, M. (1990). The influence of age and gender on the stereoselective metabolism and pharmacokinetics of mephobarbital in humans. *Clin Pharmacol Ther*, 48, 633–640.

House, J. S., Landis, K. R., and Umberson, D. (1988). Social relationships and health. *Science*, 241, 540–544.

Houston, B. K., and Kelly, K. (1986). Type A behavior in housewives: Relation to work, marital adjustment, stress, tension, health, fear-of-failure and self-esteem. *J Psychosom Res*, 31(1), 55–61.

Hudson, J., Pope, H., and Jonas, J. (1983). HPA axis hyperactivity in bulimia. *Psychiatry Res*, 8, 111–117.

Hulka, B. S. (1994). Links between hormone replacement therapy and neoplasia. *Fertil Steril*, 62, 168S–175S.

Hullett, F. J., and Bidder, T. G. (1983). Phenelzine plus triiodothyronine combination in a case of refractory depression. *J Nerv Ment Dis*, 171, 318–320.

Hunter, D. J., Spiegelman, D., Adami, H-O., et al. (1996). Cohort studies of fat intake and the risk of breast cancer–a pooled analysis. *N Engl J Med*, 334, 356–361.

Hunter, D. J., and Willett, W. C. (1993). Diet, body size, and breast cancer. *Epidemiol Rev*, 15, 110–132.

Hurt, S. W., Schnurr, P. P., Severino, S. R., et al. (1992). Late luteal phase dysphoric disorder in 670 women evaluated for premenstrual complaints. *Am J Psychiatry*, 149, 525–530.

Hurwitz, N. (1969). Predisposing factors in adverse reactions to drugs. *Br J Med*, 1, 536–539.

Hussain, M., Harinath, M., and Murphy, J. (1972). Tranquilizer-induced galactorrea. *Can Med Assoc J*, 106, 1107–1108.

ICD. (1992). *International classification of diseases – ICD 10*. Geneva: World Health Organization.

Ilnyckyj, A., Farber, J., Cheang, M. C., and Weinerman, B. H. (1994). A randomized controlled trial of psychotherapeutic intervention in cancer patients. *Ann R Coll Physicians Surg Can*, 27, 93–96.

Infante, C., Hurtado, J., Salazar, G., et al. (1991). The dose-to-mother method to measure milk intake in infants by deuterium dilution: A validation study. *Eur J Clin Nutr*, 45, 121–129.

Insel, T. (1990). Oxytocin and maternal behavior. In N. Krasnegor and R. Bridges (Eds.), *Mammalian parenting* (pp. 260–280). New York: Oxford University Press.

Inskip, P. D. (1994). Pelvic radiotherapy, sex hormones, and breast cancer. *Cancer Causes and Control*, 5, 471–478.

Institute of Medicine Committee to Review the NIH Women's Health Initiative. (1993). In S. Thaul and D. Hotra (Eds.), *An assessment of the NIH Women's Health Initiative* (pp. 25–75). Washington, DC: National Academy Press.

Irwin, M. (1993). Stress-induced immune suppression. Role of the autonomic nervous system. *Ann NY Acad Sciences*, 697, 203–218.

Irwin, M., Daniels, M., Risch, S. C., et al. (1988). Plasma cortisol and natural killer cell activity during bereavement. *Biol Psychiatry*, 24, 173–178.

Irwin, M., Daniels, M., Smith, T. L., et al. (1987). Impaired natural killer cell activity during bereavement. *Brain Behav Immun*, 1, 98–104.

Isaacs, A., Leslie, D., Gomez, J., and Bayliss, R. (1980). The effect of weight gain on gonadatrophins and prolactin in anorexia nervosa. *Acta Endocrinol*, 94, 145–150.

Isacsson, G., Wasserman, D., and Bergman, U. (1995). Self-poisonings with antidepressants and other psychotropics in an urban area of Sweden. *Ann Clin Psychiatry*, 7, 113–118.

Israel, Y., and Orrego, H. (1984). Hypermetabolic state and hypoxic liver damage. *Recent Dev Alcohol*, 2, 119–133.

Israel, Y., Walfish, P. G., Orrego, H., Blake, J., and Kalant, H. (1979). Thyroid hormones in alcoholic liver disease. *Gastroenterology*, 76, 116–122.

Ito, S., and Koren, G. (1994). A novel index for expressing exposure of the infant to drugs in breast milk. *Br J Clin Pharmacol*, 38, 99–102.

Jacobs, D. R., Meban, I. L., Bangdiwala, S. I., Criqui, M. H., and Tyroler, H. A. (1990). High density lipoprotein as a predictor of cardiovascular disease mortality in men and women: The follow-up studies of the lipid research clinics prevalence study. *Am J Epidemiol*, 131, 32–47.

Jacobson, L., and Sapolsky, R. (1991). The role of the hippocampus in feedback regulation of the hypothalamic-pituitary-adrenocortical axis. *Endocrinol Rev*, 12, 118–134.

Jaeckle, R. S., Kathol, R. G., Lopez, J. F., Meller, W. H., and Krummel, S. J. (1987). Enhanced adrenal sensitivity to exogenous ACTH stimulation in major depression. *Arch Gen Psychiatry*, 44, 233–240.

Jaffe, K., and Zisook, S. (1978). Galactorrhea in a patient treated with amoxapine. *J Clin Psychiatry*, 39, 821.

Jaffe, R. B., Plosker, S., Marshal, L., and Martin, M. C. (1990). Neuromodulatory regulation of gonadotropin-releasing hormone pulsatile discharge in women. *Am J Obstet Gynecol*, 163, 1727–1731.

Jain, V. K. (1972). A psychiatric study of hypothyroidism. *Psychiatr Clin*, 5, 121–130.

Jakacki, R., Kelch, R., Sauder, S., et al. (1982). Pulsatile secretion of luteinizing hormone in children. *J Clin Endocrinol Metab*, 55, 453–458.

Jarrett, S. R., Ramirez, A. J., Richards, M. A., and Weinman, J. (1992). Measuring coping in breast cancer. *J Psychosom Res*, 36, 593–602.

Jaszmann, L., Van Lith, N. D., and Zaat, J. C. A. (1969). The perimenopausal symptoms. *Med Gynecol Sociol*, 4, 268–277.

Jenkins, R., and Clare, A. W. (1985). Women and mental illness. *Br Med J*, 291, 1521–1522.

Jensen, A. B. (1991). Psychological factors in breast cancer and their possible impact upon prognosis. *Cancer Treat Rev*, 18, 191–210.

Jensen, M. R. (1987). Psychobiological factors predicting the course of breast cancer. *J Pers*, 55, 317–342.

Jernstrom, H., and Olsson, H. (1994). Suppression of plasma insulin-like growth factor-1 levels in healthy multiparous young women using low dose oral contraceptives. *Gynecol Obstet Invest*, 38, 261–265.

Jochemsen, R., van der Graaff, M., Boeijinga, J., and Breimer, D. (1982). Influence of sex, menstrual cycle and oral contraception on the disposition of nitrazepam. *Br J Clin Pharmacol*, 13, 319–324.

Joffe, R. T. (1987). Antithyroid antibodies in major depression. *Acta Psychiatr Scand*, 76, 598–599.

Joffe, R. T. (1988a). Triiodothyronine potentiation of the antidepressant effect of phenelzine. *J Clin Psychiatry*, 49, 409–410.

Joffe, R. T. (1988b). T_3 and lithium potentiation of tricyclic antidepressants [Letter]. *Am J Psychiatry*, 145, 1317–1318.

Joffe, R. T., Blank, D. W., Post, R. M., and Uhde, T. W. (1985). Decreased triiodothyronines in depression: A preliminary report. *Biol Psychiatry*, 20, 922–925.

Joffe, R. T., Kutcher, S., and MacDonald, C. (1988). Thyroid function and bipolar affective disorder. *Psychiatry Res*, 25, 117–121.

Joffe, R. T., and Levitt, A. J. (1992). Major depression and subclinical (grade 2) hypothyroidism. *Psychoneuroendocrinology*, 17, 215–221.

Joffe, R. T., Levitt, A. J., Bagby, R. M., MacDonald, C., and Singer, W. (1993). Predictors of response to lithium and triiodothyronine augmentation of antidepressants in tricyclic non-responders. *Br J Psychiatry*, 163, 574–578.

Joffe, R. T., and Singer, W. (1987). Effect of phenelzine on thyroid function in depressed patients. *Biol Psychiatry*, 22, 1033–1035.

Joffe, R. T., and Singer, W. (1990a). A comparison of triiodothyronine and thyroxine in the potentiation of tricyclic antidepressants. *Psychiatr Res*, 32, 241–251.

Joffe, R. T., and Singer, W. (1990b). The effect of tricyclic antidepressants on basal thyroid hormone levels in depressed patients. *Pharmacopsychiatry*, 23, 67–69.

Joffe, R. T., Singer, W., Levitt, A. J., MacDonald, C. (1993). A placebo-controlled comparison of lithium and triiodothyronine augmentation of tricyclic antidepressants in unipolar refractory depression. *Arch Gen Psychiatry*, 50, 387–393.

Johnson, C., and Connors, M. (1987). *The etiology and treatment of bulimia nervosa*. New York: Basic Books.

Jones, B., and Jones, M. (1976). Alcohol effects in women during the menstrual cycle. *Ann NY Acad Sci*, 273, 576–587.

Kagan, J., Reznick, J., and Snidman, N. (1987). The physiology and psychology of behavioral inhibition in children. *Child Dev*, 58, 1459–1473.

Kalin, N. H., Risch, S. C., Janowsky, D. S., and Murphy, D. L. (1982). Plasma ACTH and cortisol concentrations before and after dexamethasone. *Psychiatry Res*, 7, 87–92.

Kalter, H., and Warkany, J. (1983). Congenital malformations. Part I: Etiologic factors and their role in prevention. *N Engl J Med*, 308, 424–431.

Kalucy, R., Crisp, A., Chard, T., et al. (1976). Nocturnal hormonal profiles in massive obesity, anorexia nervosa and normal females. *J Psychosom Res*, 20, 595–604.

Kamen, L., Rodin, J., Seligman, M. E. P., and Dwyer, J. (1991). Explanatory style and cell-mediated immunity in elderly men and women. *Health Psychol*, 10, 229–235.

Kampen, D. L., and Sherwin, B. B. (1994). Estrogen use and verbal memory in healthy postmenopausal women. *Obstet Gynecol*, 83, 979–983.

Kanarek, R. B., and Collier, G. H. (1983). Self-starvation: A problem of overriding the satiety signal? *Physiol Behav*, 30, 307–311.

Kandel, D., and Davies, M. (1982). Epidemiology of depressive mood in adolescents. *Arch Gen Psychiatry*, 39, 1205–1212.

Kane, J. P., Malloy, M. J., Ports, T. A., et al. (1990). Regression of coronary atherosclerosis during treatment of familial hypercholesterolemia with combined drug regimens. *JAMA*, 264, 3007–3012.

Kannel, W. B. (1987). Metabolic risk factors for coronary heart disease in women: Perspective from the Framingham study. *Am Heart J*, 114, 413–419.

Kannel, W. B., and Abbott, R. D. (1987). Incidence and prognosis of myocardial infarction in women: The Framingham Study. In E. D. Eaker, B. Packer, and N. K. Wenger (Eds.), *Coronary heart disease in women* (p. 208). New York: Haymarket Doyma.

Kaplan, H. I., Sadock, B. J., and Grebb, J. A. (1994). *Synopsis of psychiatry*, 7th ed. Baltimore: Williams & Wilkins.

Karlberg, B. E., Kjellman, B. F., and Kagedol, B. (1978). Treatment of endogenous depression with oral thyrotropin. *Acta Psychiatr Scand*, 58, 389–400.

Karlsson, K., Lindstedt, G., and Lundberg, P. (1975). Transplacental lithium poisoning: Reversible inhibition of fetal thyroid. *Lancet*, 1, 1259.

Kathol, R. G., and Delahunt, J. W. (1986). The relationship of anxiety and depression to symptoms of hyperthyroidism using operational criteria. *Gen Hosp Psychiatry*, 8, 23–28.

Kathol, R. G., Jaeckle, R. S., Lopez, J. R., and Mullter, W. H. (1989). Consistent reduction of ACTH responses to stimulation with CRH, vasopressin and hypoglycaemia in patients with depression. *Br J Psychiatry*, 155, 468–478.

Kathol, R. G., Mutgi, A., Williams, J., et al. (1990). Diagnosis of major depression in cancer patients according to four sets of criteria. *Am J Psychiatry*, 147, 1021–1024.

Kathol, R. G., Noyes, R., Williams, J., et al. (1990). Diagnosing depression in patients with medical illness. *Psychosomatics*, 31, 434–440.

Kathol, R. G., Turner, R., and Delahunt, J. (1986). Depression and anxiety associated with hyperthyroidism: Response to antithyroid therapy. *Psychosomatics*, 27, 501–505.

Kato, R., and Yamazoe, Y. (1992). Sex-specific cytochrome P_{450} as a cause of sex- and species-related differences in drug toxicity. *Toxicol Lett*, 64–65, 661–667.

Katz, J., Boyar, R., Roffwarg, H., Hellman, L. D., and Weiner, H. (1978). Weight and circadian luteinizing hormone secretory pattern in anorexia nervosa. *Psychosom Med*, 40, 549–567.

Katz, M., Wetzler, S., Cloitre, M., et al. (1993). Expressive characteristics of anxiety in depressed men and women. *J Affect Disord*, 28, 267–277.

Keck, P. E., Jr., McElroy, S. L., Rugrul, K. C., and Bennett, J. A. (1993). Valproate oral loading in the treatment of acute mania. *J Clin Psychiatry*, 54, 305–308.

Keller, S. E., Weiss, J. M., Schliefer, S. J., et al. (1983). Stress-induced suppression of immunity in adrenalectomized rats. *Science*, 221, 1301–1304.

Kelley, D. (1986). The genesis of male and female brains. *Trends Neurosci*, 9, 499–502.

Kelsey, J. L., and Whittemore, A. S. (1994). Epidemiology and primary prevention of cancers of the breast, endometrium, and ovary. *Ann Epidemiol*, 4, 89–95.

Kendall, R. E., Chalmers, J. C., and Platz, C. (1987). Epidemiology of puerperal psychosis. *Br J Psychiatry*, 150, 662–673.

Kendler, K., MacLean, C., Neale, M., et al. (1991). The genetic epidemiology of bulimia nervosa. *Am J Psychiatry*, 148, 1627–1637.

Kendler, K. S., Neale, M. C., Kessler, R. C., Heath, A. C., and Eaves, L. J. (1992a). A population-based twin study of alcoholism in women. *JAMA*, 268, 1877–1882.

Kendler, K. S., Neale, M. C., Kessler, R. C., Heath, A. C., and Eaves, L. J. (1992b). Childhood parental loss and adult psychopathology in women. A twin study perspective. *Arch Gen Psychiatry*, 49, 109–116.

Kendler, K. S., Neale, M. C., Kessler, R. C., Heath, A. C., and Eaves, L. J. (1992c). Generalized anxiety disorder in women–a population-based twin study. *Arch Gen Psychiatry*, 49, 267–272.

Kendler, K. S., Neale, M. C., Kessler, R. C., Heath, A. C., and Eaves, L. J. (1992d). The genetic epidemiology of phobias in women. The interrelationship of agoraphobia, social phobia, situational phobia, and simple phobia. *Arch Gen Psychiatry*, 49, 273–281.

Kendler, K. S., Neale, M. C., Kessler, R. C., Heath, A. C., and Eaves, L. J. (1993). A longitudinal twin study of 1-year prevalence of major depression in women. *Arch Gen Psychiatry*, 50, 843–852.

Kendler, K. S., Walters, E. E., Neale, M. C., et al. (1995). The structure of the genetic and environmental risk factors for six major psychiatric disorders in women. *Arch Gen Psychiatry*, 52, 374–383.

Kennedy, D. L. C. (1980). Estrogens and endometrial cancer. *Drug Intell Clin Pharm*, 14, 406–411.

Kennedy, D. L. C. (1985). Noncontraceptive estrogens and progestins: Use patterns over time. *Obstet Gynecol*, 65, 441–446.

Kennedy, S., Brown, G., and McVey, G. (1991). Pineal and adrenal function before and after refeeding anorexia nervosa. *Biol Psychiatry*, 30, 216–224.

Kennedy, S., Kiecolt-Glaser, J. K., and Glaser, R. (1988). Immunological consequences of acute and chronic stressors: Mediating role of interpersonal relationships. *Br J Med Psychiatry*, 61, 77–85.

Kennedy, S. H., Tighe, S., McVey, G., and Brown, G. M. (1989). Melatonin and cortisol "switches" during mania, depression, and euthymia in a drug-free bipolar patient. *J Nerv Ment Dis*, 177, 300–303.

Kessler, R., Brown, R., and Boman, C. (1981). Sex differences in psychiatric help-seeking: Evidence from four large-scale surveys. *J Health Soc Behav*, 22, 49–64.

Kessler, R. C., McGonagle, K. A., Swartz, M., Blazer, D. G., and Nelson, C. B. (1993). Sex and depression in the National Comorbidity Survey I: Lifetime prevalence, chronicity and recurrence. *J Affect Disord*, 29, 85–96.

Kessler, R. C., McGonagle, K. A., Zhao, S., et al. (1994). Lifetime and 12-month prevalence of DSM-III-R psychiatric disorders in the United States: Results from the National Comorbidity Survey. *Arch Gen Psychiatry*, 51, 8–19.

Ketter, T., Flockhart, D., Post, R., et al. (1995). The emerging role of cytochrome P_{450} 3A in psychopharmacology. *J Clin Psychopharmacol*, 15, 387–398.

Keys, A., Brozek, J., Henschel, A., Mickelsen, O., and Taylor, H. (1950). *The biology of human starvation*. Minneapolis: University of Minnesota Press.

Khanna, S., and Mukherjee, D. (1992). Checkers and washers: Valid subtypes of obsessive compulsive disorder. *Psychopathology*, 25, 283–288.

Kiecolt-Glaser, J. K., Fisher, L., Ogrocki, P., et al. (1987). Marital quality, marital disruption, and immune function. *Psychosom Med*, 49, 13–34.

Kiecolt-Glaser, J. K., Glaser, R., Dyer, C., et al. (1987). Chronic stress and immunity in family caregivers of Alzheimer's disease victims. *Psychosom Med*, 49, 523–535.

Kiecolt-Glaser, J. K., Glaser, R., Strain, E. C., et al. (1986). Modulation of cellular immunity in medical students. *J Behav Med*, 9, 5–21.

Kiecolt-Glaser, J. K., and Greenberg, B. (1984). Social support as a moderator of the after effects of stress in female psychiatric inpatients. *J Abnorm Psychol*, 93, 192–199.

Kijne, B., Aggernaes, H., Fog-Moller, F., et al. (1982). Circadian variation of serum thyrotropin in endogenous depression. *Psychiatr Res*, 6, 277–282.

King, B., Camp, C. J., and Downey, A. M. (1991). *Human sexuality today*. Englewood Cliffs, NJ: Prentice Hall.

King, M. C., Rowell, S., and Love, S. M. (1993). Inherited breast and ovarian cancer: What are the risks? What are the choices? *JAMA*, 269, 1975–1980.

Kinsella, K. G. (1992). Changes in life expectancy 1900–1990. *Am J Clin Nutr*, 55, 1196S–1202S.

Kiriike, N., Izumiya, Y., Nishiwaki, S., et al. (1988). TRH test and DST in schizoaffective mania, mania, and schizophrenia. *Biol Psychiatry*, 24, 415–422.

Kiriike, N., Nishiwaki, S., and Izumiya, Y. (1987). Thyrotropin, prolactin and growth hormone responses to thyrotropin-releasing hormone in anorexia nervosa and bulimia. *Biol Psychiatry*, 22, 167–176.

Kirkegaard, C. (1981). The thyrotropin response to thyrotropin releasing hormone in endogenous depression. *Psychoneuroendocrinology*, 6, 189–212.

Kirkegaard, C., Bjorum, N., Cohn, D., et al. (1977). Studies on the influence of biogenic amines and psychoactive drugs on the prognostic value of the TRH stimulation test in endogenous depression. *Psychoneuroendocrinology*, 2, 131–136.

Kirkegaard, C., and Faber, J. (1981). Altered serum levels of thyroxine, triiodothyronines and diiodothyronines in endogenous depression. *Acta Endocrinol*, 96, 199–207.

Kirkegaard, C., and Faber, J. (1986). Influence of free thyroid hormone levels on the TSH response to TRH in endogenous depression. *Psychoneuroendocrinology*, 11, 491–497.

Kirkegaard, C., and Faber, J. (1991). Free thyroxine and 3,3',5'-triiodothyronine levels in cerebrospinal fluid in patients with endogenous depression. *Acta Endocrinol*, 124, 166–172.

Kirkegaard, C., Faber, J., Hummer, L., and Rogowski, P. (1979). Increased levels of TRH in cerebrospinal fluid from patients with endogenous depression. *Psychoneuroendocrinology*, 4, 227–235.

Kirkegaard, C., Norlem, N., Lauridsen, U. B., Bjorum, N., and Christiansen, C. (1975). Protirelin stimulation test and thyroid function during treatment of depression. *Arch Gen Psychiatry*, 32, 1115–1118.

Kirkpatrick, B., Kim, J., and Insel, T. (1994). Limbic system *fos* expression associated with paternal behavior. *Brain Res*, 658, 112–118.

Kirkwood, C., Moore, A., Hayes, P., De Vane, C., and Pelonero, A. (1991). Influence of menstrual cycle and gender on alprazolam pharmacokinetics. *Clin Pharmacol Ther*, 50, 404–409.

Kissebah, A. H., Vydelengum, N., Murray, R., et al. (1982). Relation of body fat distribution to metabolic complications of obesity. *J Clin Endocrinol Metab*, 54, 254–260.

Kjellman, B. F., Beck-Friis, J., Ljunggren, J. G., and Wetterberg, L. (1984). Twenty-four-hour serum levels of TSH in affective disorders. *Acta Psychiatr Scand*, 69, 491–502.

Kjellman, B. F., Ljunggren, J. G., Beck-Friis, J., and Wetterberg, L. (1983). Reverse T3 levels in affective disorders. *Psychiatr Res*, 10, 1–9.

Kjellman, B. F., Ljunggren, J. G., Beck-Friis, J., and Wetterberg, L. (1985). Effect of TRH on TSH and prolactin levels in affective disorders. *Psychiatry Res*, 14, 353–363.

Klaiber, E., Broverman, D., Vogel, W., and Kobayashi, Y. (1979). Estrogen therapy for severe persistent depressions in women. *Arch Gen Psychiatry*, 36, 550–554.

Kleber, H. (1996). Drugs, alcohol and cigarettes during pregnancy: A lethal combination for mother and child. In *Substance abuse and the American woman* (pp. 69–95). New York: CASA.

Kleerekoper, M., Peterson, E. L., Nelson, D. A. (1991). A randomized trial of sodium fluoride as a treatment for postmenopausal osteoporosis. *Osteoporos Int*, 1, 155–161.

Klijn, J. G., Setyono-Han, B., Sander, H. J., et al. (1994). Preclinical and clinical treatment of breast cancer with antiprogestins. *Human Reprod*, 9, 181–189.

Kling, M. A., Rubinow, D. R., Doran, A. R., et al. (1993). Cerebrospinal fluid immunoreactive somatostatin concentrations in patients with Cushing's disease and major depression: Relationship to indices of corticotropin-releasing hormone and cortisol secretion. *Neuroendocrinology*, 57, 79–88.

Klonoff-Cohen, H., Edelstein, S., Lefkowitz, E., et al. (1995). The effect of passive smoking and tobacco exposure through breast milk on sudden infant death syndrome. *JAMA*, 273, 795–798.

Knobil, E. (1990). The GnRH pulse generator. *Am J Obstet Gynecol*, 163, 1721–1727.

Kolakowska, T., and Swigar, M. E. (1977). Thyroid function in depression and alcohol abuse. *Arch Gen Psychiatry*, 34, 984–988.

Kopelman, A., McCullar, F., and Heggeness, L. (1975). Limb malformations following maternal use of haloperidol. *JAMA*, 231, 62–64.

Koppelman, M. S. C., Parry, B. L., Hamilton, J. A., Alagna, S. W., and Lariaux, L. (1987). Effect of bromocriptine on affect and libido in hyperprolactinemia. *Am J Psychiatr*, 8, 1037–1041.

Korenman, S. G., and Sherman, B. M. (1973). Further studies of gonadotropin and estradiol secretion during the pre-ovulatory phase of the human menstrual cycle. *J Clin Endocrinol Metab*, 36, 1205–1209.

Korner, A., Kirkegaard, C., and Larsen, J. K., (1987). The thyrotropin response to thyrotropin-releasing hormone as a biological marker of suicidal risk in depressive patients. *Acta Psychiatr Scand*, 76, 355–358.

Kovacs, G., and Telegdy, G. (1985). Role of oxytocin in memory, amnesia and reinforcement. In J. Amico and A. Robinson (Eds.), *Oxytocin: Clinical and laboratory studies* (pp. 359–371). New York: Elsevier.

Krieger, N. (1989). Exposure, susceptibility, and breast cancer risk: A hypothesis regarding exogenous carcinogens, breast tissue development, and social gradients, including black/white differences, in breast cancer incidence. *Breast Cancer Res Treat*, 13, 205–223.

Kreiger, N. (1990). Racial and gender discrimination: Risk factors for high school students' blood pressure? *Soc Sci Med*, 30(12), 1273–1281.

Krishnan, K. R. R., Doraiswamy, P. M., Lurie, S. N., et al. (1991). Pituitary size in depression. *J Clin Endocrinol Metab*, 72, 256–259.

Krishnan, K. R. R., France, R. D., Pelton, S., et al. (1985). What does the dexamethasone suppression test identify? *Biol Psychiatry*, 20, 957–964.

Krishnan, K. R. R., Maltbie, A. A., and Davidson, J. R. T. (1983). Abnormal cortisol suppression in bipolar patients with simultaneous manic and depressive symptoms. *Am J Psychiatry*, 140, 203–205.

Krishnan, K. R. R., Rayasam, K., Reed, D., et al. (1993). The CRF corticotropin-releasing factor stimulation test in patients with major depression: Relationship to dexamethasone suppression test results. *Depression*, 1, 133–136.

Kristensen, C. (1983). Imipramine serum protein binding in healthy subjects. *Clin Pharmacol Ther*, 34, 689–694.

Kristjansson, F., and Thorsteinsson, S. (1991). Disposition of alprazolam in human volunteers: Differences between genders. *Acta Pharm Nord*, 3, 249–250.

Kroner, K., Knudsen, U. B., Lundby, L., and Hvid, H. (1992). Long-term phantom breast syndrome after mastectomy. *Clin J Pain*, 8, 346–350.

Kuhs, H., and Toelle, R. (1991). Sleep deprivation therapy. *Biol Psychiatry*, 29, 1129–1148.

Kumar, R., Marks, M., Wiek, A., et al. (1993). Neuroendocrine and psychosocial mechanisms in postpartum psychosis. *Prog Neuropsychopharmacol Biol Psychiatry*, 17, 571–579.

Kumar, R., and Robson, K. M. (1984). A prospective study of emotional disorders in child-bearing women. *Br J Psychiatry*, 144, 35–47.

Kupperman, H. S., Blatt, M. G., Wisbader, H., and Filler, W. (1959). Comparative clinical evaluation of estrogen preparations by the menopause and amenorrheal indices. *Endocrinology*, 13, 688–703.

Kusalic, M., Engelsmann, F., and Bradwejn, J. (1993). Thyroid functioning during treatment for depression. *J Psychiatry Neurosci*, 18, 260–263.

Kvale, G., Hugdahl, K., Asbjornsen, A., et al. (1991). Anticipatory nausea and vomiting in cancer patients. *J Consult Clin Psychol*, 59, 894–898.

Lacey, J. (1983). Bulimia nervosa, binge-eating and psychogenic vomiting: A controlled treatment study and long-term outcome. *Br J Med*, 286, 1609–1613.

Lacey, J. (1993). Self-damaging and addictive behaviour in bulimia nervosa: A catchment area study. *Br J Psychiatry*, 163, 190–194.

LaCroix, A. Z. (1994). Psychosocial factors and risk of coronary heart disease in women: An epidemiologic perspective. *Fertil Steril*, 62, 133S–139S.

Laegreid, L., Hagberg, G., and Lundberg, A. (1992). Neurodevelopment in late infancy after prenatal exposure to benzodiazepines – a prospective study. *Neuropediatrics*, 23, 60–67.

Laegreid, L., Olegard, R., Wahlstrom, J., and Conradi, N. (1987). Abnormalities in children exposed to benzodiazepines in utero. *Lancet*, 1, 108–109.

Laessle, R., Zoettle, C., and Pirke, K. (1987). Meta-analysis of treatment studies for bulimia. *Int J Eating Disord*, 6, 647–654.

Lancaster, F. E. (1995). Gender differences in animal studies. Implications for the study of human alcoholism. In M. Galanter (Ed.), *Recent developments in alcoholism. Volume 12: Women and alcoholism* (pp. 209–215). New York: Plenum Press.

Lapidus, L., Bengtsson, C., Larsson, B., et al. (1984). Distribution of adipose tissue and risk of cardiovascular disease and death: A 12-year follow up of participants in the population study of women in Gothenburg, Sweden. *Br Med J*, 289, 1257–1261.

Largo, R., and Prader, A. (1983). Pubertal development in Swiss girls. *Helv Paediatr Acta*, 38, 229–243.

Larsen, P. R., and Ingbar, S. H. (1992). The thyroid gland. In J. D. Wilson and D. W. Foster (Eds.), *Textbook of endocrinology* (pp. 357–487). Philadelphia: W. B. Saunders.

Larson, R., Csikszentmihalyi, M., and Graef, R. (1980). Mood variability and the psychosocial adjustment of adolescents. *J Youth Adolesc*, 9, 469–490.

Lasègue, E. (1873). De l'anorexie hystérique. *Arch Gen Med*, 21, 885–900.

Laue, L., Loriaux, D. L., and Chrousos, G. P. (1988). Glucocorticoid antagonists and the role of glucocorticoids at the resting and stress state. *Adv Exp Med Biol*, 245, 237–247.

Lavie, C. L., and Milani, R. V. (1995). Effects of cardiac rehabilitation and exercise training on exercise capacity, coronary risk factors, behavioral characteristics, and quality of life in women. *Am J Cardiol*, 75, 340–343.

Lawler, K. A., Harralson, T. L., Armstead, C. A., and Schmied, L. A. (1993). Gender and cardiovascular responses: What is the role of hostility? *J Psychosom Res*, 37, 603–613.

Lazarus, J. H., McGregor, A. M., Ludgate, M., et al. (1986). Effect of lithium carbonate therapy on thyroid immune status in manic depressive patients: A prospective study. *J Affect Disord*, 11, 155–160.

Lazarus, R. S., and Folkman, S. (1984). *Stress, appraisal, and coping*. New York: Springer-Verlag.

Lechin, F., van der Dijs, B., Vitelli-Florez, O., et al. (1990). Psychoneuroendocrinological and immunological parameters in cancer patients: Involvement of stress and depression. *Psychoneuroendocrinology*, 15, 435–451.

Lee, C. K., Kwak, Y. S., Yamamoto, J., et al. (1990). Psychiatric epidemiology in Korea. Part I. Gender and age differences in Seoul. *J Nerv Ment Disord*, 178, 242–246.

Lee, M. S., Love, S. B., Mitchell, J. B., et al. (1993). Mastectomy or conservation for early breast cancer: Psychological morbidity. *Eur J Cancer*, 28A, 1340–1344.

Leer, E. M., Seidell, J. C., and Kromhout, D. (1994). Differences in association between alcohol consumption and blood pressure by age, gender, and smoking. *Epidemiology*, 5(6), 576–582.

Leibenluft, E. (1993). Do gonadal steroids regulate circadian rhythms in humans? *J Affect Disord*, 29, 175–181.

Leibenluft, E. (1996). Women with bipolar illness: Clinical and research issues. *Am J Psychiatry*, 153, 163–173.

Leichter, S. B., Kirstein, L., and Martin, N. D. (1977). Thyroid function and growth hormone secretion in amitriptyline-treated depression. *Am J Psychiatry*, 134, 1270–1272.

Lenton, E. A., Cooke, I. D., Sampson, G. A., and Sexton, L. (1978). Episodic secretion of oestradiol in pre-menopausal women, men and post-menopausal women. *Clin Endocrinol*, 9, 37–47.

Leon, G., Perry, C., and Mangelsdorf, C. (1989). Adolescent nutritional and psychological patterns and risk for the development of eating disorder. *J Youth Adolesc*, 181, 273–282.

Leonard, J. L. (1990). Identification and structure analysis of iodothyronine deiodinases. In M. A. Greer (Ed.), *The thyroid gland* (pp. 285–305). New York: Raven Press.

Leslie, R., Isaacs, A., Gomez, J., Raggatt, P., and Bayliss, R. (1978). Hypothalamo-pituitary-thyroid function in anorexia nervosa: Influence of weight gain. *Br Med J*, 2, 526–528.

Leslie, S. (1974). Psychiatric disorder in the young adolescents of an industrial town. *Br J Psychiatry*, 125, 113–124.

Lesperance, F., Frasure-Smith, N., and Talajic, M. (1996). Major depression before and after myocardial infarction: Its nature and consequences. *Psychosom Med*, 58, 99–110.

Levin, R. M. (1993). Osteoporosis: Prevention is key to management. *Geriatrics*, 48, 18–24.

Levy, A., Dixon, K., and Malarkey, W. (1988). Pituitary response to TRH in bulimia. *Biol Psychiatry*, 23, 476–484.

Levy, S., Herberman, R., Lippman, M., and D'Angelo, T. (1987). Correlation of stress factors with sustained depression of natural killer cell activity with predicted prognosis in patients with breast cancer. *J Clin Oncol*, 5, 348–353.

Levy, S. M., Haynes, L. T., Herberman, R. B., et al. (1992). Mastectomy versus breast conservation surgery: Mental health effects at long-term follow-up. *Health Psychol*, 11, 349–354.

Levy, S. M., Herberman, R. B., Lee, J., et al. (1990). Estrogen receptor concentration and social factors as predictors of natural killer cell activity in early-stage breast cancer patients. *Nat Immun Cell Growth Reg*, 9, 313–324.

Levy, S. M., Herberman, R. B., Lippman, M., et al. (1991). Immunological and psychosocial predictors of disease recurrence in patients with early-stage breast cancer. *Behav Med*, 17, 67–75.

Levy, S. M., Herberman, R. B., Maluish, A. M., et al. (1985). Prognostic risk assessment in primary breast cancer by behavioral and immunological parameters. *Health Psychol*, 4, 99–113.

Levy, W., and Wisniewski, K. (1974). Chlorpromazine causing extrapyramidal dysfunction in newborn infants of psychotic mothers. *NY State J Med*, 74, 684–685.

Lewine, R. R. J., and Seeman, M. V. (1995). Gender, brain, and schizophrenia. Anatomy of differences/differences of anatomy. In M. V. Seeman (Ed.), *Gender and psychopathology* (pp. 131–158). Washington, DC: American Psychiatric Press.

Lewis, B. V., and Parsons, M. (1966). Chorea gravidarum. *Lancet*, 1, 284–286.

Lewis, F. M., and Hammond, M. A. (1992). Psychosocial adjustment of the family to breast cancer: A longitudinal analysis. *J Am Med Wom Assoc*, 47, 194–200.

Lewis, S. (1992). Sex and schizophrenia: Vive la différence. *Br J Psychiatry*, 161, 445–450.

Lex, B. W. (1995). Alcohol and other psychoactive substance dependence in women and men. In M. V. Seeman (Ed.), *Gender and psychopathology* (pp. 311–358). Washington, DC: American Psychiatric Press.

Li, C., Windsor, R., Perkins, L., Goldenberg, R., and Lowe, J. (1993). The impact on birth weight and gestational age of nicotine-validated smoking reduction during pregnancy. *JAMA*, 269, 1519–1524.

Li, F. P., Correa, P., and Fraumeni, J. F., Jr. (1991). Testing for germ line p53 mutations in cancer families. *Cancer Epidemiol Biomarkers Prev*, 1, 91–94.

Li, F. P., and Fraumeni, J. F., Jr. (1982). Prospective study of a family cancer syndrome. *JAMA*, 247, 2692–2694.

Liberman, U. A., Weiss, S. R., Bröll, J., et al. (1995). Effect of oral alendronate on bone mineral density and the incidence of fractures in postmenopausal osteoporosis. *N Engl J Med*, 333, 1437–1443.

Lief, H. (Ed.). (1981). *Sexual problems in medical practice* (pp. 3–419) Chicago: AMA Press.

Lindal, E., and Stefansson, J. G. (1993). The lifetime prevalence of anxiety disorders in Iceland as estimated by the U.S. National Institute of Mental Health Diagnostic Interview Schedule. *Acta Psychiatr Scand*, 88, 29–34.

Linden, S., and Rich, C. (1983). The use of lithium during pregnancy and lactation. *J Clin Psychiatry*, 44, 358–361.

Lindhout, D., Meinardi, H., Meijer, J., and Nau, H. (1992). Antiepileptic drugs and teratogenesis in two consecutive cohorts: Changes in prescription policy paralleled by changes in pattern of malformations. *Neurology*, 42, 94–110.

Lindley, C. M., Hirsch, J. D., O'Neill, C. V., et al. (1992). Quality of life consequences of chemotherapy-induced emesis. *Qual Life Res*, 1, 331–340.

Lindsay, R. (1993). Hormone replacement for prevention and treatment of osteoporosis. *Am J Med*, 95, 37S–39S.

Lindsay, R., Hart, D. M., and Clark, D. M. (1984). The minimum effective dose of estrogen for prevention of postmenopausal bone loss. *Obstet Gynecol*, 63, 759–763.

Lindstedt, G., Lundberg, P., Hammond, G., and Vihko, R. (1985). Sex hormone binding globulin – still many questions. *Scand J Clin Lab Invest*, 45, 1–6.

Linkowski, P., Mendlewicz, J., Leclerq, R., et al. (1985). The 24-hour profile of ACTH and cortisol in major depressive illness. *J Clin Endocrinol Metab*, 61, 429–438.

Linkowski, P., Mendlewicz, J., Leclerq, R., et al. (1987). The 24-hour profile of adrenocorticotropin and cortisol in major depressive illness. *J Clin Endocrinol Metab*, 65, 141–152.

Linn, M. W., Linn, B. S., and Harris, R. (1982). Effects of counseling for late-stage cancer patients. *Cancer*, 49, 1048–1055.

Linnoila, M., Cowdry, R., Lamberg, B. A., Makinen, T., and Rubinow, D. (1983). CSF triiodothyronine (rT_3) levels in patients with affective disorders. *Biol Psychiatry*, 18, 1489–1492.

Linnoila, M., Lamberg, B. A., Rosberg, G., Karonen, S. L., and Welin, M. G. (1979). Thyroid hormones and TSH, prolactin and LH responses to repeated TRH and LRH injections in depressed patients. *Acta Psychiatr. Scand*, 59, 536–544.

Lipid Research Clinics Program. (1984). The Lipid Research clinics coronary primary prevention trial results. II: The relationship of reduction in incidence of coronary heart disease to cholesterol lowering. *JAMA*, 251, 365–374.

Lissoni, P., Barni, S., Meregalli, S., et al. (1995). Modulation of cancer endocrine therapy by melatonin: A phase II study of tamoxifen plus melatonin in metastatic breast cancer patients progressing under tamoxifen alone. *Br. J Cancer*, 71, 854–856.

Lobo, A., Perez-Echeverria, M. J., Jiminez-Aznarez, A., and Sancho, M. A. (1988). Emotional disturbances in endocrine patients. Validity of the scaled version of the General Health Questionnaire. *Br J Psychiatry*, 152, 807–812.

Lobo, R. A. (1991). Effects of hormonal replacement on lipids and lipoproteins in postmenopausal women. *J Clin Endocrinol Metab*, 73, 925–930.

Lobo, R. A., Pickar, J. H., Wild, R. A., Walsh, B., and Hirvonen, E. (1994). Metabolic impact of adding medroxyprogesterone acetate to conjugated estrogen therapy in postmenopausal women. *Obstet Gynecol*, 84, 987–995.

Lombardi, G., Panza, N., Biondi, B., et al. (1993). Effects of lithium treatment on hypothalamic-pituitary-thyroid axis: A longitudinal study. *J Endocrinol Invest*, 16, 259–263.

Longcope, C. (1986). Adrenal and gonadal steroid secretion in normal women. *J Clin Endocrinol Metab*, 15, 213–220.

Lonning, P. E., Johannessen, D. C., Lien, E. A., et al. (1995). Influence of tamoxifen on sex hormones, gonadotrophins and sex hormone binding globulin in postmenopausal breast cancer patients. *J Steroid Biochem Mol Biol*, 52, 491–516.

Loosen, P. T. (1986). Hormones of the hypothalamic-pituitary-thyroid axis: A psychoneuroendocrine perspective. *Pharmacopsychiatry*, 19, 401–415.

Loosen, P. T. (1988a). TRH: Behavioral and endocrine effects in man. *Prog Neuropsychopharm Biol Psychiatry*, 12, (Suppl), S87–S117.

Loosen, P. T. (1988b). Thyroid function in affective disorders and alcoholism. [Review]. In W. A. Brown (Ed.), *Endocrinology of neuropsychiatric disorders* (pp. 55–82). Philadelphia: W. B. Saunders.

Loosen, P. T. (1989). TRH test in psychiatric disorders. In W. E. Bunney, H. Hippius, G. Laakmann, and M. Schmaus (Eds.), *Neuropsychopharmacology* (pp. 328–336). New York: Springer-Verlag.

Loosen, P. T., Chambliss, B., DeBold, C. R., Shelton, R., and Orth, D. N. (1992). Psychiatric phenomenology in Cushing's disease. *Pharmacopsychiatry*, 5, 321–348.

Loosen, P. T., Garbutt, J. C., and Prange, A. J., Jr. (1987). Evaluation of the diagnostic utility of the TRH-induced TSH response in psychiatric disorders. *Pharmacopsychiatry, 20,* 90–95.

Loosen, P. T., Merkel, U., Amelung, U. (1976). Combined sleep deprivation and clomipramine in primary depression. *Lancet, 2,* 156–157.

Loosen, P. T., and Prange, A. J. J. (1982). The serum thyrotropin (TSH) response to thyrotropin-releasing hormone (TRH) in psychiatric patients: A review. *Am J Psychiatry, 139,* 405–416.

Loosen, P. T., and Prange, A. J. J. (1984). Hormones of the thyroid axis and behavior. In C. B. Nemeroff and A. J. Dunn, (Eds.) *Peptides, Hormones and Behavior,* (pp. 533–577). New York: Spectrum Publishers.

Loosen, P. T., Sells, S., Geracioti, T. D., and Garbutt, J. C. (1992). Thyroid hormones and alcoholism. In R. R. Watson (Ed.), *Drug and alcohol abuse reviews,* vol. 3: *Alcohol abuse treatment,* (pp. 283–306). Totowa, NJ: Humana Press.

Love, R. (1994). Prevention of breast cancer in premenopausal women. *J Nat Cancer Inst Monogr, 16,* 61–65.

Love, R. (1995). Approaches to the prevention of breast cancer. *J Clin Endocrinol and Metab, 80,* 1757–1760.

Love, R. R., Mazess, R. B., Barden, H. S., et al. (1992). Effects of tamoxifen on bone mineral density in postmenopausal women with breast cancer. *N Engl J Med, 326,* 852–856.

Love, R. R., Wiebe, D. A., Feyze, J. M., Newcomb, P. A., and Chappell, R. J. (1994). Effects of tamoxifen on cardiovascular risk factors in postmenopausal women after 5 years of treatment. *J Natl Cancer Inst, 86,* 1534–1539.

Love, S. M. (1989). Use of risk factors in counseling patients. *Hematol Oncol Clin North Am, 3,* 599–611.

Luine, V. N., Khylchevskaya, R. I., and McEwen, B. S. (1975). Effect of gonadal steroids on activities of monoamine oxidase and choline acetylase in rat brain. *Brain Res, 86,* 293–306.

Lurie, N., Slater, J., McGovern, P., et al. (1993). Preventive care for women. Does the sex of the physician matter? *N Engl J Med, 329,* 478–482.

Lurie, S. N., Doraiswamy, P. M., Husain, M. M., et al. (1990). In vivo assessment of pituitary gland volume with MRI: Effect of age. *J Clin Endocrinol Metab, 71,* 505–508.

Lynch, H. T., Watson, P., Lynch, J. F., et al. (1993). Hereditary ovarian cancer. Heterogeneity in age at onset. *Cancer, 71,* 573–581.

Lynch, J., Kaplan, G. A., Salonen, R., Cohen, R. D., and Salonen, J. T. (1995). Socioeconomic status and carotid atherosclerosis. *Circulation, 92,* 1786–1792.

Macaron, C., Wilber, J., and Green, O. (1978). Studies of growth hormone (GH), thyrotrophin (TSH) and prolactin (PRL) secretion in anorexia nervosa. *Psychoneuroendocrinology, 3,* 181–185.

Maccoby, E. E., and Jacklin, C. N. (1974). *The psychology of sex differences.* Stanford, CA: Stanford University Press.

MacDonald, P. (1981). Estrogen plus progestin in postmenopausal women. *N Engl J Med, 305,* 1644–1645.

Mack, M., and Ross, R. K. (1989). Risks and benefits of long-term treatment with estrogens. *Schweiz Med Wochenschr, 119,* 1811–1820.

MacLusky, N. J., and Naftolin, F. (1981). Sexual differentiation of the nervous system. *Science*, 211, 1294–1303.

Mahler, M. (1963). Thoughts about development and individuation. *Psychoanal Study Child*, 18, 307–324.

Majewska, M., Harrison, N., Schwartz, R., et al. (1986). Steroid hormone metabolites are barbiturate-like modulators of the GABA receptor. *Science*, 232, 1024–1027.

Majewska, M., and Schwartz, R. (1987). Pregnenolone-sulfate: An endogenous antagonist of the gamma aminobutyric acid receptor complex in brain? *Brain Res*, 404, 355–360.

Mamby, C. C., Love, R. R., and Lee, K. E. (1995). Thyroid function test changes with adjuvant tamoxifen therapy in postmenopausal women with breast cancer. *J Clin Oncol*, 13, 854–857.

Manu, P., Lane, T. J., and Mathews, D. A. (1992). The pathophysiology of chronic fatigue syndrome: Confirmations, contradictions, and conjectures. *Int J Psychiatry Med*, 22, 397–408.

Maraste, R., Brandt, L., Olsson, H., and Ryde-Brandt, B. (1992). Anxiety and depression in breast cancer patients at start of adjuvant radiotherapy. Relations to age and type of surgery. *Acta Oncol*, 31, 641–643.

Marce, L. V. (1858). Traité de la folie des femmes enceintes, des nouvelles accouchées et des nourrices. Paris: Baillière et Fils.

Marchetti, E., Romero, M., Bonati, M., and Tognoni, G., for the International Cooperative Drug Use in Pregnancy study. (1993). Use of psychotropic drugs during pregnancy. A report of the International Cooperative Drug Use in Pregnancy (DUP) study. *Eur J Clin Pharmacol*, 45, 495–501.

Marcus, R., for the PEPI Trial Investigators. (1995). Effects of hormone replacement therapies on bone mineral density results from the postmenopausal estrogen and progestin intervention trial. [Abstract] Program of the 17th Annual Marketing, American Society for Bone and Mineral Research, *J Bone Miner Res*, 1 (Suppl), 276.

Marks, M. N., Wieck, A., Checkley, S. A., and Kumar, R. (1991). Life stress and postpartum psychosis: A preliminary report. *Br J Psychiatry*, 10 (Suppl), 45–49.

Marmar, C. R. (1991). Brief dynamic psychotherapy of post-traumatic stress disorder. *Psychiatr Ann*, 21, 405–414.

Marsh, L., Lauriello, J., Sullivan, E., and Pfefferbaum, A. (1996). Neuroimaging in psychiatric disorders. In E. Bigler (Ed.), *Neuroimaging II: Clinical applications* (pp. 73–125). New York: Plenum Press.

Marshall, W., and Tanner, J. (1969). Variations in pattern of pubertal changes in girls. *Arch Dis Child*, 44, 291–303.

Mason, J. W., Kennedy, J. L., Kosten, T. R., and Giller, E. L., Jr. (1989). Serum thyroxine levels in schizophrenic and affective disorder diagnostic subgroups. *J Nerv Ment Dis*, 177, 351–358.

Massie, M. J., and Holland, J. C. (1990). Depression and the cancer patient. *J Clin Psychiatry*, 51, 12–17.

Massobrio, M., Migliardi, M., Cassoni, P., et al. (1994). Steroid gradients across the cancerous breast: An index of altered steroid metabolism in breast cancer? *J Steroid Biochem Mol Biol*, 51, 175–181.

Masters, W., and Johnson, V. (1966). *Human sexual response.* Boston: Little, Brown.

Masters, W., and Johnson, V. (1970). *Human sexual inadequacy* Boston: Little, Brown.

Masterson, J., Jr. (1968). The psychiatric significance of adolescent turmoil. *Am J Psychiatry*, 124, 1549–1554.

Mastroianni, A. C., Faden, R., and Fedeman, D. (1994). Women's participation in clinical studies. In A. C. Mastroianni, R. Faden, and D. Federman (Eds.), *Women and health research,* vol. I (pp. 36–74). Washington, DC: National Academy Press.

Mattes, R. D., Curran, W. J., Jr., Alavi, J., et al. (1992). Clinical implications of learned food aversions in patients with cancer treated with chemotherapy or radiation therapy. *Cancer*, 70, 192–200.

Matthews, K. A., Kelsey, S. F., Meilahn, E. N., Kuller, L. H., and Wing, R. R. (1989). Educational attainment and behavioral and biologic risk factors for coronary heart disease in middle-aged women. *Am J Epidemiol*, 129, 1132–1144.

Maunsell, E., Brisson, J., and Deschenes, L. (1992). Psychological adaptation to facial disfigurement in a female head and neck cancer patient. *Psychooncology*, 1, 247–251.

Maynard, C. N., Every, N., Litwin, P. E., Martin, J. S., and Weaver, W. D., for the MITI Project Investigators. (1993). Characteristics of black women admitted to coronary care units with suspected acute myocardial infarction: Results from the MITI registry [Abstract 0253]. *Circulation*, 88(4), I, 50.

McArdle, J. M., George, W. D., McArdle, C. S., et al. (1996). Psychological support for patients undergoing breast cancer surgery: A randomised study. *Br Med J*, 312, 813–816.

McClay, E. F., Albright, K. D., Jones, J. A., et al. (1994). Tamoxifen delays the development of resistance to cisplatin in human melanoma and ovarian cancer cell lines. *Br J Cancer*, 70, 449–452.

McClintock, M. (1971). Menstrual synchrony and suppression. *Nature (London)*, 229, 244–245.

McDonald, C. C., Alexander, F. E., Whyte, B. W., Forrest, A. P., and Stewart, H. J. (1995). Cardiac and vascular morbidity in women receiving adjuvant tamoxifen for breast cancer in a randomized trial. *Br Med J*, 311, 977–980.

McElhatton, P. (1994). The effects of benzodiazepine use during pregnancy and lactation. *Reprod Toxicol*, 8, 461–475.

McElroy, S. L., Keck, P. E. Jr, Tugrul, K. C., and Bennett, J. A. (1993). Valproate as a loading treatment in acute mania. *Neuropsychobiology*, 27, 146–149.

McEwen, B. S. (1981). Neural gonadal steroid actions. *Science*, 211, 1303–1310.

McEwen, B. S. (1991). Nongenomic and genomic effects of steroids on neural activity. *Trends Pharmacol Sci*, 12, 141–147.

McMillen, M. (1979). Differential mortality by sex in fetal and neonatal deaths. *Science*, 204, 89–91.

McNeil, T. F. (1987). A prospective study of postpartum psychoses in a high-risk group. *Acta Psychiatr Scand*, 75, 35–43.

McNeil, T. F., Kaij, L., Malmquist-Larsson, A. (1984). Women with non-organic psychoses: Pregnancy's effect on mental health during pregnancy. *Acta Psychiatr Scand*, 75, 140–148.

Mead, M. (1949). *Male and female.* New York: William Morrow.

McLltin, G. J., Brockington, I. F., Lynch, S., and Jones, S. R. (1995). Dopamine supersensitivity and hormonal status in postpartum. *Br J Psychiatry*, 166, 73–79.

Mecklenburg, R., Loriaux, D, and Thompson, R. (1974). Hypothalamic dysfunction in patients with anorexia nervosa. *Medicine*, 53, 147–159.

Menkes, D. B., Coates, D. C., and Fawcett, J. P. (1994). Acute tryptophan depletion aggravates premenstrual syndrome. *J Affect Disord*, 32, 37–44.

Menkes, D. B., Taghavi, E., Mason, P. A., Spears, G. F. S., and Howard, R. C. 1992. Fluoxetine treatment of severe premenstrual syndrome. *Br Med J*, 305, 346–347.

Mercer, P. W., and Khavari, K. A. (1990). Are women drinking more like men? An empirical examination of the convergence hypothesis. *Alcohol Clin Exp Res*, 14, 461–466.

Metz, A., Sichel, D. A., Goff, D. (1988). Postpartum panic disorder. *J Clin Psychiatry*, 49, 278–279.

Meyerhoff, J. L., Oleshansky, M. A., Kalogeras, K. T., et al. (1990). Neuroendocrine responses to emotional stress: Possible interactions between circulating factors and anterior pituitary hormone release. In J. C. Porter and D. Jezova (Eds.), *Circulating regulatory factors and neuroendocrine function* (pp. 91–111). New York: Plenum Press.

Michna, H., Nishino, Y., Neef, G., et al. (1992). Progesterone antagonists: Tumor-inhibiting potential and mechanism of action. *J Steroid Biochem Mol Biol*, 41, 339–348.

Midgely, A. R., and Jaffee, R. B. (1971). Regulation of human gonadotropins: Episodic fluctuation of LH across the menstrual cycle. *J Clin Endocrinol Metab*, 33, 962–969.

Midmer, D., Wilson, L., and Cummings, S. (1995). A randomized, controlled trial of the influence of prenatal parenting education on postpartum anxiety and marital adjustment. *Family Med*, 27, 200–205.

Miller, L. J. (1994). Psychiatric medication during pregnancy: Understanding and minimizing the risks. *Psychiatr Ann*, 24, 69–75.

Misri, S, and Sivertz, K. (1991). Tricyclic drugs in pregnancy and lactation: A preliminary report. *Int J Psychiatry Med*, 21, 157–171.

Mitchell, J., and Bantle, J. (1983). Metabolic and endocrine investigations in women of normal weight with bulimia syndrome. *Biol Psychiatry*, 18, 355–365.

Mitchell, J., Pyle, R., Eckert, E., et al. (1990). A comparison study of antidepressants and structured intensive group psychotherapy in the treatment of bulimia nervosa. *Arch Gen Psychiatry*, 47, 149–157.

Miyai, K., Yamamoto, T., Azukizawa, M., Tshibashi, K., and Kumahara, Y. (1975). Serum thyroid hormones and thyrotrophin in anorexia nervosa. *J Clin Endocrinol Metab*, 40, 334–338.

Monjan, A. A. (1984). Effects of acute and chronic stress upon lymphocyte blastogenesis in mice and humans. In E. L. Cooper (Ed.), *Stress, immunity, and aging* (pp. 81–108). New York: Marcel Dekker.

Moos, R. H. (1968). The development of a menstrual distress questionnaire. *Psychosom Med*, 30, 853–867.

Morgenstern, H., Glazer, W., and Doucette, J. (1996). Handedness and the risk of tardive dyskinesia. *Biol Psychiatry*, 40, 35–42.

Morley, J. E. (1981). Neuroendocrine control of thyrotropin secretion. *Endocr Rev*, 2, 396–436.

Morrison, J. (1989). Childhood sexual histories of women with somatization disorder. *Am J Psychiatry*, 146, 239–241.

Morrow, A., Suzdak, P., and Paul, S. (1987). Steroid hormone metabolites potentiate GABA receptor mediated chloride ion flux with nanomolar potency. *Eur J Pharmacol*, 142, 483–485.

Morrow, G. R., Linde, J., and Black, P. M. (1991). Anticipatory nausea in cancer patients: Replication and extension of a learning model. *Br J Psychol*, 82, 61–72.

Morse, C. A., and Dennerstein, L. (1988). The factor structure of symptom reports in premenstrual syndrome. *J Psychosom Res*, 32, 93–98.

Moshang, T., and Utiger, R. (1977). Low triiodothyronine euthyroidism in anorexia nervosa. In R. Vigersky (Ed.), *Anorexia nervosa* (pp. 263–270). New York: Raven Press.

Moshang, T. J., Parks, J., and Balsor, L. (1975). Low serum triiodothyronine in patients with anorexia nervosa. *J Clin Endocrinol Metab*, 40, 470–473.

Mugge, A., Riedel, M., Barton, M., Kuhn, M., and Lichtlen, P. R. (1993). Endothelium independent relaxation of human coronary arteries by 17β-oestradiol in vitro. *Cardiovasc Res*, 27, 1939–1942.

Muller, B., and Boning, J. (1988). Changes in the pituitary-thyroid axis accompanying major affective disorders. *Acta Psychiatr Scand*, 77, 143–150.

Mumma, G. H., Mashberg, D., and Lesko, L. M. (1992). Long-term psychosexual adjustment of acute leukemia survivors: Impact of marrow transplantation versus conventional chemotherapy. *Gen Hosp Psychiatry*, 14, 43–55.

Murabito, J. M., Anderson, K. M., Kannel, W. B., Evans, J., and Levy, D. (1990). Risk of coronary disease in subjects with chest discomfort: The Framingham Heart Study. *Am J Med*, 89, 297–302.

Murphy, B. E., Dhar, V., Ghadirian, A. M., Chouinard, G., and Keller, R. (1991). Response to steroid suppression in major depression resistant to antidepressant therapy. *J Clin Psychopharmacol*, 11, 121–126.

Murray, L., and Seger, D. (1994). Drug therapy during pregnancy and lactation. *Emerg Med Clin North Am*, 12, 129–149.

Muse, K., Cetel, N., Futterman, L., et al. (1984). The premenstrual syndrome: Effects of "medical ovariectomy." *N Engl J Med*, 311, 1345–1349.

Musisi, S., and Garfinkel, P. (1985). Comparative Dexamethasone Suppression Test measurements in bulimia, depression and normal controls. *Can J Psychiatry*, 30, 190–194.

Myers, A. H., Rosner, B., Abbey, H., et al. (1987). Smoking behavior among participants in the nurses' health study. *Am J Public Health*, 77, 628–630.

Myers, D. H., Carter, R. A., Burns, B. H., et al. (1985). A prospective study of the effects of lithium on thyroid function and on the prevalence of antithyroid antibodies. *Psychol Med*, 15, 55–61.

Myers, J. K., Weissman, M. M., Tischler, G. L., et al. (1984). Six-month prevalence of psychiatric disorders in three communities. *Arch Gen Psychiatry*, 41, 959–966.

Myers, L. S. (1995). Methodological review and meta-analysis of sexuality and menopause research. *Neurosci Biobehav Rev*, 19, 331–341.

Myers, L. S., Dixen, J., Morrissette, D., Carmichael, M., and Davidson, J. M. (1990). The effects of estrogen, androgen and progestin on sexual psychophysiology and behavior in postmenopausal women. *J Clin Endocrinol Metab*, 70, 1124–1131.

Naito, Y., Tamai, S., Shingu, K., et al. (1992). Responses of plasma adrenocorticotropic hormone, cortisol, and cytokines during and after upper abdominal surgery. *Anesthesiology*, 77, 426–431.

National Institute on Drug Abuse. (1994). *National health and pregnancy survey*. Rockville, MD: National Institute on Drug Abuse.

National Surgical Adjuvant Breast and Bowel Project (NSABP). (1992). NSABP Protocol P-1: A clinical trial to determine the worth of tamoxifen for preventing breast cancer. Pittsburgh, PA: National Surgical Adjuvant Breast and Bowel Project, January 24, 1992.

Nayfield, S. G., Karp, J. E., Ford, L. G., Dorr, F. A., and Kramer, B. S. (1991). Potential role of tamoxifen in prevention of breast cancer. *J Natl Cancer Inst*, 83, 1450–1459.

NCEP II, The Expert Panel. (1993). *The second report of the expert panel on: Detection, evaluation and treatment of high blood cholesterol in adults*. Washington, DC: National Institutes of Health, Publication No. 93-3095.

Nemeroff, C. B., Bissette, G., Akil, H., and Fin, M. (1991). Neuropeptide concentrations in the cerebrospinal fluid of depressed patients treated with electroconvulsive therapy: Corticotropin-releasing factor, β-endorphin and somatostatin. *Br J Psychiatry*, 158, 59–63.

Nemeroff, C. B., and Evans, D. L. (1984). Correlation between the dexamethasone suppression test in depressed patients and clinical response. *Am J Psychiatry*, 141, 247–249.

Nemeroff, C. B., Krishnan, K. R. R., Reed, D., et al. (1992). Adrenal gland enlargement in major depression: A computed tomographic study. *Arch Gen Psychiatry*, 49, 384–387.

Nemeroff, C. B., Owens, M. J., Bissette, G., Andorn, A. C., and Stanley, M. (1988). Reduced corticotropin-releasing factor (CRF) binding sites in the frontal cortex of suicides. *Arch Gen Psychiatry*, 45, 577–579.

Nemeroff, C. B., Simon, J. S., Haggerty, J. J., Jr., and Evans, D. L. (1985). Antithyroid antibodies in depressed patients. *Am J Psychiatry*, 142, 840–843.

Nemeroff, C. B., Widerlov, E., Bissette, G., et al. (1984). Elevated concentrations of CSF corticotropin-releasing factor-like immunoreactivity in depressed patients. *Science*, 226, 1342–1344.

Neuhaus, W., Zok, C., Gohring, U. J., and Scharl, A. (1994). A prospective study concerning psychological characteristics of patients with breast cancer. *Arch Gynecol Obstet*, 255, 201–209.

Newcomb, P. A., Longnecker, M. P., Storer, B. E., et al. (1995). Long-term hormone replacement therapy and risk of breast cancer in postmenopausal women. *Am J Epidemiol*, 142, 788–795.

Neziroglu, F., Anemone, R., and Yaryura-Tobias, J. A. (1994). Onset of obsessive compulsive disorder in pregnancy. *Am J Psychiatry*, 149, 947–950.

Nickel, J. T., and Chirikos, T. N. (1990). Functional disability of elderly patients with long-term coronary heart disease: A sex-stratified analysis. *J Gerontol*, 45, S60–S68.

Nielsen, S. (1990). The epidemiology of anorexia nervosa in Denmark from 1973 to 1987: A nationwide register study of psychiatric admission. *Acta Psychiatr Scand*, 81, 507–514.

Nolan-Hoeksema, S. (1995). Epidemiology and theories of gender differences in unipolar depression. In M. V. Seeman (Ed.), *Gender and psychopathology* (pp. 63–87). Washington, DC: American Psychiatric Press.

Nolten, W. E., and Rueckert, P. A. (1981). Elevated free cortisol index in pregnancy: Possible regulatory mechanisms. *Am J Obstet Gynecol*, 139, 492–498.

Nora, J., Nora, A., and Toews, W. (1974). Lithium, Ebstein's anomaly and other congenital heart defects. *Lancet*, 1, 594–595.

Nora, J., Nora, A., and Way, G. (1975). Cardiovascular maldevelopment associated with maternal exposure to amantadine (Letter). *Lancet*, 2, 607.

Nordstrom, G. M., and Nyman, C. R. (1992). Male and female sexual function and activity following ileal conduit urinary diversion. *Br J Urol*, 70, 33–39.

Northcott, C. J., and Stein, M. B. (1994). Panic disorder in pregnancy. *J Clin Psychiatry*, 55, 539–542.

Noshirvani, H. F., Kasvikis, Y., Marks, I. M., Tsakiris, F., and Monteiro, W. O. (1991). Gender-divergent aetiological factors in obsessive-compulsive disorder. *Br J Psychiatry*, 158, 260–263.

Nott, P. N., Franklin, M., Armitage, C., and Gelder, M. G. (1976). Hormonal changes in the puerperium. *Br J Psychiatry*, 128, 379–383.

Nottebohm, F., and Arnold, A. (1976). Sexual dimorphism in vocal control areas of the songbird brain. *Science*, 194, 211–213.

Nowotny, B., Teuber, J., an der Heiden, W., et al. (1990). The role of TSH psychological and somatic changes in thyroid dysfunctions. *Klin Wochenschr*, 68, 964–970.

Nulman, I., Rovet, J., Stewart, D. E., Wolpin, J., Gardner, H. A., Theis, J., Kulin, N., Koren, G. (1997). Neurodevelopment of children exposed in utero to antidepressant drugs. *N Engl J Med*, 336, 258–262.

O'Brien, T. (1974). Excretion of drugs in human milk. *Am J Hosp Pharm*, 31, 844–854.

O'Callaghan, W. G., Teo, K. K., O'Riordan, J., et al. (1984). Comparative response of male and female patients with coronary artery disease to exercise rehabilitation. *Eur Heart J*, 5, 649–651.

O'Dowd, M., and Philipp, E. (1994). *The history of obstetrics and gynaecology*. New York: Parthenon Publishing Group.

O'Hara, M. (1987). Post-partum "blues," depression, and psychosis: A review. *J Psychosom Obstet Gynaecol*, 7, 205–227.

O'Hara, M. A. (1986). Social support, life events and depression during pregnancy and the puerperium. *Arch Gen Psychiatry*, 43, 569–573.

O'Hara, M. S., Zekoski, E. M., Phillips, L. H., and Wright, E. J. (1990). Controlled prospective study of postpartum mood disorders: Comparison of childbearing and non-childbearing women. *J Abnorm Psychol*, 99, 3–15.

O'Hara, M. W., Schlechte, J. A., Lewis, D. A., and Wright, E. J. (1991). Prospective study of postpartum blues. *Arch Gen Psychiatry*, 48, 801–806.

O'Malley, K., Crooks, J., Duke, E., and Stevenson, I. (1971). Effect of age and sex on human drug metabolism. *Br Med J*, 3, 607–609.

O'Shanick, G. J., and Ellinwood, E. H., Jr. (1982). Persistent elevation of thyroid-stimulating hormone in women with bipolar affective disorder. *Am J Psychiatry*, 139, 513–514.

Ochoa, L., Beck, A. T., and Steer, R. A. (1992). Gender differences in comorbid anxiety and mood disorders (Letter). *Am J Psychiatry*, 149, 1409–1410.

Ochs, H., Greenblatt, D., and Otten, H. (1981). Disposition of oxazepam in relation to age, sex, and cigarette smoking. *Klin Wochenschr*, 59, 899–903.

Offer, D., Ostrov, E., and Howard, K. (Eds.). (1981). *The adolescent: A psychological self-portrait*. New York: Basic Books.

Ogilvie, K. M., and Rivier, C. (1996). Gender difference in alcohol-evoked hypothalamic-pituitary-adrenal activity in the rat: Ontogeny and role of neonatal steroids. *Alcohol Clin Exp Res*, **20**, 255–261.

Ogura, C., Okuma, T., Uchida, Y., et al. (1974). Combined thyroid (triiodothyronine)-tricyclic antidepressant treatment in depressive states. *Folia Psychiatr Neurol Jpn*, **28**, 179–186.

Ohkura, T., Isse, K., Akazawa, K., et al. (1994). Evaluation of estrogen therapy of female patients with dementia of Alzheimer type. *Endocr J*, **41**, 367–371.

Ohkura, T., Isse, K., Akazawa, K., et al. (1995). Long-term replacement therapy in female patients with dementia of the Alzheimer type: 7 case reports. *Dementia*, **6**, 99–107.

Omne-Ponten, M., Holmberg, L., Burns, T., et al. (1992). Determinants of the psychosocial outcome after operation for breast cancer. Results of a prospective comparative interview study following mastectomy and breast conservation. *Eur J Cancer*, **28A**, 1062–1067.

Ontiveros, A., Fontaine, R., Breton, G., et al. (1989). Correlation of severity of panic disorder and neuroanatomical changes on magnetic resonance imaging. *J Neuropsychiatry*, **1**, 404–408.

Orencia, A., Bailey, K., Yawn, B. P., and Kottke, T. M. E. (1993). Effect of gender on long-term outcome of angina pectoris and myocardial infarction/sudden unexpected death. *JAMA*, **269**, 2392–2397.

Ornish, D. M., Scherwitz, L. W., Brown, S. E., et al. (1990). Can lifestyle changes reverse atherosclerosis? *Lancet*, **336**, 129–133.

Orsulak, P. J., Crowley, G., Schlesser, M. A., et al. (1985). Free triiodothyronine (T$_3$) and thyroxine (T$_4$) in a group of unipolar depressed patients and normal subjects. *Biol Psychiatry*, **20**, 1047–1054.

Osborne, C. K., Jarman, M., McCague, R., et al. (1994). The importance of tamoxifen metabolism in tamoxifen-stimulated breast tumor growth. *Cancer Chemother Pharmacol*, **34**, 89–95.

Overgaard, K., Hansen, M. A., Jenson, S. B., and Christiansen, C. (1992). Effect of salcatonin given intranasally on bone mass and fracture rates in established osteoporosis: A dose-response study. *Br Med J*, **305**, 556–561.

Owens, J. F., Matthews, K. A., Wing, R. R., and Kuller, L. H. (1992). Can physical activity mitigate the effects of aging in middle aged-women? *Circulation*, **85**, 1265–1270.

Ozasa, H., Kita, M., Inoue, T., and Mori, T. (1990). Plasma dehydroepiandrosterone to cortisol ratios as an indicator of stress in gynecologic patients. *Gynecol Oncol*, **37**, 178–182.

Packard, B., and Eaker, E. (1987). Forward. In E. Eaker, B. Packer, N. K. Wenger, T. B. Clarkson, and H. A. Tyroler (Eds.), *Coronary heart disease in women* (p. iii). New York: Haymarket Doyma.

Paganini-Hill, A., and Henderson V. W. (1994). Estrogen deficiency and risk of Alzheimer's disease in women. *Am J Epidemiol*, **140**, 256–261.

Pagel, M. D., Bicher, J., and Cappel, D. B. (1985). Loss of control, self-blame and depression: An investigation of spouse caregivers of Alzheimer's disease patients. *J Abnorm Psychol*, **94**, 169–182.

Pagley, P. R., and Goldberg, R. J. (1995). Coronary artery disease in women: A population-based perspective. *Cardiology*, **86**, 265–269.

Pajer, K. (1995). New strategies in the treatment of depression in women. *J Clin Psychiatry*, **56** (Suppl 2), 30–37.

Pak, C. Y. C., Sakhaee, K., Piziak, V., et al. (1994). Slow-release sodium fluoride in the management of postmenopausal osteoporosis. A randomized controlled trial. *Ann Intern Med*, 120, 625–632.

Pansini, F., Albertazzi, P., Bonaccorsi, G. (1994). The menopausal transition: A dynamic approach to the pathogenesis of neurovegetative complaints. *Obstet Gynecolo Reprod Bio*, 7, 103–109.

Parish, R., and Spivey, C. (1991). Influence of menstrual cycle phase on serum concentration of alpha 1-acid glycoprotein. *Br J Clin Pharmacol*, 31, 1991.

Parker, L. N., Levin, E. R., and Lifrak, E. T. (1985). Evidence for adrenocortical adaptation to severe illness. *J Clin Endocrinol Metab*, 60, 947–952.

Parry, B. L., Berga, S. L., Kripke, D. F., et al. (1990). Altered waveform of plasma nocturnal melatonin secretion in premenstrual depression. *Arch Gen Psychiatry*, 47, 1139–1145.

Parry, B. L., Cover, H., Mostofi, N., et al. (1995). Early versus late partial sleep deprivation in patients with premenstrual dysphoric disorder and normal comparison subjects. *Am J Psychiatry*, 152, 404–412.

Parry, B. L., Gerner, R. H., Wilkins, J. N., et al. (1991). CSF and endocrine studies of PMS. *Neuropsychopharmacology*, 8, 127–137.

Pastuszak, A., Schick-Boschetto, B., and Zuber, C. (1993). Pregnancy outcome following first-trimester exposure to fluoxetine (Prozac). *JAMA*, 269, 2246–2248.

Pavlov, E. P., Harman, S. M., Chrousos, G. P., Loriaux, D. C., and Blackman, M. R. (1986). Responses of plasma adrenocorticotropin, cortisol, and dihydroepiandrosterone of ovine corticotropin-releasing hormone in healthy aging men. *J Clin Endocrinol Metab*, 62, 767–772.

Paykel, E. S. (1991). Depression in women. *Br J Psychiatry*, 158, 22–29.

Paykel, E. S., Emms, E. M., Fletcher, J., et al. (1980). Life events and social support in puerperal depression. *Br J Psychiatry*, 136, 339–346.

Pearce, K. J., and Hawton, (1996). Psychological and sexual aspects of the menopause and HRT. *Baillière's Clin Obstet Gynec*, 10, 385–399.

Pearce, J., Hawton, K., and Blake, F., (1995). Psychological and sexual symptoms associated with the menopause and the effects of hormone replacement therapy. *Br J Psych*, 167, 162–173.

Pearlstein, T. B., and Stone, A. B. (1994). Long-term fluoxetine treatment in late luteal phase dysphoric disorder. *J Clin Psychiatry*, 55, 332–335.

Pearlstein, T. Y., Frank, E., Rivera-Tovar, A., et al. (1991). Prevalence of Axis I and Axis II disorder in late luteal phase dysphoric disorder. *J Affect Disord*, 20, 129–134.

Pedersen, C., and Prange, A., Jr. (1987). Evidence that central oxytocin plays a role in the activation of maternal behavior. In N. Krasnegor, E. Blass, M. Hofer, and W. Smotherman (Eds.), *Prenatal development: A psychobiological perspective* (pp. 299–320). New York: Academic Press.

Pennebaker, J. W., Kiecolt-Glaser, J. K., and Glaser, R. (1988). Disclosure of traumas and immune function: Health implications for psychotherapy. *J Consult Clin Psychol*, 56, 239–245.

Petersen, A., Sarigiani, P., and Kennedy, R. (1991). Adolescent depression: Why more girls? *J Youth Adolesc*, 20, 247–271.

Petrovic, S. I., McDonald, J. K., De Castro, G., Snyder, C. K., and McCann, S. M. (1983). Regulation of anterior pituitary and brain beta-adrenergic receptors by ovarian steroids. *Life Sci*, 37, 1563–1570.

Phillips, L., and Vassilopoulou-Sellin, R. (1980). Somatomedins. *N Engl J Med*, 302, 438–446.

Phillips, S. M., and Sherwin, B. B. (1992). Effects of estrogen on memory function in surgically menopausal women. *Psychoneuroendocrinology*, 17, 485–495.

Pickens, R. W., Svikis, D. S., McGue, M., et al. (1991). Heterogeneity in the inheritance of alcoholism: A study of male and female twins. *Arch Gen Psychiatry*, 48, 19–28.

Pike, M. C., Ross, R. K., Lobo, R. A., et al. (1989). LHRH agonists and the prevention of breast and ovarian cancer. *Br J Cancer*, 60, 142–148.

Pike, M. C., Spicer, D. V., Dahmoush, L., and Press, M. F. (1993). Estrogens, progestogens, normal breast cell proliferation, and breast cancer risk. *Epidemiol Rev*, 15, 17–35.

Pilote, L., and Hlatky, M. (1995). Attitudes of women toward hormone therapy and prevention of heart disease. *Am Heart J*, 129, 1237–1238.

Pimstone, B., Barbezat, G., and Hansen, J. P. L. (1968). Studies on growth hormone secretion in protein caloric malnutrition. *Am J Clin Nutr*, 21, 482–487.

Pine, D., Cohen, P., and Brook, J. (1996). Emotional problems during youth as predictors of stature during early adulthood: Results from a prospective epidemiologic study. *Pediatrics*, 97, 856–863.

Pinsky, J. L., Jette, A. M., Branch, L. G., Kannel, W. B., and Feinlab, M. (1990). The Framingham disability study: Relationship of various coronary heart disease manifestations to disability in older persons living in the community. *Am J Public Health*, 80, 1363–1368.

Pirke, K., Fichter, M., and Chlond, C. (1987). Disturbances of the menstrual cycle in bulimia nervosa. *Clin Endocrinol*, 27, 245–251.

Pirke, K., Pahl, J., and Schweiger, U. (1985). Metabolic and endocrine indices of starvation in bulimia: A comparison with anorexia nervosa. *Psychiatry Res*, 15, 33–39.

Pirke, K. M., Trimborn, P., Platte, P., and Fichter, M. (1991). Average total energy expenditure in anorexia nervosa, bulimia nervosa, and healthy young women. *Biol Psychiatry*, 30, 711–718.

Pistrang, N., and Barker, C. (1992). Disclosure of concerns in breast cancer. *Psychooncology*, 1, 183–192.

Pistrang, N., and Barker, C. (1995). The partner relationship in psychological response to breast cancer. *Soc Sci Med*, 40, 789–797.

Pitt, B. (1975). Psychiatric illness following childbirth. *Br J Psychiatry Spec Publ*, 9, 409–415.

Pitts, A. F., Samuelson, S. D., Meller, W. H., et al. (1995). Cerebrospinal fluid corticotropin-releasing hormone, vasopressin, and oxytocin concentrations in treated patients with major depression and controls. *Biol Psychiatry*, 38, 330–335.

Plu-Bureau, G., Le, M. G., Sitruk-Ware, R., et al. (1994). Progestogen use and decreased risk of breast cancer in a cohort study of premenopausal women with benign breast disease. *Br J Cancer*, 70, 270–277.

Pokorny, A. D., and Overall, J. E. (1970). Relationships of psychopathology to age, sex, ethnicity, education and marital status in state hospital patients. *J Psychiatry Res*, 7, 143–152.

Pons, G., Rey, E., and Matheson, I. (1994). Excretion of psychoactive drugs into breast milk. Pharmacokinetic principles and recommendations. *Clin Pharmacokinet*, 27, 270–289.

Pope, H. G., Jr., McElroy, S. L., Keck, P. E., and Hudson, J. I. (1991). Valproate in the treatment of acute mania. A placebo-controlled study. *Arch Gen Psychiatry*, 48, 62–68.

Pope, H. J., and Hudson, J. (1992). Is childhood sexual abuse a risk factor for bulimia nervosa. *Am J Psychiatry*, 149, 455–463.

Post, R. M., Gold, P., Rubinow, D. R., et al. (1982). Peptides in cerebrospinal fluid of neuropsychiatric patients: An approach to central nervous system peptide function. *Life Sci*, 31, 1–15.

Potter, J. D., Slattery, M. L., Bostick, R. M., and Gastur, S. M. (1993). Colon cancer: A review of the epidemiology. *Epidemiol Rev*, 15, 499–505.

Powell, G., Brasel, J., and Blizzard, R. (1967). Emotional deprivation and growth retardation simulating idiopathic hypopituitarism I. Clinical evaluation of the syndrome. *N Engl J Med*, 276, 1271–1278.

Powell, L. H., Shaker, L. A., Jones, B. A., et al. (1993). Psychosocial predictors of mortality in 83 women with premature acute myocardial infarction. *Psychosom Med*, 55, 426–433.

Powles, T. J. (1992). The case for clinical trials of tamoxifen for prevention of breast cancer. *Lancet*, 340, 1145–1147.

Powles, T. J., Hickish, T., Kanis, J. A., Tidy, A., and Ashley, S. (1996). Effect of tamoxifen on bone mineral density measured by dual-energy x-ray absorptiometry in healthy premenopausal and postmenopausal women. *J Clin Oncol*, 14, 78–84.

Pozo, C., Carver, C. S., Noriega, V., et al. (1992). Effects of mastectomy versus lumpectomy on emotional adjustments to breast cancer: A prospective study of the first year postsurgery. *J Clin Oncol*, 10, 1292–1298.

Prader, A., Tanner, J., and von Harnack, G. (1963). Catch-up growth following illness or starvation. *J Pediatr*, 62, 646–659.

Prange A. J. (1972). Estrogen may well affect response to antidepressant. *J Am Med Assoc*, 219, 143–144.

Prange, A. J., Jr., Haggerty, J. J., Jr., Browne, J. L., and Rice, J. D. (1990). Marginal hypothyroidism in mental illness: Preliminary assessments of prevalence and significance. In W. E. Bunney, H. Hippius, G. Laakmann, and M. Schmauss (Eds.), *Neuropsychopharmacology* (pp. 352–361). Berlin: Springer-Verlag.

Prange, A. J. J., Loosen, P. T., and Nemeroff, C. B. (1979). Peptides: Application to research in nervous and mental disorders. In S. Fielding (Ed.), *New frontiers of psychotropic drug research* (pp. 117–189). Mount Kisco, NY: Futura Publishing.

Prange, A. J. J., Nemeroff, C. B., and Loosen, P. T. (1978). Behavioral effects of hypothalamic peptides. In J. Hughes (Ed.), *Centrally acting peptides* (pp. 99–118). Basingstroke, UK: Macmillan.

Prange, A. J. J., Wilson, I. C., Rabon, A. M., and Lipton, M. A. (1969). Enhancement of imipramine antidepressant activity by thyroid hormone. *Am J Psychiatry*, 126, 457–469.

Price, W. A., and Heil, D. (1988). Estrogen induced panic attacks. *Psychosomatics*, 29, 433–435.

Prien, R. F., and Kupfer, D. J. (1986). Continuation drug therapy for major depressive episodes: How long should it be maintained? *Am J Psychiatry*, 143, 18–23.

Pritchard, J. (1992). Ondansetron metabolism and pharmacokinetics. *Semin Oncol*, 19, 9–15.

Raádsheer, F. C., Hoogendijk, W. J. G., Stam, F. C., Tilders, F. J., and Swaab, D. F. (1994). Increased numbers of corticotropin releasing hormone expressing neurons in the hypothalamic paraventricular nucleus of depressed patients. *Neuroendocrinology*, 60, 436–444.

Raadsheer, F. C., Van Heerikhuize, J. J., Lucassen P. J., et al. (1995). Increased corticotropin releasing hormone (CRH) mRNA in the paraventricular nucleus of patients with Alzheimer's disease and depression. *Am J Psychiatry*, 152, 1372–1376.

Ramirez, A. J. (1989). Stress and relapse of breast cancer. *Br Med J*, 98, 291–293.

Rapaport, M. H., Thompson, P. M., Kelsoe, J. R., et al. (1995). Gender differences in outpatient research subjects with affective disorders: A comparison of descriptive variables. *J Clin Psychiatry*, 56, 67–72.

Rappaport, R., Prevot, C., and Czernichow, P. (1980). Somatomedin activity and growth hormone secretion. *Acta Pediatr Scand*, 69, 37–41.

Rapkin, J., Edelmuth, E., Chang, A., et al. (1987). Whole blood serotonin in premenstrual syndrome. *Obstet Gynecol*, 70, 533–537.

Rapola, J. M., Virtamo, J., Haukka, J. K., et al. (1996). Effect of Vitamin E and beta carotene on the incidence of angina pectoris. *JAMA*, 275, 693–698.

Raskin, A. (1974). Age-sex differences in response to antidepressant drugs. *J Nerv Ment Dis*, 159, 120–130.

Rasmussen, S. A., and Eisen, J. L. (1992). The epidemiology and clinical features of obsessive compulsive disorder. In M. A. Jenike (Ed.), *Obsessional disorders* (pp. 743–758). Philadelphia: W. B. Saunders.

Rastam, M., Gillberg, C., and Gillberg, I. (1996). A six-year follow-up study of anorexia nervosa with teenage onset. *J Youth Adolesc*, 25, 439–453.

Ratko, T. A., Detrisac, C. J., Mehta, R. G., Kelloff, G. J., and Moon, R. C. (1991). Inhibition of rat mammary gland chemical carcinogenesis by dietary dehydroepiandrosterone or a fluorinated analogue of dehydroepiandrosterone. *Cancer Res*, 51, 481–486.

Ratnasuriya, R., Eisler, I., Szmukler, G., and Russell, G. (1991). Anorexia nervosa: Outcome and prognostic factors after 20 years. *Br J Psychiatry*, 158, 495–502.

Ravindranath, V., and Boyd, M. (1995). Xenobiotic metabolism in brain. *Drug Metab Rev*, 27, 419–448.

Ray, W., Griffin, M., Schaffner, W., Baugh, D., and Melton, L., III. (1987). Psychotropic drug use and the risk of hip fracture. *N Engl J Med*, 316, 363–369.

Rayter, Z., Gazet, J. C., Shepherd, J., et al. (1994). Gynaecological cytology and pelvic ultrasonography in patients with breast cancer taking tamoxifen compared with controls. *Eur J Surg Oncol*, 20, 134–140.

Reame, N., Sauder, S. E., Kelch, R. P., and Marshal, J. C. (1984). Pulsatile gonadotropin secretion during the human menstrual cycle: Evidence for altered pulse frequency of gonadotropin releasing hormone secretion. *J Clin Endocrinol Metab*, 59, 328–337.

Recchione, C., Venturelli, E., Manzari, A., et al. (1995). Testosterone, dihydrotestosterone and oestradiol levels in postmenopausal breast cancer tissues. *J Steroid Biochem Mol Biol*, 52, 541–546.

Redd, W. (1989). Management of anticipatory nausea and vomiting. In J. C. Holland and J. H. Rowland (Eds.), *The handbook of psychooncology* (pp. 423–433). New York: Oxford University Press.

Regier, D. A., Meyer, J. K., Kramer, M., et al. (1984). The NIMH Epidemiological Catchment Area (ECA) Program: Historical context, major objective, and study population characteristics. *Arch Gen Psychiatry*, 41, 934–941.

Rehavi, M., Sepcuti, H., and Weizman, A. (1987). Up regulation of imipramine binding and serotonin uptake by estrogen in female rat brain. *Brain Res*, 410, 135–139.

Reich, T., and Winokur, G. (1970). Postpartum psychoses in patients with manic depressive disease. *J Nerv Ment Disord*, 152, 60–68.

Reimherr, F., Ward, M., and Byerly, W. (1989). The introductory placebo washout: A retrospective evaluation. *Psychiatry Res*, 30, 191–199.

Reinberg, A., Bicakova-Rocher, A., Gorciex, A., Ashkenaxi, I., and Smolensky, M. (1994). Placebo effect on the circadian rhythm period tau of temperature and hand-grip strength rhythms: Interindividual and gender-related difference. *Chronobiol Int*, 11, 45–53.

Reiss, D., and Johnson-Sabine, E. (1995). Bulimia nervosa: 5-year social outcome and relationship to eating pathology. *Int J Eating Disord*, 18, 127–133.

Reiter, E., Biggs, D., Veldhuis, I., and Bietins, I. (1987). Pulsatile release of bioactive luteinizing hormone in prepubertal girls: Discordance with immunoreactive luteinizing hormone pulses. *Pediatr Res*, 21, 409–413.

Renshaw, D. C. (1981). Sexual problems in old age, illness, and disability. *Psychosomatics*, 22(11), 975–985.

Renshaw, D. C. (1983a). Communication in marriage. *Medical Aspects of Human Sexuality*, 17(6), 199–220.

Renshaw, D. C. (1983b). Relationship therapy for sex problems. *Compr Ther*, 9(6), 32–36.

Renshaw, D. C. (1989). The unconsummated marriage. *Medical Aspects of Human Sexuality*, 23(8), 74–79.

Rey, E., d'Athis, P., Gineux, P., et al. (1979). Pharmacokinetics of clorazepate in pregnant and non-pregnant women. *Eur J Clin Pharmacokinet*, 15, 175–180.

Reynolds, P., and Kaplan, G. A. Social connections and risk for cancer: Prospective evidence from the Alameda County Study. *Behav Med*, 16, 101–110.

Richards, M., Casper, R., and Larson, R. (1990). Weight and eating concerns among pre- and young adolescent boys and girls. *J Adolesc Health Care*, 11, 203–209.

Richardson, J., Shelton, D., Krailo, M., and Levine, A. (1990). The effect of compliance with treatment on survival among patients with hematologic malignancies. *J Clin Oncol*, 8, 356–364.

Richardson, J. L., Marks, G., and Levine, A. (1988). The influence of symptoms of disease and side effects of treatment on compliance with cancer therapy. *J Clin Oncol*, 6, 1746–1752.

Rich-Edwards, J. W., Manson, J. E., Hennekens, C. H., and Buring, J. E. (1995). The primary prevention of coronary heart disease in women. *N Engl J Med*, 332, 1758–1766.

Rich-Edwards, J. W., Manson, J. E., Stampfer, M. J., et al. (1995). Height and the risk of cardiovascular disease in women. *Am J Epidemiol*, 142, 909–917.

Rickels, K. (1965). Some comments on non-drug factors in psychiatric therapy. *Psychosomatics*, 6, 303–309.

Rickels, K., Freeman, E., Sondheimer, S., et al. (1989). Buspirone in the treatment of premenstrual syndrome (Letter). *Lancet*, 1, 777.

Rickels, K., Freeman, E., Sondheimer, S., et al. (1990). Fluoxetine in the treatment of premenstrual syndrome. *Curr Ther Res*, 48, 161–166.

Riecher-Roessler, A., and Haefner, H. (1993). Schizophrenia and estrogens—Is there an association? *Eur Arch Psychiatry Clin Neurosci*, 242, 323–328.

Riggs, B. L., Hodgson, S., O'Fallon, W. M., et al. (1990). Effect of fluoride treatment on the fracture rate in postmenopausal women with osteoporosis. *N Engl J Med*, 322, 802–809.

Rigotti, N., Nussbaum, S., Herzog, D., and Neer, R. (1984). Osteoporosis in women with anorexia nervosa. *N Engl J Med*, 311, 1601–1606.

Rijken, M., de Kruif, A. T., Komproe, I. H., and Roussel, J. G. (1995). Depressive symptomatology of post-menopausal breast cancer patients: A comparison of women recently treated by mastectomy or by breast-conserving therapy. *Eur J Surg Oncol*, 21, 498–503.

Riley, V. (1981). Psychoneuroendocrine influences on immunocompetence and neoplasia. *Science*, 212, 1100–1109.

Rinieris, P. M., Christodoulou, G. N., Souvatzoglou, A., Koutras, D. A., and Stefanis, C. N. (1978a). Free thyroxine index in mania and depression. *Compr Psychiatry*, 19, 561–564.

Rinieris, P. M., Christodoulou, G. N., Souvatzoglou, A., Koutras, D. A., and Stefanis, C. N. (1978b). Free-thyroxine index in psychotic and neurotic depression. *Acta Psychiatr Scand*, 58, 56–60.

Risch, S. C., Lewine, R. J., Kalin, N. H., et al. (1992). Limbic-hypothalamic-pituitary-adrenal axis activity and ventricular-to-brain ratio studies in affective illness and schizophrenia. *Neuropsychopharmacology*, 6, 95–100.

Ritchie, J. C., Belkin, B. M., Krishnan, K. R. R., Nemeroff, C. B., and Carroll, B. J. (1990). Plasma dexamethasone concentrations and the dexamethasone suppression test. *Biol Psychiatry*, 27, 159–173.

Rivera-Tovar, A., and Frank, E. (1990). Late luteal phase dysphoric disorder in young women. *Am J Psychiatry*, 147, 1634–1636.

Roberts, C. S., Rossetti, K., Cone, D., and Cavanagh, D. (1992). Psychosocial impact of gynecologic cancer: A descriptive study. *J Psychosoc Oncol*, 10, 99–109.

Robertson, A. G., Tricou, B. J., Fang, V. S., and Meltzer, H. Y. (1982). Biological markers for depressive illness. *Psychopharmacol Bull*, 18, 120–122.

Robinson, D., Friedman, L., Marcus, R., Tinklenberg, J., and Yesavage, J. (1991). Estrogen replacement therapy and memory in older women. *AGS*, 42, 919–922.

Rockel, M., Teuber, J., Schmidt, R., et al. (1987). Correlation of "latent hyperthyroidism" with psychological and somatic changes. *Klin Wochenschr*, 65, 264–273.

Rockey, P. H., and Griep, R. J. (1980). Behavioral dysfunction in hyperthyroidism. Improvement with treatment. *Arch Intern Med*, 140, 1194–1197.

Rodrigue, J. R., Boggs, S. R., Weiner, R. S., and Behen, J. M. (1993). Mood, coping style, and personality functioning among adult bone marrow transplant candidates. *Psychosomatics*, 34, 159–165.

Rojansky, N., Halbreich, U., Zander, K., Barkai, A., and Goldstein, S. (1991). Imipramine receptor binding and serotonin uptake in platelets of women with premenstrual changes. *Gynecol Obstet Invest*, 31, 146–152.

Romero, L. M., Raley-Susman, K. M., Redish, D. M., et al. (1992). Possible mechanism by which stress accelerates growth of virally derived tumors. *Proc Natl Acad Sci USA*, 89, 1084–1087.

Rosano, G. M. C., Sarrel, P. M., Poole-Wilson, P. A., and Collins, P. (1993). Beneficial effects of oestrogen on exercise-induced myocardial ischaemia in women with coronary artery disease. *Lancet*, 342, 133–136.

Rosenblatt, J. (1994). Psychobiology of maternal behavior: Contribution to the clinical understanding of maternal behavior among humans. *Acta Paediatr* (Suppl), 397, 3–6.

Rosensweig, N., and Pearsall, F. P. (1978). Sex education for the health professional. New York: Grune & Stratton.

Rosenzweig, P., Broheir, S., and Zipfel, A. (1993). The placebo effect in healthy volunteers: Influence of experimental conditions on the adverse events profile during phase I studies. *Clin Pharmacol Ther*, 54, 578–583.

Ross, D. S. (1991). Subclinical hypothyroidism. In L. E. Braverman and R. D. Utiger (Eds.), *The thyroid* (pp. 1256–1262). Philadelphia: J. B. Lippincott.

Rossouw, J. E., Finnegan, L. P., Harlan, W. R., et al. (1995). The evolution of the Women's Health Initiative: Perspectives from the NIH. *J Am Med Wom Assoc*, 50, 50–55.

Rounsaville, B. J., Dolinsky, Z. S., Babor, T. F., and Meyer, R. E. (1987). Psychopathology as a predictor of treatment outcome in alcoholics. *Arch Gen Psychiatry*, 44, 505–513.

Rousseau, G. G., Baxter, J. D., and Tomkins, G. M. (1972). Glucocorticoid receptors: Relations between steroid binding and biological effects. *Mol Biol*, 67, 99–115.

Rowland, J. H., Holland, J. C., Chaglassian, T., and Kinne, D. (1993). Psychological response to breast reconstruction: Expectations for and impact on postmastectomy functioning. *Psychosomatics*, 34, 241–250.

Roy, A., Pickar, D., Paul, S., et al. (1987). CSF corticotropin-releasing hormone in depressed patients and normal control subjects. *Am J Psychiatry*, 144, 641–645.

Roy, A., Wolkowitz, O. M., Bissette, G., and Nemeroff, C. B. (1994). Differences in CSF concentrations of thyrotropin-releasing hormone in depressed patients and normal subjects: Negative findings. *Am J Psychiatry*, 151, 600–602.

Roy, M., Neale, M., and Kendler, K. (1995). The genetic epidemiology of self-esteem. *Br J Psychiatry*, 166, 813–820.

Roy-Byrne, P. P., Joffe, R. T., Uhde, T. W., and Post, R. M. (1984). Carbamazepine and thyroid function in affectively ill patients. Clinical and theoretical implications. *Arch Gen Psychiatry*, 41, 1150–1153.

Rubin, R. T., Phillips, J. J., Sadow, T. F., and McCracken, J. T. (1995). Adrenal gland volume in major depression: Increase during the depressive episode and decrease with successful treatment. *Arch Gen Psychiatry*, 52, 213–218.

Rubin, R. T., Poland, R. E., Lesser, I. M., and Martin, D. J. (1989). Neuroendocrine aspects of primary endogenous depression, V: Serum prolactin measures in patients and matched controls. *Biol Psychiatry*, 25, 4–21.

Rubin, R. T., Poland, R. E., Lesser, I. M., et al. (1987). Neuroendocrine aspects of primary endogenous depression, I: Cortisol secretory dynamics in patients and matched controls. *Arch Gen Psychiatry*, 44, 328–336.

Rubinow, D. R., Hoban, M. C., Grover, G. N., et al. (1988). Changes in plasma hormones across the menstrual cycle in patients with menstrually related mood disorder and in control subjects. *Am J Obstet Gynecol*, 158, 5–11.

Rudolph, B., Larson, G. L., Sweeny, S., et al. (1990). Hospitalized pregnant psychotic women: Characteristics and treatment issues. *Hosp Community Psychiatry*, 41, 159–163.

Rugstad, H., Hundal, O., Holme, I., et al. (1986). Piroxicam and naproxen plasma concentrations in patients with osteoarthritis: Relation to age, sex, efficacy and adverse events. *Clin Rheumatol*, 5, 389–398.

Rumeau-Roquette, C., Goujard, J., and Heul, G. (1977). Possible teratogenic effect of phenothiazines in human beings. *Teratology*, 15, 57–64.

Rupprecht, R., Rupprecht, C., Rupprecht, M., Noder, M., and Mahlstedt, J. (1989). Triiodothyronine, thyroxine, and TSH response to dexamethasone in depressed patients and normal controls. *Biol Psychiatry*, 25, 22–32.

Rush, A. J., Schlesser, M. A., Roffwarg, H. P., et al. (1983). Relationships among the TRH, REM latency, and dexamethasone suppression tests: Preliminary findings. *J Clin Psychiatry*, 44, 23–29.

Russell, G. (1977). The present status of anorexia nervosa. *Psychol Med*, 7, 363–367.

Russell, G. (1979). Bulimia nervosa: An ominous variant of anorexia nervosa. *Psychol Med*, 9, 429–448.

Rutqvist, L. E., Cerdermak, B., Glas, U., et al. (1991). Contralateral primary tumors in breast cancer patients in a randomized trial of adjuvant tamoxifen therapy. *J Natl Cancer Inst*, 83, 1299–1306.

Rutqvist, L. E., Johansson, H., Signomklao, T., et al., for the Stockholm Breast Cancer Study Group (1995). Adjuvant tamoxifen therapy for early stage breast cancer and second primary malignancies. *J Natl Cancer Inst*, 87, 645–651.

Rutqvist, L. E., and Mattsson, A. (1993). Cardiac and thromboembolic morbidity among postmenopausal women with early-stage breast cancer in a randomized trial of adjuvant tamoxifen. *J Natl Cancer Inst*, 85, 1398–1406.

Rybakowski, J., and Sowinski, J. (1973). Free thyroxine index and absolute free thyroxine in affective disorders. *Lancet*, 1, 889.

Sabbioni, M. E., and Bovbjerg, D. H., Jacobsen, P. B., et al. (1992). Treatment related psychological distress during adjuvant chemotherapy as a conditioned response. *Ann Oncol*, 3, 393–398.

Sachar, E., Hellman, L., Fukushima, D., and Gallagher, T. (1970). Cortisol production in depressive illness. *Arch Gen Psychiatry*, 23, 289–298.

Sachar, E. J., Schalch, D. S., Reichlin, S., and Platman, S. S. (1972). Plasma gonadotrophins in depressive illness: A preliminary report. In T. A. Williams, M. M. Katz, and J. A. Shield, Jr. (Eds.), *Recent advances in the psychobiology of the depressive illnesses* (pp. 229–233). Washington, DC: DHEW.

Sachar, E. O., Hellman, L., Roffwarg, H., et al. (1973). Disrupted 24-hour patterns of cortisol secretion in psychotic depression. *Arch Gen Psychiatry*, 28, 19–24.

Sachs, G., Rasoul-Rockenschaub, S., Aschauer, H., et al. (1995). Lytic effector cell activity and major depressive disorder in patients with breast cancer: A prospective study. *J Neuroimmunology*, 59, 83–89.

Saletu, B., Brandstatter, N., Metka, M., et al. (1995). Double blind, placebo-controlled, hormonal, syndromal and EEG mapping studies with transdermal oestradiol therapy in menopausal depression. *Psychopharmacology*, 122, 321–329.

Sallis, J. F., Hovell, M. F., and Hofstetter, C. R. (1992). Predictors of adoption and maintenance of vigorous physical activity in men and women. *Prev Med*, 21, 237–251.

Salokangas, R. K. R. (1995). Gender and the use of neuroleptics in schizophrenia. Further testing of the oestrogen hypothesis. *Schizophr Res*, 16, 7–16.

Saltonstall, R. (1993). Healthy bodies, social bodies: Men's and women's concepts and practices of health in everyday life. *Soc Sci Med*, 36, 7–14.

Samuels, M. H., Kramer, P., Wilson, D., and Sexton, G. (1994). Effects of naloxone infusions on pulsatile thyrotropin secretion. *J Clin Endocrinol Metab*, 78, 1249–1252.

Sands, R., and Studd, J. (1995). Exogenous androgens in postmenopausal women. *Am J Med*, 98, 76S–79S.

Sapolsky, R. M., and Donnelly, T. M. (1985). Vulnerability to stress-induced tumor growth increases with age in rats: Role of glucocorticoids. *Endocrinology*, 117, 662–665.

Sapolsky, R. M., Krey, L. C., and McEwen, B. S. (1983). The adrenocortical stress-response in the aged male rat: Impairment of recovery from stress. *Exp Gerontol*, 18, 55–64.

Sapolsky, R. M., Krey, L. C., and McEwen, B. S. (1986). The neuroendocrinology of stress and aging: The glucocorticoid cascade hypothesis. *Endocr Rev*, 7, 284–304.

Sarno, A. P., Miller, E. J., and Lunblad, E. G. (1987). Premenstrual syndrome: Beneficial effects of periodic, low dose danazol. *Obstet Gynecol*, 70, 33–36.

Savard, P., Merand, Y., Di Paolo, T., and Dupont, A. (1983). Effects of thyroid state on serotonin, 5-hydroxyindoleacetic acid and substance P in discrete brain nuclei of adult rat. *Neuroscience*, 10, 1399–1404.

Saxen, I., and Saxen, L. (1975). Association between maternal intake of diazepam and oral clefts (Letter). *Lancet*, 2, 498.

Scanlon, F. (1969). Use of antidepressant drugs during the first trimester. *Med J Austr*, 2, 1077.

Schag, C. A., Ganz, P. A., Polinsky, M. L., et al. (1993). Characteristics of women at risk for psychosocial distress in the year after breast cancer. *J Clin Oncol*, 11, 783–793.

Schairer, C., Byrne, C., Keyl, P. M., et al. (1994). Menopausal estrogen and estrogen-progestin replacement therapy and risk of breast cancer (United States). *Cancer Causes Control*, 5, 491–500.

Schatzberg, A., Kornstein, S., Keitner, G., and Thase, M. (1995). Gender and treatment response in chronic depression. ACNP 34th Annual Meeting, San Juan, Puerto Rico.

Schatzberg, A. F., Rothschild, A. J., Bond, T. C., and Cole, J. O. (1984). The DST in psychotic depression: Diagnostic and pathophysiologic implications. *Psychopharmacol Bull*, 20, 362–364.

Schedlowski, M., Jung, C., Schimanski, G., et al. (1994). Effects of behavioral intervention on plasma cortisol and lymphocytes in breast cancer patients: An exploratory study. *Psychooncology*, 3, 181–187.

Scheibe, G., and Albus, M. (1992). Age at onset, precipitating events, sex distribution, and co-occurrence of anxiety disorders. *Psychopathology*, 25, 11–18.

Scheier, M. F., and Bridges, M. W. (1995). Person variables and health: Personality predispositions and acute psychological states as shared determinants for disease. *Psychosom Med*, 57, 255–268.

Schiff, I., Regestein, Q., Tulchinsky, D., and Ryan, K. (1979). Effects of estrogens on sleep and psychological state of hypogonadal women. *JAMA*, 242, 2405–2407.

Schilder, P. (1935). *The image and appearance of the human body.* London: Kegan, Paul, Trench, Trubner and Co.

Schleifer, S. J., Keller, S. E., Camerino, M., et al. (1983). Suppression of lymphocyte stimulation following bereavement. *JAMA*, 250, 374–377.

Schleifer, S. J., Macari-Hinson, M. M., Coyle, D. A., et al. (1989). The nature and course of depression following myocardial infarction. *Arch Intern Med*, 149, 1785–1789.

Schmidt, P. J., Grover, G. N., and Rubinow, D. R. (1993). Alprazolam in the treatment of premenstrual syndrome: A double blind placebo controlled trial. *Arch Gen Psychiatry*, 50, 467–473.

Schmidt, P. J., Grover, G. N., and Rubinow, D. R. (1993). Alprazolam in the treatment of PMS. A double blind placebo controlled trial. *Arch Gen Psychiatry*, 50, 467–473.

Schmidt, P. J., and Rubinow, D. R. (1991). Menopause-related affective disorders: A justification for further study. *Am J Psychiatry*, 148, 844–852.

Schneider, H. P., and Birkhauser, M. (1995). Does HRT modify risk of gynecological cancers? *Int J. Fertil Menopausal Studies*, 40, 40–53.

Schneider, L. F., Small, G. W., Hamilton, J., et al. (In press). Estrogen replacement and response to fluoxetine in a multicenter geriatric depression trial. *Am J Geriatr Psychiatry*.

Schneider, M. A., Brotherston, P. L., and Hailes, J. (1977). The effect of exogenous oestrogens on depression in menopausal women. *Med J Australia*, 2, 162–163.

Schneider, P. G., Jackisch, C., and Brandt, B. (1994). Endocrine management of breast cancer. *Int J Fertil Menopausal Studies*, 39, 115–127.

Scholl, J. M., Veau, P., Benacerraf, A., et al. (1988). Long-term prognosis of medically treated patients with vasospastic angina and no fixed significant coronary atherosclerosis. *Am Heart J*, 115, 559–564.

Schopf, J., Rust, B. (1994). Follow-up and family study of postpartum psychoses. Part I: Overview. *Eur Arch Psychiatry Clin Neurosci*, 244, 101–111.

Schou, M. (1976). What happened to the lithium babies? A follow-up study of children born without malformations. *Acta Psychiatr Scand*, 54, 193–197.

Schou, M., Goldfield, M., Weinstein, M., and Villeneuve, A. (1973). Lithium and pregnancy. I. Report from the Register of Lithium Babies. *Br Med J*, 2, 135–136.

Schukit, M. A. (1988). Trait (and state) markers of a predisposition to psychopathology. In R. Michaels, J. O. Cavenar, A. M. Cooper, et al. (Eds.), *Psychiatry* (pp. 1–19). Philadelphia: J. B. Lippincott.

Schukit, M. A., Irwin, M., and Smith, T. L. (1994). One-year incidence rate of major depression and other psychiatric disorders in 239 alcoholic men. *Addiction*, 89, 441–445.

Schuler, G., Hambrecht, R., Schlierf, G., et al. (1992). Regular physical exercise and low-fat diet: Effects on progression of coronary artery disease. *Circulation*, 86, 1–11.

Schuster, P. M., and Waldron, J. (1991). Gender differences in cardiac rehabilitation patients. *Rehabil Nursing*, 16, 248–253.

Schuurman, A. G., van den Brandt, P. A., and Goldbohm, R. A. (1995). Exogenous hormone use and the risk of postmenopausal breast cancer: Results from the Netherlands Cohort Study. *Cancer Causes Control*, 6, 416–424.

Schwarcz, G., Halaris, A., Baxter, L., et al. (1984). Normal thyroid function in desipramine nonresponders converted to responders by the addition of L-tri-iodothyronine. *Am J Psychiatry*, 141, 1614–1616.

Schweizer, E. (1995). Generalized anxiety disorder: Longitudinal course and pharmacologic treatment. In M. H. Pollack and M. W. Otto (Eds.), *Anxiety disorders. Longitudinal course and treatment* (pp. 843–857). Philadelphia: W. B. Saunders.

Sclafani, L. (1991). Management of the high-risk patient. *Semin Surg Oncol*, 7, 261–266.

Seeman, M. (1983). Interaction of sex, age and neuroleptic dose. *Compr Psychiatry*, 24, 125–128.

Seeman, M. V. (1995). Gender differences in treatment response in schizophrenia. In M. V. Seeman (Ed.), *Gender and psychopathology* (pp. 227–251). Washington, DC: American Psychiatric Press.

Seeman, M. V. (1996). The role of estrogen in schizophrenia. *J Psychiatry Neurosci*, 21, 123–127.

Seeman, M. V., and Lang, M. (1990). The role of estrogens in schizophrenia gender differences. *Hosp Community Psychiatry*, 16, 185–194.

Segerson, T. P., Kauer, J., Wolfe, H. C., et al. (1987). Thyroid hormone regulates TRH biosynthesis in the paraventricular nucleus of the rat hypothalamus. *Science*, 238, 78–80.

Seguin, L., Potvin, L., St. Denis, M., and Loiselle, J. (1994). Chronic stressors, social support and depression during pregnancy. *Obstet Gynecol*, 85, 583–589.

Selling, L. S., and Ferraro, M. A. (1945). *The psychology of diet and nutrition.* New York: Norton.

Selvini-Palazzoli, M. (1978). *Self-starvation – from individual to family therapy in the treatment of anorexia nervosa.* New York: Jason Aronson.

Serdula, M. K., Byers, T., Mokdad, A. H., et al. (1996). The association between fruit and vegetable intake and chronic disease risk factors. *Epidemiology*, 7, 161–165.

Severino, S. K., and Moline, M. L. (1989). Premenstrual syndrome. A clinician's guide. New York: Guilford Press.

Shannon, R., Fraser, G., Aitken, R., and Harper, J. (1972). Diazepam in preeclamptic toxaemia with special reference to its effect on the newborn infant. *Br J Clin Pract*, 26, 271–275.

Shariff, S., Cumming, C. E., Lees, A., et al. (1995). Mood disorder in women with early breast cancer taking tamoxifen, an estradiol receptor antagonist. An expected or unexpected effect? *Ann NY Acad Sci*, 761, 365–368.

Sharp, N. C., and Koutedakis, Y. (1992). Sport and the overtraining syndrome: Immunological aspects. *Br Med Bull*, 48, 518–533.

Shaver, J. L. F., Giblin, E., and Paulsen, V. (1991). Sleep quality subtypes in midlife women. *Sleep*, 14, 18–23.

Shaw, J., Kennedy, S. H., and Joffe, R. T. (1995). Gender differences in mood disorders. A clinical focus. In M. V. Seeman (Ed.), *Gender and psychopathology* (pp. 89–111). Washington, DC: American Psychiatric Press.

Shekelle, R. B., Raynor, W. J., Jr., Ostfeld, A., et al. (1981). Psychological depression and 17-year risk of death from cancer. *Psychosom Med*, 43, 117–125.

Sheldon, J. M., Fetting, J. H., and Siminoff, L. A. (1993). Offering the option of randomized clinical trials to cancer patients who overestimate their prognoses with standard therapies. *Cancer Invest*, 1, 57–62.

Shelton, R. C., Winn, S., Ekhatore, N., and Loosen, P. T. (1993). The effects of antidepressants on the thyroid axis in depression. *Biol Psychiatry*, 33, 120–126.

Shen, W. H., Hsu, C. H., Chen, Y. S., Jeng, C. Y., and Fuh, M. M. (1994). Prospective evaluation of insulin resistance and lipid metabolism in women receiving oral contraceptives. *Clin Endocrinol*, 40, 249–255.

Shenfield, G., and Griffin, J. (1991). Clinical pharmacokinetics of contraceptive steroids: An update. *Clin Pharmacokinet*, 20, 15–37.

Sherman, B., and Halmi, K. (1977). Effect of nutritional rehabilitation on hypothalamic-pituitary function in anorexia nervosa. In R. Vigersky (Ed.), *Anorexia nervosa* (pp. 211–223). New York: Raven Press.

Sherwin, B. B. (1988). Affective changes and estrogen and androgen replacement therapy in surgically menopausal women. *J Affect Disord*, 14, 177.

Sherwin, B. B. (1995). Changes in sexual behavior as a function of plasma sex steroid levels in post-menopausal women. *Maturitas*, 7, 225–233.

Sherwin, B. B., and Gelfand, M. M. (1985). Sex steroids and affect in the surgical menopause: A double blind, crossover study. *Psychoneuroendocrinology*, 10, 325–335.

Sherwin, B. B., and Gelfand, M. M. (1987). The role of androgen in the maintenance of sexual functioning in oophorectomized women. *Psychosom Med*, 49, 397–409.

Sherwin, B. B., Gelfand, M. M., and Brender, W. (1985). Androgen enhances sexual motivation in females: A prospective crossover study of sex steroid administration in the surgical menopause. *Psychosom Med*, 47, 339–351.

Shi, Y. E., Liu, Y. E., Lippman, M. E., and Dickson, R. B. (1994). Progestins and antiprogestins in mammary tumour growth and metastasis. *Hum Reprod*, 9, 162–173.

Shively, C. A., Clarkson, T. B., and Kaplan, J. R. (1989). Social deprivation and coronary artery atherosclerosis in female cynomolgus monkeys. *Atherosclerosis*, 77, 69–76.

Sholomskas, D. E., Wickamoratne, P. J., Dogolo, L., et al. (1993). Postpartum onset of panic disorder: A coincidental event? *J Clin Psychiatry*, 54, 476–480.

Sichel, D., A., Cohen, L. S., Dimmock, J. A., and Rosenbaum, R. F. (1993). Postpartum obsessive compulsive disorder: A case series. *J Clin Psychiatry*, 54, 156–159.

Sichel, D. A., Cohen, L. S., Robertson, L. M., et al. (1995). Prophylactic estrogen in recurrent postpartum affective disorder. *Biol Psychiatry*, 38, 814–818.

Sieber, W. J., Rodin, J., Larson, L., et al. (1992). Modulation of human natural killer cell activity by exposure to uncontrollable stress. *Brain Behav Immun*, 6, 141–156.

Siegel, B. S. (1986). *Love, medicine and miracles* (pp. 127–225). New York: Harper & Row.

Simmonds, M. (1914). Hypophysisschwund mit toedlichem Ausgang. *Dtsch Med Wochenschr*, 40, 322.

Simpson, G., Yadalam, K., Levinson, D., et al. (1990). Single dose pharmacokinetics of fluphenazine after fluphenazine decanoate administration. *J Clin Psychophamacol*, 10, 417–421.

Sims, M. (1972). Imipramine and pregnancy. *Br Med J*, 2, 45.

Sklar, L. S., and Anisman, H. (1979). Stress and coping factors influence tumor growth. *Science*, 205, 513–515.

Slavney, P. R., and Teitelbaum, M. L. (1985). Patients with medically unexplained symptoms: DSM-III diagnoses and demographic characteristics. *Gen Hosp Psychiatry*, 7, 21–25.

Slone, D., Siskind, V., Heinonen, O., et al. (1977). Antenatal exposure to the phenothiazines in relation to congenital malformations, perinatal mortality rate, birth weight, and intelligence quotient score. *Am J Obstet Gynecol*, 128, 486–488.

Smith, D. C., Prentice, R., Thompson, D. J., and Hermann, W. L. (1975). Association of exogenous estrogen and endometrial carcinoma. *N Engl J Med*, 293, 1164–1167.

Smith, G. R., Monson, R. A., and Livingston, R. L. (1985). Somatization disorder in men. *Gen Hosp Psychiatry*, 7, 4–8.

Smith, J., and Dunn, D. (1979). Sex differences in the prevalence of severe tardive dyskinesia. *Am J Psychiatry*, 136, 1080–1082.

Smith, N. (1980). Excessive weight loss and food aversion in athletes simulating anorexia nervosa. *Pediatrics*, 66, 139–142.

Smith, S., Rhinehart, J. S., Ruddock, V. E., and Schiff, E. (1987). Treatment of premenstrual syndrome with alprazolam: Results of a double blind, placebo-controlled randomized cross over clinical trial. *Obstet Gynecol*, 70, 37–43.

Smith, T. (1992). Hostility and health: Current status of a psychosomatic hypothesis. *Health Psychol*, 11, 193–150.

Sneeuw, K. C., Aaronson, N. K., Yarnold, J. R., et al. (1992). Cosmetic and functional outcomes of breast conserving treatment for early stage breast cancer, 2. Relationship with psychosocial functioning. *Radiother Oncol*, 25, 160–166.

Sobel, D. (1960). Fetal damage due to ECT, insulin coma, chlorpromazine or reserpine. *Arch Gen Psychiatry*, 2, 606–611.

Sokol, R. (1989). The CAGE questions: Practical prenatal detection of risk drinking. *Am J Obstet Gynecol*, 160, 863–870.

Sokol, R., Miller, S., and Reed, G. (1980). Alcohol abuse during pregnancy: An epidemiologic study. *Alcohol Clin Exp Res*, 4, 135–145.

Sokolov, S. T., Kutcher, S. P., and Joffe, R. T. (1994). Basal thyroid indices in adolescent depression and bipolar disorder. *J Am Acad Child Adolesc Psychiatry*, 33, 469–475.

Soma, M. R., Osnago-Gadda, I., Paoletti, R., et al. (1993). The lowering of lipoprotein (a) induced by estrogen plus progesterone replacement therapy in postmenopausal women. *Arch Intern Med*, 153, 1462–1468.

Sorger, D., Schenck, S., and Schneider, D. (1992). Effect of various contraceptives on laboratory parameters in the diagnosis of thyroid gland function with special reference to the free hormones FT_4 and FT_3. *Z Gesamte Inn Med*, 47, 58–64.

Souetre, E., Salvati, E., Belugou, J. L., et al. (1989). Circadian rhythms in depression and recovery: Evidence for blunted amplitude as the main chronobiological abnormality. *Psychiatr Res*, 28, 263–278.

Souetre, E., Salvati, E., Wehr, T. A., et al. (1988). Twenty-four-hour profiles of body temperature and plasma TSH in bipolar patients during depression and during remission and in normal control subjects. *Am J Psychiatry*, 145, 1133–1137.

Southwick, S., Mason, J. W., Giller, E. L., and Kosten, T. R. (1989). Serum thyroxine change and clinical recovery in psychiatric inpatients. *Biol Psychiatry*, 25, 67–74.

Sovner, R., and Orsulak, P. (1979). Excretion of imipramine and desipramine in human breast milk. *Am J Psychiatry*, 136, 451–452.

Spicer, D. V., Pike, A., Rude, R., Shoupe, D., and Richardson, J. (1993). Pilot trial of a gonadotropin hormone agonist with replacement hormones as a prototype contraceptive to prevent breast cancer. *Contraception*, 47, 427–444.

Spicer, D. V., Ursin, G., Parinsky, Y. R., et al. (1994). Changes in mammographic densities induced by a hormonal contraceptive designed to reduce breast cancer risk. *J Natl Cancer Inst*, 86, 431–436.

Spiegel, D. (1992). Conserving breasts and relationships (Editorial). *Health Psychol*, 11, 347–348.

Spiegel, D. (1993). Psychosocial intervention in cancer. *J Natl Cancer Inst*, 85, 1198–1205.

Spiegel, D. (1996). Cancer and depression. *Br J Psychiatry*, 168, 109–116.

Spiegel, D., and Bloom, J. R. (1983). Group therapy and hypnosis reduce metastatic breast cancer pain. *Psychosom Med*, 45, 333–339.

Spiegel, D., Bloom, J., Kraemer, H. C., and Gottheil, E. (1989). The beneficial effect of psychosocial treatment on survival of metastatic breast cancer patients: A randomized prospective outcome study. *Lancet*, 14, 888–891.

Spiegel, D., Bloom, J., and Yalom, I. D. (1981). Group support for patients with metastatic breast cancer. *Arch Gen Psychiatry*, 38, 527–533.

Spiegel, D., Sands, S., and Koopman, C. (1994). Pain and depression in patients with cancer. *Cancer*, 74, 2570–2578.

Stampfer, M. J., Walter, C. W., Colditz, G. A., et al. (1995). A prospective study of postmenopausal estrogen therapy and coronary heart disease. *N Engl J Med*, 313, 1044–1049.

Stanford, J. L., Weiss, N. S., Voigt, L. F., et al. (1995). Combined estrogen and progestin hormone replacement therapy in relation to risk of breast cancer in middle-aged women. *JAMA*, 274, 137–142.

Starkey, T., and Lee, R. (1969). Menstruation and fertility in anorexia nervosa. *Am J Obstet Gynecol*, 105, 374–379.

Steege, J. F., Stout, A. L., Knight, D. L., et al. (1992). Reduced platelet tritium labeled imipramine binding sites in women with PMS. *Am J Obstet Gynecol*, 167, 168–172.

Steering Committee of the Physicians' Health Study Research Group. (1989). Final report on the aspirin component of the ongoing Physicians' Health Study. *N Engl J Med*, 321, 129–135.

Stein, G., and Bernadt, M. (1993). Lithium augmentation therapy in tricyclic-resistant depression. A controlled trial using lithium in low and normal doses. *Br J Psychiatry*, 162, 634–640.

Steinberg, S., Annable, L., Young, S. N., and Belanger, M. C. (1994). Tryptophan in the treatment of late luteal phase dysphoric disorder: A pilot study. *J Psychiatry Neurosci*, 19, 114–119.

Steiner, M., Radwan, M., Elizur, A., et al. (1978). Failure of L-triiodothyronine (T_3) to potentiate tricyclic antidepressant response. *Curr Ther Res*, 23, 655–659.

Steiner, M., Steinberg, S., Stewart, D., et al. (1995). Fluoxetine in the treatment of premenstrual dysphoria. *N Engl J Med*, 332, 1529–1534.

Steingart, R. M., Packer, M., and Hamm, P. (1991). Sex differences in the management of coronary artery disease. *N Engl J Med*, 325, 226–230.

Steinhausen, H., Rauss-Mason, C., and Seidel, R. (1991). Follow-up studies of anorexia nervosa: A review of four decades of outcome research. *Psychol Med*, 21, 447–454.

Sternberg, E. M., Chrousos, G. P., Wilder, R. L., and Gold, P. W. (1992). The stress response and the regulation of inflammatory disease. *Ann Intern Med*, 117, 854–866.

Sternberg, E. M., Wilder, R. L., Gold, P. W., and Chrousos, G. P. (1990). A defect in the central component of the immune system – hypothalamic-pituitary-adrenal axis feedback loop is associated with susceptibility to experimental arthritis and other inflammatory diseases. *Ann NY Acad Sci*, 594, 289–292.

Stewart, D., Raskin, J., and Garfinkel, P. (1987). Anorexia nervosa, bulimia and pregnancy. *Am J Obstet Gynecol*, 157, 1194–1198.

Stewart, D. E., Addison, A. M., Robinson, G. E., et al. (1996). Thyroid function in psychosis following childbirth. *Am J Psychiatry*, 145, 1579–1581.

Stewart, D. E., and Boydell, K. M. (1993). Psychological distress during menopause: Associations across the reproductive life cycle. *Intl J Psychiatry Med*, 23, 157–162.

Stewart, D. E., Klompenhauwer, J. L., Kendell, R. E., and Brockington, I. (1991). Prophylactic lithium in puerperal psychosis. The experience of three centers. *Brit J Psychiatry*, 158, 393–397.

Stewart, R., and Cluff, L. (1974). Gastrointestinal manifestations of adverse drug reactions. *Am J Dig Dis*, 19, 1–7.

Stokes, P. E., and Sikes, C. R. (1987). Hypothalamic-pituitary-adrenal axis in affective disorders. In H. Y. Meltzer (Ed.), *Psychopharmacology: The third generation of progress* (pp. 589–607). New York: Raven Press.

Stone, A. A., Cox, D. S., Valdimarsdottir, H., et al. (1987). Evidence that secretory IgA antibody is associated with daily mood. *J Pers Soc Psychol*, 52, 988–993.

Stone, A. B., and Pearlstein, T. B. (1994). Evaluation and treatment of changes in mood, sleep, and sexual functioning associated with menopause. *Obstet Gynecol Clin North Am*, 21, 391–402.

Stone, A. B., Pearlstein, T. B., and Brown, W. A. (1991). Fluoxetine in the treatment of late luteal phase dysphoric disorder. *J Clin Psychiatry*, 52, 290–293.

Stowe, Z. N., and Nemeroff, C. B. (1995). Women at risk for postpartum-onset major depression. *Am J Obstet Gynecol*, 173, 639–645.

Strang, P. (1992). Emotional and social aspects of cancer pain. *Acta Oncol*, 31, 323–326.

Streissguth, A., and Dehaene, P. (1993). Fetal alcohol syndrome in twins of alcoholic mothers: Concordance of diagnosis and IQ. *Am J Med Genet*, 47, 857–861.

Strober, M., Freeman, R., Bower, S., and Rigali, J. (1996). Binge eating in anorexia nervosa predicts later onset of substance use disorder: A ten-year prospective, longitudinal follow-up of 95 adolescents. *J Youth Adolesc*, 25, 519–532.

Stroebe, M., and Stroebe, W. (1983). Who suffers more? Sex differences in health risks of the widowed. *Psychol Bull*, 93, 279–301.

Strouse, T. B., Szuba, M. P., and Baxter, L. R. (1992). Response to sleep deprivation in three women with postpartum psychosis. *J Clin Psychiatry*, 53, 204–206.

Stuart, S., and O'Hara, M. S. (1995). Interpersonal psychotherapy for postpartum depression: A treatment program. *J Psychother Pract Res*, 4, 18–29.

Studd, J., Chakravarti, S., and Oram, D. (1977). The climacteric. *Clin Obestet Gynecol*, 4, 3–29.

Styra, R., Joffe, R., and Singer, W. (1991). Hyperthyroxinemia in major affective disorders. *Acta Psychiatr Scand*, 83, 61–63.

Sunblad, C., Modigh, K., Andersch, B., et al. (1992). Clomipramine effectively reduces premenstrual irritability and dysphoria: A placebo controlled study. *Acta Psychiatr Scand*, 85, 39–47.

Susman, E., Dorn, L., and Chrousos, G. (1991). Negative affect and hormone levels in young adolescents. *J Youth Adolescence*, 20, 167–190.

Suthers, M. B., Presley, L. S., and Funder, J. W. (1976). Glucocorticoid receptors: Evidence for a second non-glucocorticoid binding site. *Endocrinology*, 9, 260–269.

Svec, F. (1988). Differences in the interaction of RU 486 and ketoconazole with the second binding site of the glucocorticoid receptor. *Endocrinology*, 123, 1902–1906.

Swann, A. C., Stokes, P. E., Casper, R., et al. (1992). Hypothalamic-pituitary-adrenocortical function in mixed and pure mania. *Acta Psychiatr Scand*, 85, 270–274.

Swanson, L. W., Sawchenko, P. E., Rivier, J., and Vale, W. (1983). Organization of ovine corticotropin-releasing factor immunoreactive cells and fibers in the rat brain: An immunohistochemical study. *Neuroendocrinology*, 36, 165–186.

Swift, W. (1982). The long-term outcome of early onset anorexia nervosa: A critical review. *J Am Acad Child Psychiatry*, 21, 38–46.

Sykes, P., Quarrie, J., and Alexander, F. (1976). Lithium carbonate and breast-feeding. *Br Med J*, 2, 1299.

Szigethy, E., Conwell, Y., Forbes, N. T., Cox, C., and Caine, E. D. (1994). Adrenal weight and morphology in victims of completed suicide. *Biol Psychiatry*, 36, 374–380.

Szmukler, G., Brown, S., and Parsons, V. (1985). Premature loss of bone in chronic anorexia nervosa. *Br Med J Clin Res Educ*, 290, 26–27.

Tabar, L., Pagerberg, G., Day, N. E., et al. (1992). Breast cancer treatment and natural history: New insights from results of screening. *Lancet*, 339, 412–414.

Talbott, E., Kuller, L., Detre, K., et al. (1977) Biologic and psychosocial risk factors of sudden death from coronary disease in white women. *Am J Cardiol*, 39, 858–864.

Tanner, J. (1981). *History of the study of human growth*, vol. 289–298. Cambridge, UK: Cambridge University Press.

Tanner, J., Whitehouse, R., and Marshall, W. (1975). *Assessment of skeletal maturity and prediction of adult height: TW 2 method*. New York: Academic Press.

Tappy, L., Randin, J. P., Schwed, P., Wertheimer, J., and Lemarchand Beraud, T. (1987). Prevalence of thyroid disorders in psychogeriatric inpatients. A possible relationship of hypothyroidism with neurotic depression but not with dementia. *J Am Geriatr Soc*, 35, 526–531.

Targum, S. D., Greenberg, R. D., Harmon, R. L., et al. (1984). Thyroid hormone and the TRH stimulation test in refractory depression. *J Clin Psychiatry*, 45, 345–346.

Taylor, D., Mathew, R. J., Ho, H., and Weinman, M. L. (1984). Serotonin levels and platelet uptake during premenstrual tension. *Neuropsychobiology*, 12, 16–18.

Temoshok, L. (1985). Biopsychosocial studies on cutaneous malignant melanoma: Psychosocial factors associated with prognostic indicators, progression, psychophysiology and tumor-host response. *Soc Sci Med*, 20, 833–840.

Temoshok, L., and Dreher, H. (1992). *The Type C connection: The behavioral links to cancer and your health*. New York: Random House.

Temoshok, L., Heller, B. W., Sagebiel, R. W., et al. (1985). The relationship of psychosocial factors to prognostic indicators in cutaneous malignant melanoma. *J Psychosom Med*, 29, 139–154.

Thase, M. E., Kupfer, D. J., and Jarrett, D. B. (1989). Treatment of imipramine-resistant recurrent depression, I: An open clinical trial of adjunctive L-triiodothyronine. *J Clin Psychiatry*, 50, 385–388.

Theander, S. (1970). Anorexia nervosa: A psychiatric investigation of 94 female cases. *Acta Psychiatr Scand*, 214, 1–194.

Theander, S. (1985). Outcome and prognosis in anorexia nervosa and bulimia: Some results of previous investigations, compared with those of a Swedish long-term study. *J Psychiatr Res*, 19, 493–508.

Theorell, T., Orth-Gomer, K., and Eneroth, P. (1990). Slow-reacting immunoglobulin in relation to social support and changes in job strain: A preliminary note. *Psychosom Med*, 52, 511–516.

Thompson, J., and Oswald, I. (1977). Effects of estrogen on the sleep, mood and sexuality of menopausal women. *Br Med J*, 2, 1317–1319.

Thoresen, C. E., and Graff-Low, K. (1990). Women and the Type A behavior pattern: Review and commentary. *J Soc Behav Pers*, 5, 117–133.

Tien, R. D., Kucharczyk, J., Bessette, J., and Middleton, M. (1992). MR imaging of the pituitary gland in infants and children: Changes in size, shape, and MR signal with growth and development. *Am J Roentgenol*, 158, 1151–1154.

Tikkanen, M. J., Kuusi, T., Nikkila, E. A., and Sipinen, S. (1986). Post-menopausal hormone replacement therapy: Effects of progestogens on serum lipids and lipoproteins: A review. *Maturitas*, 8, 7–17.

Tizabi, Y., Aguilera, G., and Gilad, G. M. (1992). Age-related reduction in pituitary corticotropin-releasing hormone receptors in two rat strains. *Neurobiol Aging*, 13, 227–230.

Tolstrup, K., Brinch, M., Isagen, T., et al. (1985). Long-term outcome of 151 cases of anorexia nervosa. *Acta Psychol Scand*, 71, 380–387.

Torrey, E. F. (1992). Are we overestimating the genetic contribution to schizophrenia? *Schizophr Bull*, 18, 159–170.

Troutman, W. (1979). *Drugs in pregnancy*. Washington, DC: Drug Intelligence Publications.

Trouton, D. S. (1957). Placebos and their psychological effects. *J Ment Sci*, 103, 344–354.

Tsutsui, S., Yamazaki, Y., Namba, Y., Tsushima, M. (1979). Combined therapy of T_3 antidepressants in depression. *J Int Med Res*, 7, 138–146.

Tunbridge, W. M. G., and Caldwell, G. (1991). The epidemiology of thyroid diseases. In L. E. Braverman and R. D. Utiger (Eds.), *The thyroid gland* (pp. 578–587). Philadelphia: J. B. Lippincott.

Turner, B. B., and Weaver, D. A. (1985). Sexual dimorphism of glucocorticoid binding in rat brain. *Brain Res*, 343, 16–23.

Uhlenhuth, E. H., and Paykel, E. S. (1973). Symptom intensity and life events. *Arch Gen Psychiatry*, 28, 744–748.

Uhlir, F., and Ryznar, J. (1973). Appearance of chlorpromazine in mothers' milk. *Act Nerv Super*, 15, 106.

Unden, F., Ljunggren, J. G., Beck-Friis, J., Kjellman, B. F., and Wetterberg, L. (1988). Hypothalamic-pituitary-gonadal axis pulse detection. *Am J Physiol*, 250, E486–E493.

Unden, F., Ljunggren, J. G., Kjellman, B. F., Beck-Friis, J., Wetterberg, L. (1986). Twenty-four-hour serum levels of T_4 and T_3 in relation to decreased TSH serum levels and decreased TSH response to TRH in affective disorders. *Acta Psychiat Scand*, 73, 358–365.

U.S. Bureau of the Census. (1990). *Statistical abstract of the United States: 1990*. Washington, DC.

U.S. Department of Health and Human Services (DHSS). (1988). Mortality, part B, in *Vital statistics of the United States, 1986* (pp. 170–195). Washington, DC: Publication PHS 88-1114.

Vagenakis, A., Burger, A., Portnary, G., et al. (1975). Diversion of peripheral thyroxine metabolism from activating pathways during complete fasting. *J Clin Endocrinol Metab*, 41, 191–194.

Vale, W., Spiess, J., Rivier, C., and Rivier, J. (1981). Characterization of a 41 residue ovine hypothalamic peptide that stimulates secretion of corticotropin of β-endorphin. *Science*, 213, 1394–1397.

Van Gent, E. M., and Verhoeven, W. M. (1992). Bipolar illness, lithium prophylaxis and pregnancy. *Pharmacopsychiatry*, 26, 187–191.

Van Hartesveldt, C., and Joyce, J. N. (1986). Effects of estrogen on the basal ganglia. *Neurosci Biobehav Rev*, 10, 1–14.

VanHulle, R., and Demol, R. (1976). A double blind study into the influence of estriol on a number of psychological tests in postmenopausal women. In P. A. Van Kemp, R. B. Greenblatt, and E. Albeaux-Fernet (Eds.), *Consensus on menopause research*. London: MTP Press.

Veith, I. J. (1965). *Hysteria: The history of a disease*. Chicago: University of Chicago Press.

Veith, R. C., Lewis, N., Langohr, J. I., et al. (1992). Effect of desipramine on cerebrospinal fluid concentrations of corticotropin-releasing factor in human subjects. *Psychiatry Res*, 46, 1–8.

Verburg, C., Griez, C., and Meijer, J. (1994). Increase of panic disorder during second half of pregnancy. *Eur Psychiatry*, 9, 260–261.

Videbech, P., and Gouliaev, G. (1995). First admission with puerperal psychosis: 7–14 years of follow-up. *Acta Psychiatr Scand*, 91, 167–173.

Vigersky, R., Andersen, A., Thompson, R., and Loriaux, D. (1977). Hypothalamic dysfunction in secondary amenorrhea associated with simple weight loss. *N Engl J Med*, 297, 1141–1145.

Vigersky, R., Loriaux, D., and Andersen, A. (1976). Delayed pituitary hormone response to LRF, TRF in patients with anorexia nervosa and with secondary amenorrhea associated with simple weight loss. *J Clin Endocrinol Metab*, 43, 898–900.

Villeneuve, A., Langelier, P., and Bedard, P. (1980). Estrogens, dopamine and dyskinesias. *Can Psychiatr Assoc J*, 23, 68–70.

Villeponteaux, V. A., Lydiard, R. B., Laraia, M. T., Stuart, G. W., and Ballinger, J. C. (1992). The effects of pregnancy on preexisting panic disorder. *J Clin Psychiatry*, 53, 201–203.

Vinogradov, S., and Csernansky, J. G. (1990). Postpartum psychosis with abnormal movements: Dopamine supersensitivity unmasked by withdrawal of endogenous estrogens? *J Clin Psychiatry*, 51, 365–366.

Von Schoultz, B. (1986). Climacteric complaints as influenced by progestogens. *Maturitas*, 8, 107–112.

Wagner, J. D., Clarkson, T. B., St. Clair, R. W., et al. (1991). Estrogen and progesterone replacement therapy reduces low density lipoprotein in the coronary arteries of surgically postmenopausal cynomologus monkeys. *J Clin Invest*, **88**, 1995–2002.

Wahby, V., Ibrahim, G., Friedenthal, S., et al. (1989). Serum concentrations of circulating thyroid hormones in a group of depressed men. *Neuropsychobiology*, **22**, 8–10.

Wakeling, A., DeSouza, V., Gore, M., et al. (1979). Amenorrhea, body weight and serum hormone concentration, with particular reference to prolactin and thyroid hormones in anorexia nervosa. *Psychol Med*, **9**, 265–272.

Wald, A., Van Thiel, D., Hoeshtetter, L., et al. (1981). Gastrointestinal transit: The effect of the menstrual cycle. *Gastroenterology*, **80**, 1497–1500.

Walford, G., and McCune, N. (1991). Long-term outcome in early-onset anorexia nervosa. *Br J Psychiatry*, **159**, 383–389.

Wallace, J. E., and McCrimmon, D. J. (1980). Acute hyperthyroidism: Cognitive and emotional correlates. *J Abnorm Psychol*, **89**, 519–527.

Walle, T., Walle, U., Fagan, T., Topmiller, M., and Conradi, E. (1993). Influence of gender and sex steroid hormones on plasma binding of the propanalol enantiomers. *Clin Pharmacol Ther*, **53**, 183.

Walsh, B., Katz, J., Levin, J., et al. (1978). Adrenal activity in anorexia nervosa. *Psychosom Med*, **40**, 499–506.

Walsh, B., Roose, S., and Katz, J. (1987). Hypothalamic-pituitary-adrenal-cortical activity in anorexia nervosa and bulimia. *Psychoneuroendocrinology*, **12**, 131–140.

Walsh, B., Stewart, J., Roose, S., Gladis, M., and Glassman, A. (1984). Treatment of bulimia with phenelzine: A double-blind, placebo-controlled study. *Arch Gen Psychiatry*, **41**, 1105–1109.

Walsh, B. W., Schiff, I., Rosner, B., et al. (1991). Effects of postmenopausal estrogen replacement on the concentrations and metabolism of plasma lipoproteins. *N Engl J Med*, **325**, 1196–1204.

Wang, Z., and de Vries, G. (1993). Testosterone effects on paternal behavior and vasopressin immunoreactive projections in prairie voles. *Brain Res*, **631**, 156–160.

Ward, S., Leventhal, H., Easterling, D., et al. (1992). Social support, self-esteem, and communication in patients receiving chemotherapy. *J Psychosoc Oncol*, **9**, 95–116.

Ware, M., and DeVane, C. (1990). Imipramine treatment of panic disorder during pregnancy. *J Clin Psychiatry*, **51**, 482–484.

Warren, M., and Vande Wiele, R. (1973). Clinical and metabolic features of anorexia nervosa. *Am J Obstet Gynecol*, **117**, 435–449.

Washburn, S. A., Adams, M. R., Clarkson, T. B., and Adelman, S. J. (1993). A conjugated equine estrogen with differential effects on uterine weight and plasma cholesterol in the rat. *Am J Obstet Gynecol*, **169**, 251–256.

Waters, D., Higginson, L., Gladstone, P., et al., for the CCAIT Study Group. (1995). Effects of cholesterol lowering on the progression of coronary atherosclerosis in women. *Circulation*, **92**, 2404–2410.

Watson, S. J., Lopez, J. F., Young, E. A., et al. (1986). Effects of low dose ovine corticotropin-releasing hormone in humans: Endocrine relationships and beta-endorphin/beta-lipotropin responses. *J Clin Endocrinol Metab*, **66**, 10–15.

Watts, G. F., Lewis, B., Brunt, J. N. H., et al. (1992). Effects on coronary artery disease of lipid-lowering diet, or diet plus cholestyramine, in the St Thomas' Atherosclerosis Regression Study (STARS). *Lancet*, **339**, 563–569.

Watts, J. F., Butts, W. R., and Edwards, R. L. (1987). Clinical trial using danazol for the treatment of premenstrual tension. *Br J Obstet Gynaecol*, 94, 30–34.

Watts, J. F., Butts, W. R., Edwards, R. I., and Holder, G. (1985). Hormonal studies in women with premenstrual tension. *Br J Obstet Gynaecol*, 92, 247–255.

Watts, J. F., Edwards, R. L., Butts, W. R. (1985). Treatment of premenstrual syndrome using danazol: Preliminary report of a placebo-controlled, double-blind, dose ranging study. *J Int Med Res*, 13, 127–128.

Watts, N. B., Harris, S. T., Genant, H. K., et al. (1990). Intermittent cyclical etidronate treatment of postmenopausal osteoporosis. *N Engl J Med*, 323, 73–79.

Waxler-Morrison, N., Hislop, T. G., Mears, B., and Kan, L. (1992). Effects of social relationships on survival for women with breast cancer: A prospective study. *Soc Sci Med*, 33, 177–183.

Webster, P. (1973). Withdrawal symptoms in neonates associated with maternal antidepressant therapy. *Lancet*, 2, 318–319.

Weeke, A., and Weeke, J. (1978). Disturbed circadian variation of serum thyrotropin in patients with endogenous depression. *Acta Psychiatr Scand*, 57, 281–289.

Weeke, A., and Weeke, J. (1980). The 24-hour pattern of serum TSH in patients with endogenous depression. *Acta Psychiatr Scand*, 62, 69–74.

Wehr, T. A. (1990). Manipulations of sleep and phototherapy: Nonpharmacological alternatives in the treatment of depression. *Clin Neuropharmacol*, 13 (Suppl 1), S54–S65.

Wehr, T. A., and Goodwin, F. K. (1979). Rapid cycling in manic-depressives induced by tricyclic antidepressants. *Arch Gen Psychiatry*, 36, 555–559.

Wehr, T. A., Sack, D. A., Rosenthal, N. E., and Cowdry, R. W. (1988). Rapid cycling affective disorder: Contributing factors and treatment responses in 51 patients. *Am J Psychiatry*, 145, 179–184.

Wei, G., and Heppner, G. (1987). Natural killer activity of lymphoxytic infiltrates in mouse mammary lesions. *Br J Cancer*, 55, 589–594.

Wei, W. Z., Fulton, A., Winkelhake, J., et al. (1989). Correlation of natural killer activity with tumorigenesis of a preneoplastic mouse mammary lesion. *Cancer Res*, 49, 2709–2715.

Weidner, G., Sexton, G., McLellarn, R., Connor, S. L., and Matarazzo, J. D. (1987). The role of Type A behavior and hostility in an elevation of plasma lipids in adult women and men. *Psychosom Med*, 49, 136–145.

Weinstein, M. R., and Goldfield, M. D. (1975). Cardiovascular malformations with lithium use during pregnancy. *Am J Psychiatry*, 132, 529–531.

Weisse, C. S., Pato, C. N., McAllister, C. G., et al. (1990). Differential effects of controllable and uncontrollable acute stress on lymphocyte proliferation and leukocyte percentages in humans. *Brain Behav Immun*, 4, 339–351.

Weissman, M. M. (1993). Family genetic studies of panic disorder. *J Psychiatr Res*, 27 (Suppl 1), 69–78.

Weissman, M. M., Bland, R., Joyce, P. R., et al. (1993). Sex differences in rates of depression: Cross-national perspectives. *J Affect Disord*, 29, 77–84.

Weissman, M. M., and Klerman, G. L. (1977). Sex differences and the epidemiology of depression. *Arch Gen Psychiatry*, 34, 98–111.

Weissman, M. M., Klerman, G. L., Markowitz, J. S., and Ouellette, R. (1989). Suicidal ideation and suicide attempts in panic disorder and attacks. *N Engl J Med*, 321, 1209–1214.

Weller, L., Weller, A., and Avinir, O. (1995). Menstrual synchrony: Only in roommates who are close friends? *Physiol Behav*, 58, 883–889.

Weltzin, T., McConaha, C., McKee, M., et al. (1991). Circadian patterns of cortisol, prolactin, and growth hormonal secretion during binging and vomiting in normal weight bulimic patients. *Biol Psychiatry*, 30, 37–48.

Wenger, N. K. (1985). Coronary disease in women. *Annu Rev Med*, 36, 285–294.

Wenger, N. K., Speroff, L., and Packard, B. (1993). Cardiovascular health and disease in women. *N Engl J Med*, 329, 247–256.

Werne, J., and Yalom, I. (Eds.). (1996). *Treating eating disorders*. San Francisco: Jossey-Bass.

West, C. P., and Hillier (1994). Ovarian suppression with the gonadotrophin-releasing hormone agonist goserelin (Zoladex) in management of the premenstrual tension syndrome. *Human Repro*, 9, 1058–1063.

Wheathley, D. (1972). Potentiation of amitryptyline by thyroid hormone. *Arch Gen Psychiatry*, 26, 229–233.

Whitehead, P. C., and Layne, N. (1987). Young female Canadian drinkers: Employment, marital status and heavy drinking. *Br J Addict*, 82, 169–174.

Whybrow, P. C. (1991). Behavioral and psychiatric aspects of hypothyroidism. In L. E. Braverman and R. D. Utiger (Eds.), *The thyroid* (pp. 1078–1083). Philadelphia: J. B. Lippincott.

Whybrow, P. C., Coppen, A., Prange, A. J. J., Noguera, R., and Bailey, J. E. (1972). Thyroid function and the response to liothyronine in depression. *Arch Gen Psychiatry*, 26, 242–245.

Whybrow, P. C., Prange, A. J., Jr., and Treadway, C. R. (1969). The mental changes accompanying thyroid gland dysfunction. *Arch Gen Psychiatry*, 20, 48–63.

Wieck, A. (1989). Endocrine aspects of postnatal depression. *Baillieres Clin Obstet Gynaecology*, 3, 857–877.

Wieck, A., and Kumar, R. (1991). Increased sensitivity of dopamine receptors and recurrence of affective psychosis after childbirth. *Br Med J*, 613–616.

Wiklund, I., Johansson, S., Bengtson, A., Karlson, B. W., and Persson, N. J. (1993). Subjective symptoms and well-being differ in women and men after myocardial infarction. *Eur Heart J*, 14, 1315–1319.

Wilbush, J. (1980). Tilt, E. J., and the change of life (1857) – the only work in the English language. *Maturitas*, 2, 259–267.

Wilhelm, K., and Parker, G. (1994). Sex differences in lifetime depression rates: Fact or artifact? *Psychol Med*, 24, 97–111.

Wilkie, D. J., Keefe, F. J., Dodd, M. J., and Copp, L. A. (1992). Behavior of patients with lung cancer: Description and associations with oncologic and pain variables. *Pain*, 51, 231–240.

Williams, J. B. W., Spitzer, R. L., Linzer, M., et al. (1995). Gender differences in depression in primary care. *Am J Obstet Gynecol*, 173, 654–659.

Williams, J. K., Adams, M. R., and Klopfenstein, H. S. (1990). Estrogen modulates responses of atherosclerotic coronary arteries. *Circulation*, 81, 1680–1687.

Williams, K. E. (1990). Hysteria in seventeenth century case records and unpublished manuscripts. *Hist Psychiatry*, 1, 383–401.

Williams, R. B., Barefoot, J. C., Califf, R. M., et al. (1992). Prognostic importance of social and economic resources among patients with angiographically documented coronary artery disease. *JAMA*, 267, 520–524.

Wilsnack, S. C., and Wilsnack, R. W. (1995). Drinking and problem drinking in U.S. women. In M. Galanter (Ed.), *Recent developments in alcoholism. Volume 12: Women and alcoholism* (pp. 29–60). New York: Plenum Press.

Wilson, H. (1992). A critical review of menstrual synchrony. *Psychoneuroendocrinology*, 17, 565–591.

Wilson, I. C., Prange, A. J. J., McClane, T. K., Rabon, A. M., and Lipton, M. A. (1970). Thyroid hormone enhancement of imipramine in nonretarded depression. *N Engl J Med*, 282, 1063–1067.

Wilson, K. (1984). Sex-related differences in drug disposition in man. *Clin Pharmacokinet*, 9, 189–202.

Wilson, W. H., and Jefferson, J. W. (1985). Thyroid disease, behavior, and psychopharmacology. *Psychosomatics*, 26, 481–492.

Wilson, W. P., Johnson, J. E., and Feist, F. W. (1996). Thyroid hormone and brain function. 2. Changes in photically elicited EEG responses following the administration of triiodothyronine to normal subjects. *Electroencephalogr Clin Neurophysiol*, 16, 329–331.

Wilson, W. P., Johnson, J. E., and Smith, R. B. (1962). Affective change in thyrotoxicosis and experimental hypermetabolism. In *Recent advances in biological psychiatry*. New York: Plenum Press.

Wingard, J. R., Curbow, B., Baker, F., Zabora, J., and Piantadosi, S. (1992). Sexual satisfaction in survivors of bone marrow transplantation. *Bone Marrow Transplant*, 9, 185–190.

Winokur, A., Amsterdam, J., Caroff, S., Snyder, P. J., and Brunswick, D. (1982). Variability of hormonal responses to a series of neuroendocrine challenges in depressed patients. *Am J Psychiatry*, 139, 39–44.

Winokur, G. (1979). Unipolar depression. It is divisible into autonomous subtypes? *Arch Gen Psychiatry*, 36, 47–52.

Winokur, G. (1983). Alcoholism and depression. *Subst Alcohol Actions-Misuse*, 4, 111–119.

Wisner, K., and Perel, J. (1991). Serum nortriptyline levels in nursing mothers and their infants. *Am J Psychiatry*, 148, 1234–1236.

Wisner, K. L., and Wheeler, S. B. (1994). Prevention of recurrent postpartum major depression. *Hosp Community Psychiatry*, 45, 1191–1196.

Witelson, S. F., and Kigar, D. L. (1992). Sylvian fissure morphology and asymmetry in men and women—Bilateral differences in relation to handedness in men. *J Comp Neurol*, 323, 326–340.

Wittchen, H.-U., and Essau, C. A. (1993). Epidemiology of panic disorder: Progress and unresolved issues. *J Psychiatr Res*, 27, 47–68.

Wittchen, H.-U., Esssau, C. A., von Zerssen, D., Krieg, J.-C., and Zaudig, M. (1992). Lifetime and six-month prevalence of mental disorders in the Munich follow-up study. *Eur J Psychiatry Neurosci*, 241, 247–258.

Wolf, S., and Pinsky, R. (1954). Effects of placebo administration and occurrence of toxic reactions. *JAMA*, 155, 339–341.

Wolkowitz, O. M., Reus, V. I., Manfredi, F., et al. (1993). Ketoconazole administration in hypercortisolemic depression. *Am J Psychiatry*, 150, 810–813.

Wood, S. H., Mortola, J. F., Chan, Y. F., Moossazdeh, F., and Yen, S. S. (1992). Treatment of premenstrual syndrome with fluoxetine: A double-blind, placebo-controlled, cross-over study. *Obstet Gynecol*, 80, 339–444.

Wool, C. A., and Barsky, A. J. (1994). Do women somatize more than men? *Psychosomatics*, 35, 445–452.

Wooster, R., Bignell, G., Lancaster, J., et al. (1995). Identification of the breast cancer susceptibility gene BRCA2. *Nature*, 378, 789–792.

Writing Group for the PEPI Trial. (1995). Effects of estrogen or estrogen/progestin regimens on heart disease risk factors in postmenopausal women. The Postmenopausal Estrogen/Progestin Interventions (PEPI) Trial. *JAMA*, 237, 199–208.

Wu, J. C., and Bunney, W. E. (1990). The biological basis of an antidepressant response to sleep deprivation and relapse: Review and hypothesis. *Am J Psychiatry*, 147, 14–21.

Wyeth-Ayerst, L. (1996). Letter re: Teratogenicity of Effexor. Wyeth-Ayerst Laboratories, Philadelphia, PA.

Wynn, P. C., Aguilera, G., Morell, J., and Catt, K. J. (1983). Properties and regulation of high-affinity pituitary receptors for corticotropin-releasing factor. *Biochem Biophys Res Commun*, 110, 602–608.

Wynn, P. C., Harwood, J. P., Catt, K. J., and Aguilera, G. (1988). Corticotropin-releasing factor (CRF) induces sensitization of the rat pituitary CRF receptor-adenylase cyclase complex. *Endocrinology*, 122, 351–358.

Wynn, P. C., Hauger, R. L., Holmes, M. C., et al. (1984). Brain and pituitary receptors for corticotropin-releasing factor: Localization and differential regulation after adrenalectomy. *Peptides*, 5, 1077–1084.

Wyshak, G., and Frisch, R. (1982). Evidence for a secular trend in age of menarche. *N Engl J Med*, 306, 1033–1035.

Yalom, I. D. (1985). *The theory and practice of group psychotherapy*, 3rd ed. New York: Basic Books.

Yates, A., Leehey, K., and Shisslak, C. (1983). Running – an analogue of anorexia? *N Engl J Med*, 308, 251–255.

Yatham, L. N. (1994). Is 5-HT$_{1A}$ receptor subsensitivity a trait marker for late luteal phase dysphoric disorder? A pilot study. *Can J Psychiatry*, 37, 662–664.

Yonkers, K. A., and Gurguis, G. (1995). Gender differences in the prevalence and expression of anxiety disorders. In M. V. Seeman (Ed.), *Gender and psychopathology* (pp. 113–130). Washington, DC: American Psychiatric Press.

Yonkers K. A., Halbreich, U., Freeman, E. W., et al. (1996). Sertraline in the treatment of premenstrual dysphoric disorder. *Psychopharm Bull*, 32, 41–46.

Yonkers, K. A., Kando, J. C., Cole, J. O., and Blumenthal, S. (1992). Gender differences in pharmacokinetics and pharmacodynamics of psychotropic medication. *Am J Psychiatry*, 149, 587–595.

Yoshikawa, T., Sugiyama, Y., Sawada, Y., et al. (1984). Effect of late pregnancy of salicylate, diazepam, warfarin, and propranolol binding: Use of fluorescent probes. *Clin Pharmacol Ther*, 36, 201–208.

Young, B. C., Walton, L. A., Ellenberg, S. S., et al. (1990a). Adjuvant therapy in stage I and stage II epithelial ovarian cancer. *N Engl J Med*, 322, 1021–1027.

Young, E. A. (1995). Glucocorticoid cascade hypothesis revisited: Role of gonadal steroids. *Depression*, 3, 20–27.

Young, E. A., Kotun, J., Haskett, R. F., et al. (1993). Dissociation between pituitary and adrenal suppression to dexamethasone in depression. *Arch Gen Psychiatry*, 50, 395–403.

Young, E. A., Watson, S. J., Kotun, J., et al. (1990). Beta-lipotropin-beta-endorphin response to low-dose ovine corticotropin-releasing factor in endogenous depression. *Arch Gen Psychiatry*, 47, 449–457.

Zacharias, L., Rand, M., and Wurtman, R. (1976). A prospective study of sexual development in American girls: The statistics of menarche. *Obstet Gynecol Surv*, 31, 325–327.

Zalzstein, E., Koran, G., Einarson, T., and Freedom, R. (1990). A case-control study on the association between first trimester exposure to lithium and Ebstein's anomaly. *Am J Cardiol*, 65, 817–818.

Zerbe, K. J. (1995). Anxiety disorders in women. *Bull Menninger Clin*, 59 (Suppl. A), A38–A52.

Ziel, H. K., and Finkle, W. D. (1975). Increased risk of endometrial carcinoma among users of conjugated estrogens. *N Engl J Med*, 293, 1167–1170.

Ziolko, H. U. (1985). Bulimie. *Fortschr Neurol Psychiatr*, 53, 231–258.

Zis, K. D., and Zis, A. (1987). Increased adrenal weight in victims of violent suicide. *Am J Psychiatry*, 144, 1214–1215.

Zonderman, A. B., Costa, P. T., Jr., and McCrae, R. R. (1989). Depression as a risk for cancer morbidity and mortality in a nationally representative sample. *JAMA*, 262, 1191–1195.

Zuckerman, B., Amaro, H., Bauchner, H., and Cabral, H. (1989). Depressive symptoms during pregnancy: Relationship to poor health behaviors. *Am J Obstet Gynecol*, 160, 1107–1111.

Zumoff, B. (1994). Hormonal profiles in women with breast cancer. *Obstet Gynecol Clin North Am*, 21, 751–772.

Zumoff, B., Walsh, B., Katz, J., et al. (1983). Subnormal plasma dehydroisoandrosterone to cortisol ratio in anorexia nervosa: A second hormonal parameter of ontogenic regression. *J Clin Endocrinol Metabo*, 56, 668–672.

Zurawski, V. R., Jr., Orjaseter, H. I., Andersen, A., and Jellum, E. (1988). Elevated serum CA 125 levels prior to diagnosis of ovarian neoplasia: Relevance for early detection of ovarian cancer. *Int J Cancer*, 48, 677–680.

INDEX

Human growth hormone, 135,
138–139, 149
Hymenotomy, 45
Hyperactivity, and anorexia nervosa,
127
Hypercortisolemia, 70
Hypersexuality, 49
Hypertension, 122, 154–155
Hyperthyroidism, 73, 85
primary (Graves' disease), 88–89
Hypnosis, 175–176
Hypnotics, 41
Hypoactive sexual desire disorder,
42–44
Hypokalemia, 132
Hypomania, 24
Hypothalamic-pituitary-adrenal
(HPA) axis, 63, 70, 109–120,
180
adaptations in, 136–137
age-related changes in, 116–117
and human growth hormone regulation in anorexia nervosa, 135
imaging studies, 118–119
influence of gonadal steroids on,
115–118
pathophysiology of, 110–113
Hypothalamic-pituitary-gonadal
(HPG) axis, 113–115
adaptations in, 133–134
and human growth hormone
regulation in anorexia nervosa,
135
regulatory changes in, 134–136
Hypothalamic-pituitary-thyroid
(HPT) axis, 83, 84
adaptations in, 137–138
and human growth hormone regulation in anorexia nervosa, 135
Hypothalamus, 15, 57
Hypothyroidism, 42, 45, 85
adult, 85–88

fetal, infantile, and child, 86,
104
grades of, 87
in pregnancy, 90
subclinical, 88, 92, 95, 102–105
Hysterectomy, 41
Hysteria (*see* Somatization disorder)

Imipramine, 195, 209, 215–216
Immunosuppression:
age-related, 183
stress-induced, 178–182
Infanticide, 26
Infertility, 36, 37
Insulin-like growth factor-I
(IGF-I), 6
International Classification of Diseases
(ICD), 46
Interpersonal influences on depres-
sion, 65
Intervention trials, 219–242
Breast Cancer Prevention Trial,
219, 230–232, 240
Fracture Intervention Trial (FIT),
237
Heart Estrogen/Progestin Replace-
ment Study (HERS), 219,
229–230, 241
Nurses' Health Study, 220,
239–240
osteoporosis and, 235–239
Physicians' Health Study, 233
Postmenopausal Estrogen/Progestin
Intervention (PEPI) Trial, 219,
222–224, 240, 241
Women's Health Initiative, 219,
224–229, 237, 240, 241
Women's Health Study, 220,
232–234
Involutional melancholia, 28
Isomers, 192
IUD, painful orgasms and, 41–42

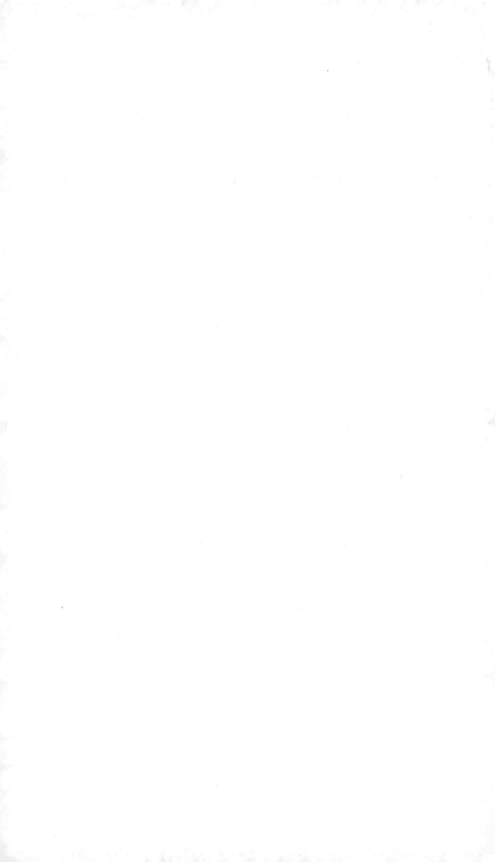